swap & drop DIET

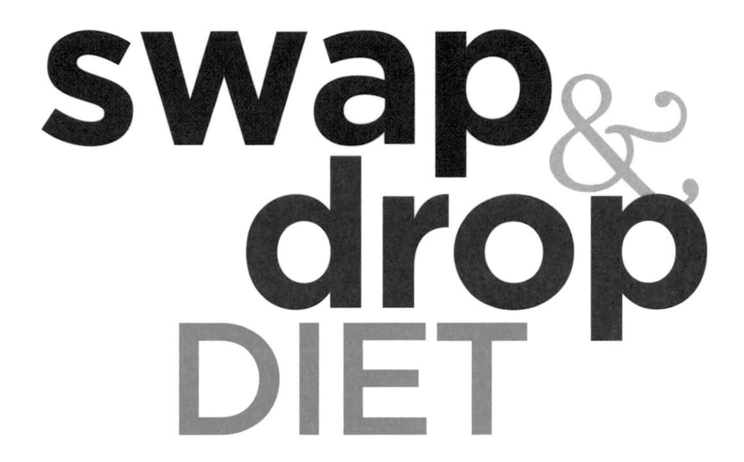

THE NEW CANADIAN
NO-DIET DIET REVOLUTION!

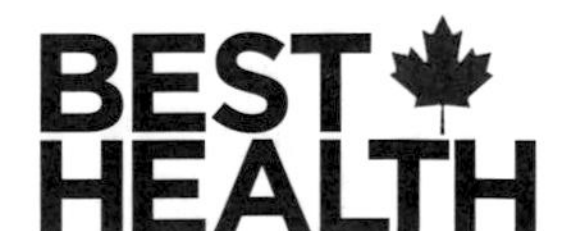

Reader's Digest Association (Canada) ULC
Montreal • Toronto

Swap & Drop Diet is published by *Best Health*, an imprint of Reader's Digest Association (Canada) ULC, 1100 René-Lévesque Blvd. West, Montreal, QC H3B 5H5

ISBN: 978-1-55475-095-5

We are committed both to the quality of our products and the service we provide to our customers. To order additional copies of this book, please contact us at 1-800-465-0780. For more information about our products, please visit us at our website at www.besthealthmag.ca

If you have any comments or suggestions about the content of our books, please write to the Book Editor at the address above.

Library and Archives Canada Cataloguing in Publication
Best Health swap & drop diet : get slim, stay slim / from the editors of Best Health.

ISBN 978-1-55475-095-5
1. Reducing diets--Canada. 2. Weight loss--Canada. I. Title: Best Health swap and drop diet.

RM222.2.B475 2011 613.2'5 C2011-906708-0

PRINTED IN THE UNITED STATES OF AMERICA

Credits: t - top, c - center, m - middle, b - bottom, l - left, c - center, r - right, tl - top left, tc - top center, tr - top right, ml - middle left, mc - middle center, mr - middle right, cl - center left, cc - center center, cr - center right, bl - bottom left, bc - bottom center, br - bottom right

All photos RDA, except: **front cover** David Muir/Masterfile; **5** Kevin Clark (hair & makeup: Tricia Clark); **6** Amy Walters/Fotolia; **7** vgstudio/Fotolia; **8** ant236/Fotolia; **12** Brenda Carson/Fotolia; **13** Michael Alberstat (hair & makeup: Laura Szucs/Tresemmé Hair Care/MAC Cosmetics/Plutino Group); **15** Pixland/Jupiter Images; **16** Gorilla/Fotolia; **19** Ryan Szulc; **21** Ryan Szulc; **22-23** Angus Fergusson; **23** r, food pictures studio/Fotolia; **25** Jodi Pudge; **26-27** Angus Fergusson; **13** Michael Alberstat; **29** Michael Alberstat; **31** rafer76/Fotolia; **32** tl, tr, iStockphoto; **32** cl, cr, Christopher Stevenson; **32** bl, rantasha/Fotolia; **32** br, AlexAranda/Fotolia; **35** tl, tc, tr, cl, cc, cl, ml, Michael Alberstat; **35** mc, mr, bl, bc, br, Tammy Dery; **37** Monkey Business/Fotolia; **38** tl, bl, br, Christopher Stevenson; **38** tr, GooDAura/Fotolia; **38** cl, cr, iStockphoto **41** Michael Gray/Fotolia; **43** Valua Vitaly/Fotolia; **44** tl, tr, cl, cr, iStockphoto **44** ml, mr, bl, br, Christopher Stevenson; **47** tl, Gorilla/Fotolia; **47** r, Christopher Stevenson; **49** Dash/Fotolia; **50** tl, tr, ml, mr, Christopher Stevenson; **50** cl, cr, bl, br, iStockphoto; **53** WavebreakMediaMicro/Fotolia; **55** webphotographeer/Getty Images; **59** iceteastock/Fotolia; **61** Ariel Skelley/Getty Images; **67** Maridav/Shutterstock; **71** Gorilla/Fotolia; **73** mangostock/Fotolia; **79** Yuri Arcurs/Fotolia; **83** Yuri Arcurs/Fotolia; **85** Yuri Arcurs/Fotolia; **89** Yuri Arcurs/Fotolia; **91** John Giustina/Getty Images; **95** Supri Suharjoto/Shutterstock; **106** Creativel/iStockphoto; **110** James McQuillan/iStockphoto; **113** b, Studiovd1/iStockphoto; **115** Marika/iStockphoto; **116** rojoimages/iStockphoto; **120** t, ozgurdonmaz/iStockphoto; **122** NightAndDayImages/iStockphoto; **124** l, Tammy Dery; **125** Comrocker/iStockphoto; **128** Eric Delmar/iStockphoto; **132** kryczka/iStockphoto; **137** arkady/iStockphoto; **138** Ryan Szulc; **139** adlifemarketing/iStockphoto; **141** r, Anna Chelnokova/iStockphoto; **146** Petrina Tinslay; **154** b, KT Tsuji/iStockphoto; **157** r, Ann Braga/iStockphoto; **158** Ryan Szulc; **159** robynmac/iStockphoto; **160** janeff/iStockphoto; **161** Angus Fergusson; **162** l, Juanmonino/iStockphoto; **162** r, Floortje/iStockphoto; **163** r, Robyn Mackenzie/iStockphoto; **164** Ryan Szulc; **165** stock.cam/iStockphoto; **166** Ryan Szulc; **168** alainolympus/iStockphoto; **169** Jodi Pudge; **171** chictype/iStockphoto; **174** PicturePartners/iStockphoto; **176** Floortje/iStockphoto; **178** Vitalina/iStockphoto; **179** l, sarsmis/Shutterstock; **180** Petrina Tinslay; **181** t, pp76/iStockphoto; **181** b, migleon/iStockphoto; **182** Netfalls/Fotolia; **184-188** Elizabeth Watt; **189** photos 1-10, Elizabeth Watt; **189** photos 11-12, Tammy Dery; **190-209** Tammy Dery; **210** Jacobs Stock Photography/Jupiter Images; **213** Gorilla/Fotolia; **215** Mark Andersen/Rubberball; **217** Jose Luis Pelaez/Getty Images; **218** Anthony-Masterson/Getty Images; **221** Jordan Siemens/Getty Images; **227** Samuelsson, Kristofer/Getty Images; **228** Gino Santa Maria/Fotolia; **230** Jurgen Magg/Getty Images; **232-249** Jill Wachter; **back cover** iQoncept/Fotolia.

NOTE TO READERS

We pledge that the information and advice inside *Swap & Drop Diet* has been checked carefully for accuracy and is supported by leading health experts and up-to-date research. However, each person's health and healing regimens are unique. Even the best information should not be substituted for, or used to alter, medical therapy without your doctor's advice.

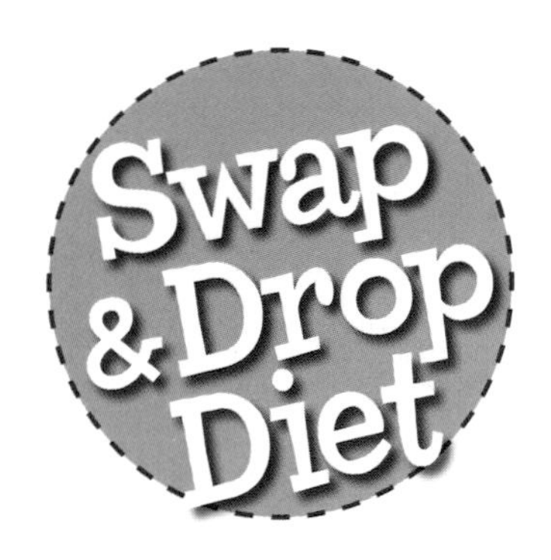

FOREWORD

by Dr. Susan Biali, M.D.

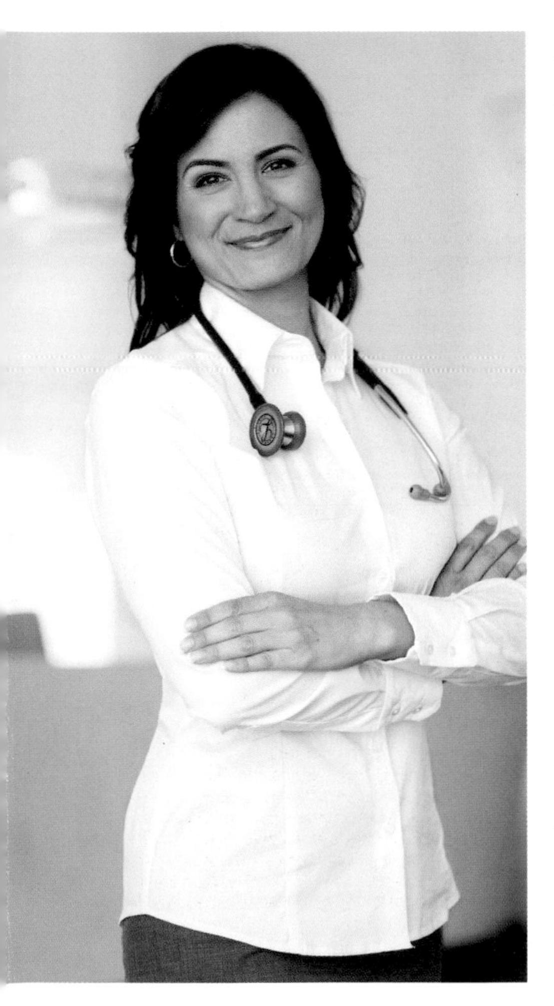

Dr. Susan Biali is a Canadian medical doctor, wellness expert and life coach who has spent over 20 years studying health, happiness, nutrition, psychology and self-development. She dedicates this extensive knowledge to helping people take back their health and enjoy a more fulfilling life than they ever imagined.

I started dieting when I was 10 years old. I still remember my aunt coming up to me, waving her favourite women's magazine in front of my face. "Just look at this, it's so easy!" she exclaimed. "You only eat grapes, and they say you'll lose at least 10 pounds in the first week. Let's do it together!"

I'd never really thought of dieting before, but was painfully aware that my parents saw me as adorably "chubby." I also felt flattered and excited by my aunt's invitation to join her in this very grown-up game. More than anything, I remember the thrill. The idea of eating nothing but grapes made me feel superior, disciplined and even noble. It also held an unspoken magical promise: If I could do this, everything else in my life would be perfect, too.

We only lasted six hours, but for years afterwards I yo-yo dieted to various extremes. Only in the last few years, after also struggling with compulsive overeating, have I finally made peace with food. That peace is what the **Swap & Drop** concept, at its core, is really about.

Our national obesity epidemic

A recent poll by the Heart & Stroke Foundation found that almost two-thirds of Canadians have tried losing weight in the past five years. Most of those who succeeded ended up gaining the weight right back. And more than a third of dieters followed a regimen which, like my aunt's grape diet, restricted or eliminated essential food groups or types.

Fad diets—extreme diet prescriptions that promise quick weight loss—don't work and never will. Sure, you'll probably lose weight in the short-term, but it won't last. It can't. These diets aren't designed for

A word about fad diets

What's most important when it comes to losing weight is following the diet, no matter which weight-loss program you choose. That's what a study in the *Journal of the American Medical Association* found. Researchers compared the effectiveness of various commercial diets. The scientists found that sticking with the plan was more important than the plan itself. However, researchers also found that none of the participants stuck with their fad diets long-term, with 21 percent quitting before two months, and 42 percent quitting before six months.

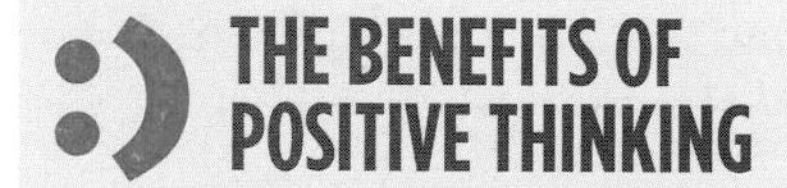

THE BENEFITS OF POSITIVE THINKING

"Whether you think you can, or you can't, you're probably right," observed car manufacturer Henry Ford. In other words, people's thoughts tend to determine how well or how badly they function. Successful people state that having "a positive attitude" is an essential component of their success. In other words, we are what we think. Remember that!

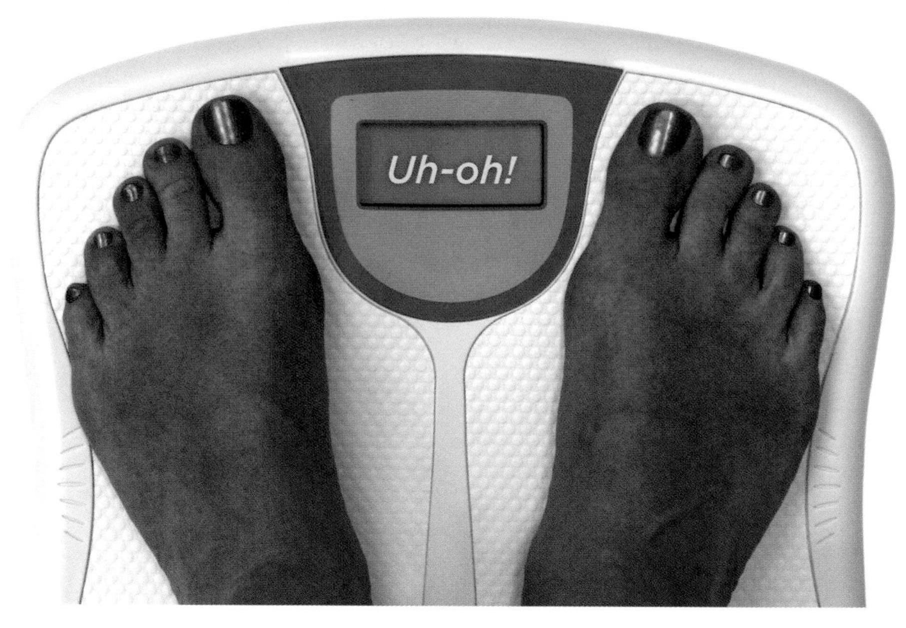

the long-term, and you would likely harm your health if you tried.

Diet pills aren't the solution either. Any time a patient shows up in my medical office requesting this kind of prescription, they get a conversation with me instead. It's human nature to want a quick fix with no effort, but it will never get you where you really want to go.

Despite the huge number of Canadians trying to lose weight, we're more overweight than ever. Additional data from the Heart & Stroke Foundation indicates that almost 60 percent of adults over 18–that's 14.1 million Canadians–are overweight or obese. The numbers of obese and overweight children are also increasing at a terrifying rate.

The financial costs are rising, too. Statistics collected a few years ago indicated that obesity-related chronic conditions accounted for $4.3 billion in direct and indirectly related costs. That doesn't include the cost of failed diets; the poll I mentioned earlier found that 42 percent of adults spend more than $500 per year on their weight-loss attempts.

Canada doesn't need another fad diet. We need to transform our relationship to food. We also need to permanently change our lifestyles.

Why a no-diet diet is best

When Bonnie Munday, Editor-in-Chief of **Best Health,** first shared with me the fundamentals of **Swap & Drop,** I was pleased to see that it was based on solid wellness principles. In fact, it's not really a "diet." Well, okay: It *is* a diet in the sense that if you are overweight and you follow it, you are very likely to lose weight. But more than anything this is a guide to creat-

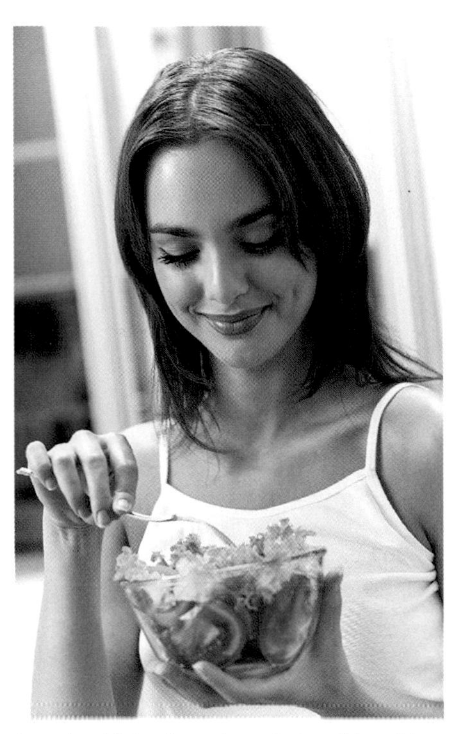

ing a healthier, happier relationship with food–and your body–that lasts a lifetime.

It's time to stop being afraid of food. The day I hit the lowest point in my dieting life, the deli where I bought my daily low-fat no-fun lunch didn't have their usual whole-wheat bread. Instead, they made my sandwich using a multigrain loaf studded with sunflower seeds. Terrified that the fat-rich seeds would irreparably damage my calorie limit for the day, I picked the seeds out, one by one.

Soon after, the man I was dating at the time insisted I visit his sister's dietitian. Her advice was about making a simple change, and it transformed my relationship to food, and my body, forever. She gave me a radically simple prescription: "Eat when you're hungry and stop when you're full." She assured me that as long as I followed this principle and generally made healthy choices, there was plenty of room for treats, too.

As you'll learn in this book, your body takes 20 minutes to turn on satiety signals, so this won't work if you shovel in first and second helpings in a rushed 15-minute meal. Take the time to enjoy your food slowly, really tasting it, and check in with your body every few forkfuls. You'll be amazed how well this works.

When the dietitian first explained this to me, I didn't believe her. Wouldn't I gain weight, instead of losing it? She assured me that I had to learn to trust my body. I had studied nutrition since I was a teen (and later went on to get a degree in dietetics), so I knew how to make healthy food choices. And over the years, as long as I followed this principle and engaged

Researchers at Harvard Medical School and Brigham and Women's Hospital in Boston studied people on two weight-loss diets. Both diets contained the same number of calories, but one was low in fat while the other was higher in monounsaturated fats such as olive oil and nuts. The researchers found that those on the higher-fat regimen (with 45 to 60 g more fat per day) were able to stay on their diet longer and better maintain their weight loss.

UNHEALTHY RISE IN CHILDHOOD OBESITY

Over the last 25 years, obesity levels in children have almost tripled. Almost 26 percent of Canadian kids between the ages of two and 17 are currently overweight or obese.

Check it!

Calories are not created equal—it does matter where they come from. Those from fat or refined carbohydrates are more likely to end up on your thighs.

"Eat when you're hungry and stop when you're full . . . take time to enjoy your food slowly, really tasting it, and check in with your body every few forkfuls. You'll be amazed how well this works."

–Dr. Susan Biali

regularly in moderate exercise, I was able to maintain a healthy weight.

How connected are you to your body? Do you pay attention to when you start to get full? Are you able to tell the difference between a craving and true hunger?

It's time to heal your relationship with food

In my work as a life and wellness coach I frequently help people heal their relationship to food, in addition to helping them transform other key areas of their lives. I'm regularly amazed by how distorted and disconnected people's interactions with food are. One client might skip breakfast, then blame her lack of will when she binges on sweet snacks instead of eating a healthy lunch. Another might regularly eat every bite of a supersized restaurant meal with enough fat to last a week. Typically, she'll have no idea how many calories are in this favourite dish and is more focused on cleaning her plate than checking in to see if she's full.

Eating three healthy, tasty, wisely-portioned meals a day, along with the right kind of enjoyable, well-chosen snacks, is a powerful "dieting" strategy. If you faithfully follow the **Swaps** and the other principles described in this program, building new habits around healthy foods and activities you love, you'll be amazed by how easily you can succeed.

Most diets also fail because it's incredibly hard to change a lifetime of habits overnight. My coaching clients have big goals and dreams, but we focus on getting there one small step at a time. This is another reason why the **Swap & Drop** concept works where many other plans flop. Small and steady victories, with minimal sacrifice and suffering, are the best way to create lasting change in your weight, your health and your life.

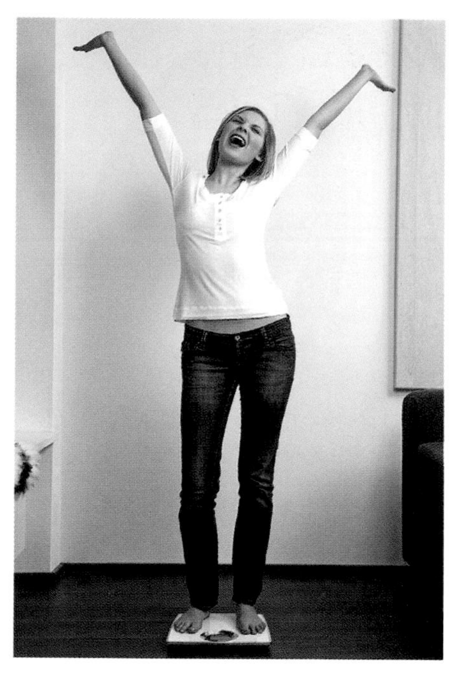

Some people say that no piece of cake tastes as good as thin feels. In my experience, slim should not be the main goal, but a nice bonus. Because nothing compares to how good *healthy* feels, when you follow nutrition and lifestyle practices that honour and respect the needs of your body. Learn to love and trust food, your body and yourself again. I am cheering you on!

Dr. Susan Biali, M.D., B.Sc. (Dietetics) is a Medical Doctor and Life Coach. She is an Embrace Life Expert for ***Best Health.***

"I often wonder what the world would be like, if we all simply did what truly moved us, what we felt calling to us–no matter how 'ridiculous' or 'impractical.' Imagine how much less depression, anger, hopelessness and stress-related illness there might be in your own life, and in the world around you."

–Dr. Susan Biali

Just do it

According to respected Canadian sociologist John Porter, "People underestimate their capacity for change. There is never a right time to do a difficult thing." Indeed, changing lifelong habits will be difficult, but with determination, you can do it. Just tell yourself that every single day.

swap & drop DIET

CONTENTS

Foreword by Dr. Susan Biali, M.D. 5

Letter from the Editor-in-Chief of *Best Health* 12

What is the Swap & Drop diet? 14

PART 1 ■ Your 12-week step-by-step plan 16

Swap 1 Right-size your portions 18

Swap 2 Eat a proper breakfast 30

Swap 3 Reinvent lunch 36

Swap 4 Learn to snack well 42

Swap 5 Eat nutritious, delicious dinners 48

Swap 6 Dine out twice a week 54

Swap 7 Be social, but eat smart 60

Swap 8 Stay motivated & engaged 66

Swap 9 Fixing your kitchen 72

Swap 10 Stress relief 78

Swap 11 Keeping on track 84

Swap 12 **Swap & Drop** for life! 90

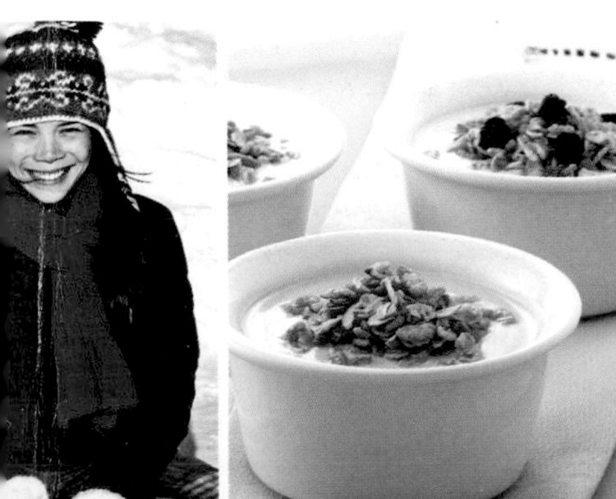
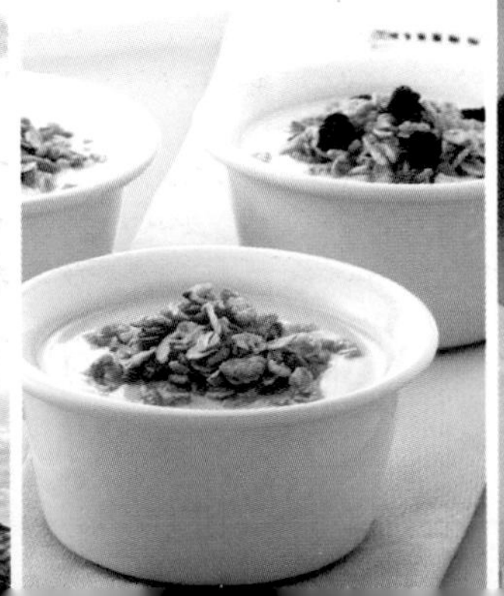
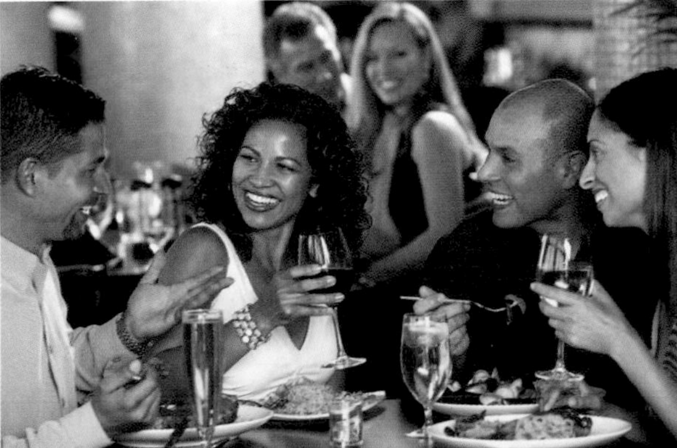
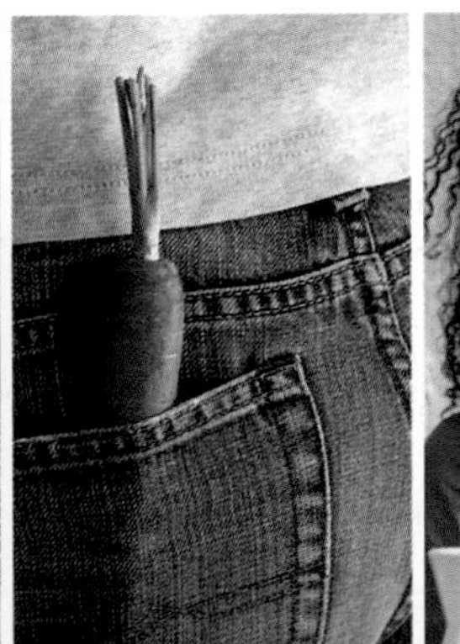
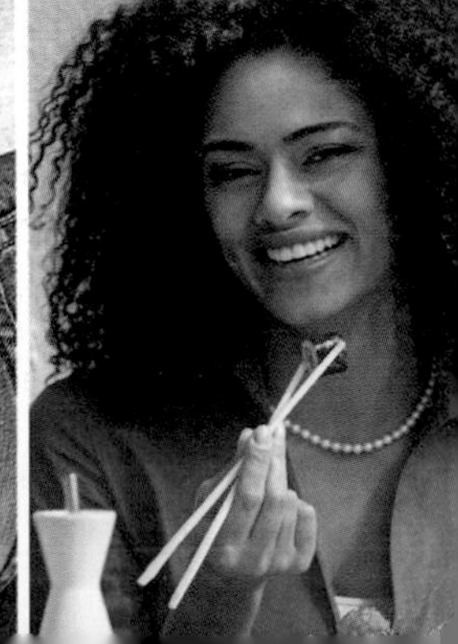

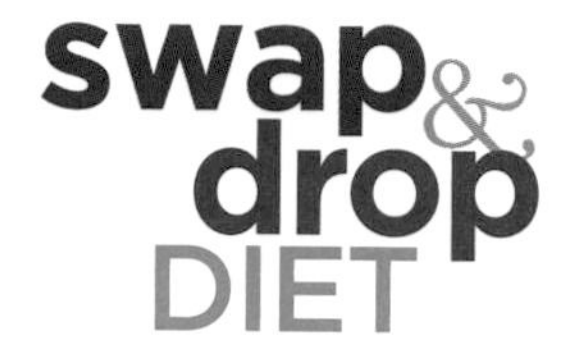

CONTENTS

PART 2 ■ Meal planner and recipes 96

A 12-week plan with 100+ healthy recipes

Meal planner Weekly guides....98
Meal planner Breakfast recipes....104
Meal planner Lunch recipes....108
Meal planner Dinner recipes....112
Meal planner Snack & dessert recipes....122
Additional recipes Breakfasts....126
Additional recipes Lunches....138
Additional recipes Dinners....152
Additional recipes Snacks & desserts....170

PART 3 ■ Swap & Drop meal makeovers 182

Switch up the food you prepare at home

Swap & Drop Breakfasts....184
Swap & Drop Lunches....185
Swap & Drop Dinners....186
Swap & Drop Desserts....188
Swap & Drop Snacks....189

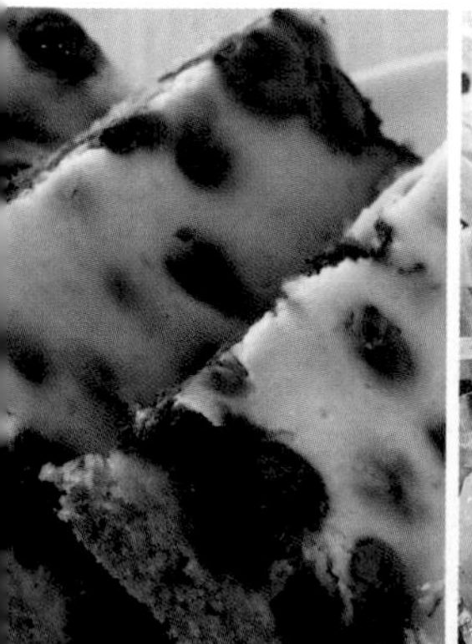
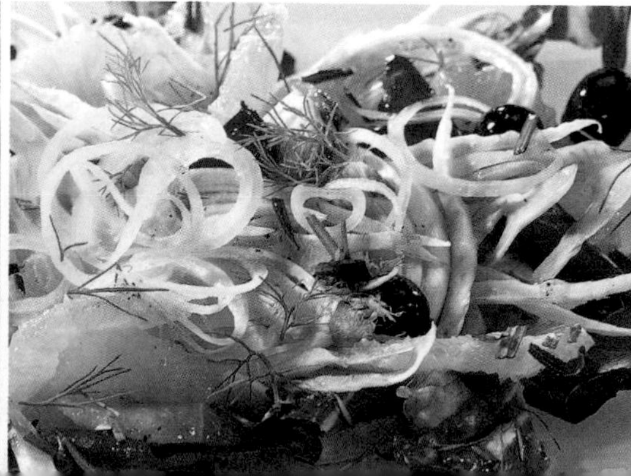
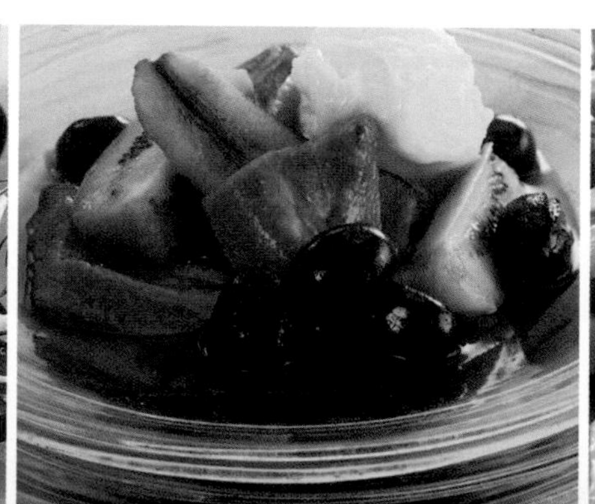
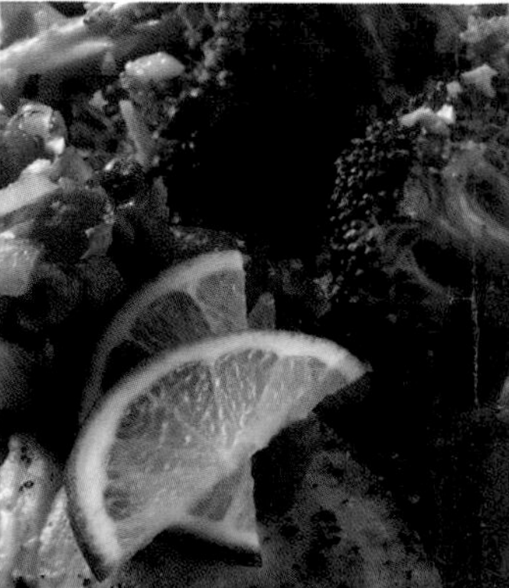

swap & drop DIET

CONTENTS

Ordering right at Canada's restaurants

Boston Pizza 190
East Side Mario's 192
Harvey's 194
The Keg 196
KFC 198
McDonald's 200
Starbucks 202
Subway 204
Taco Bell 206
Tim Hortons 208

PART 4 ■ Walk it off 210

Take walking to the next level

Why walking works 212
The mechanics of walking 215
10,000 steps to a new you 216
Get started on your journey 220
Sneak in more steps 223
A 12-week walking plan 224
Step it up 228
Aim to be flexible 232
Easy moves for belly, hips and butt 238

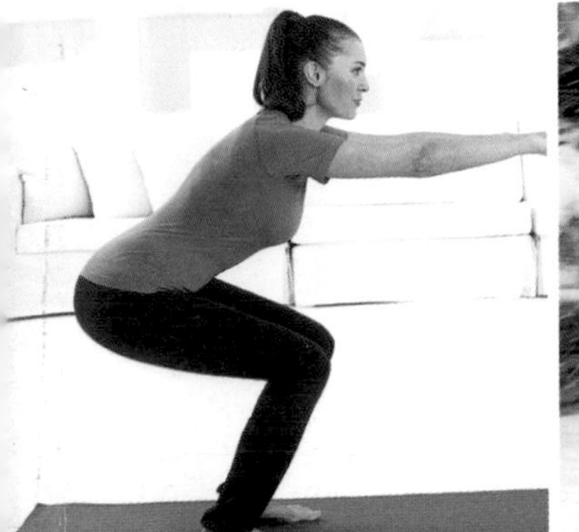
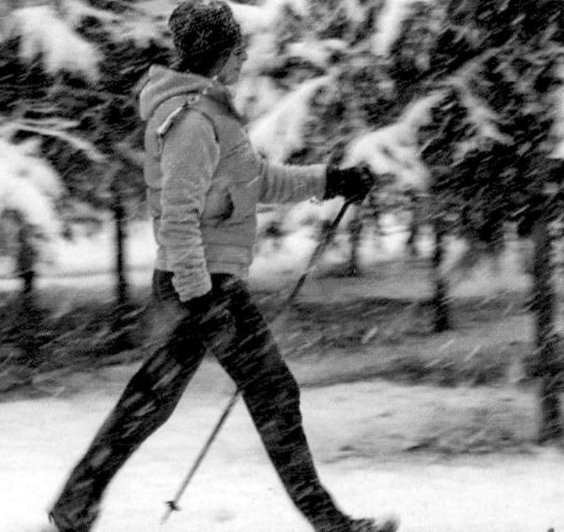
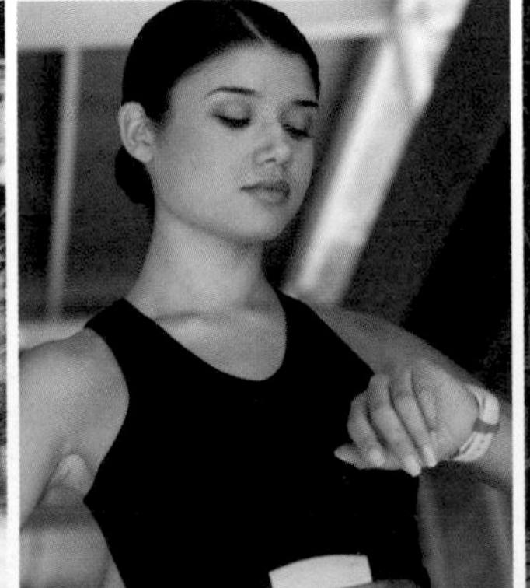
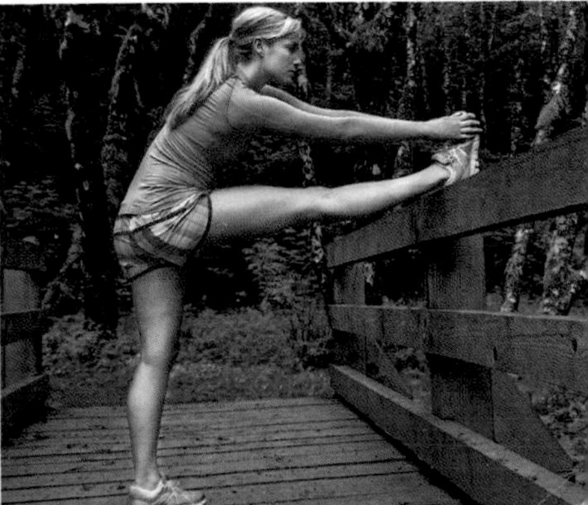

Small changes make a big difference.

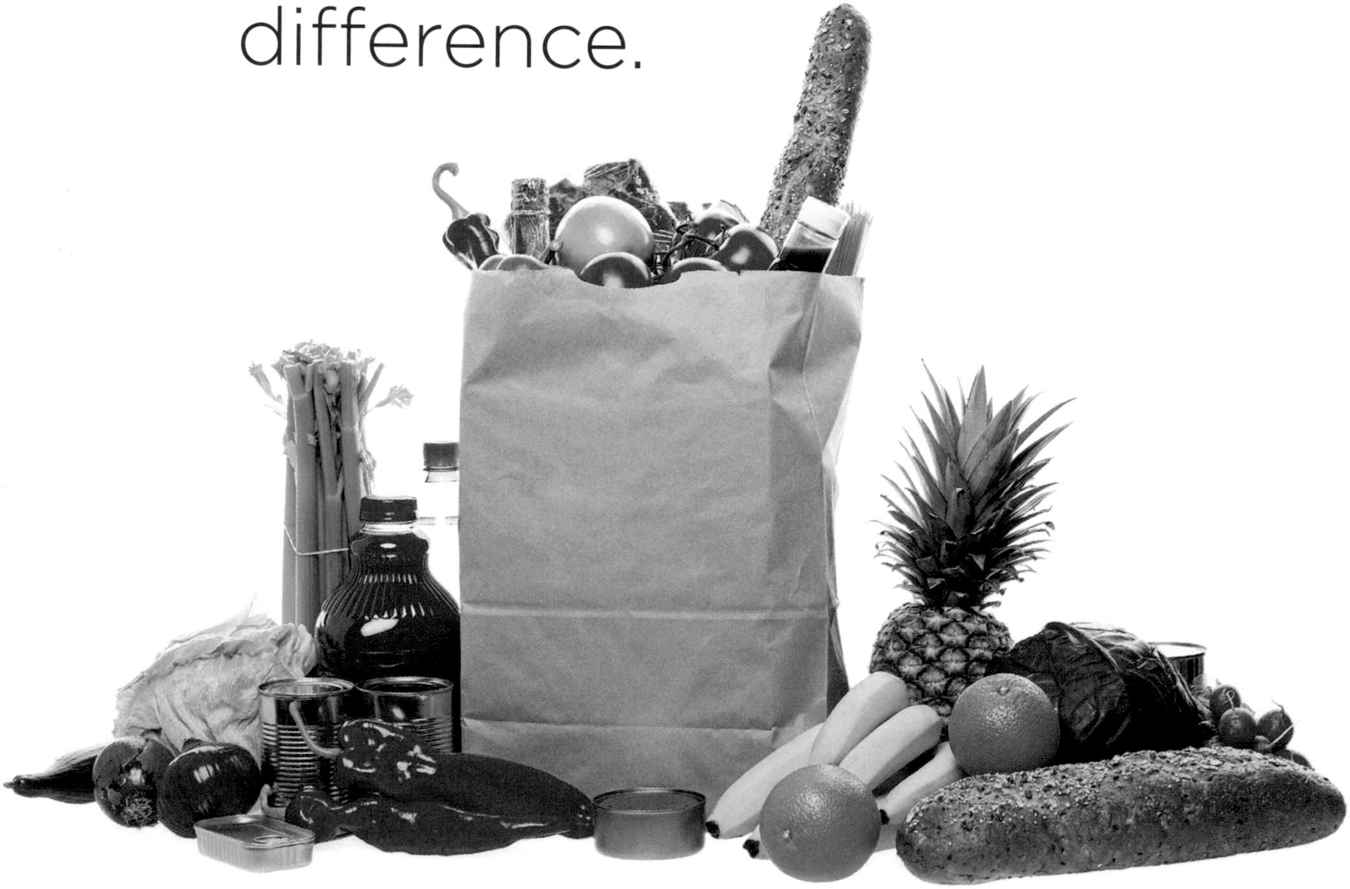

LETTER from the Editor-in-Chief of Best Health

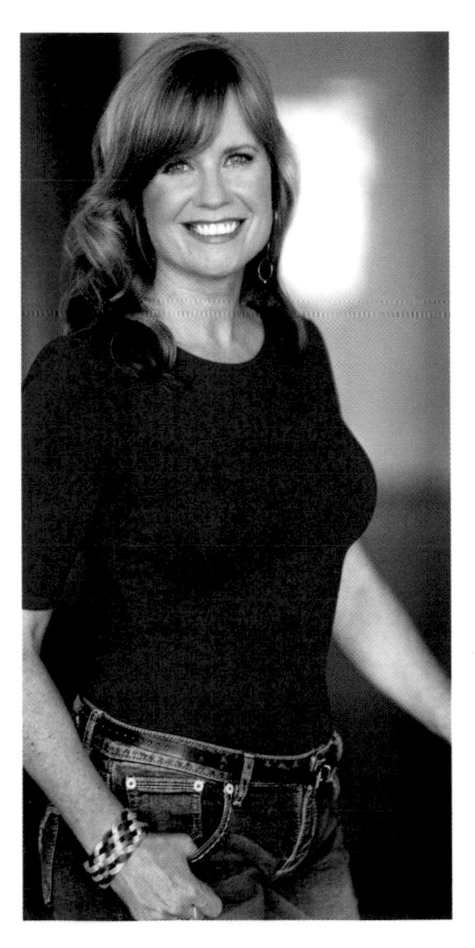

My parents are both 70, and still healthy and active. When my sister, two brothers and I were growing up, Mom and Dad were the ones encouraging us to join team sports and get moving. They set the example by taking up "jogging" (remember when running was called that?) and going to evening aerobics classes. As for family meals, dessert was only an occasional treat, and our packed lunches didn't include the can of pop, chocolate bar or Twinkie extras that I was so jealous of other kids having in their lunches. Instead, we were signed up for the school milk program and got apples and oatmeal cookies as snacks.

I'm so fortunate to have had my parents' example to follow, but today, in this not-a-minute-to-spare phase of my life, I sometimes don't make the healthiest choices. And I'm not the only one. As Editor-in-Chief of Best Health, *I'm constantly hearing from readers who tell me that weight loss tops their list of health goals—yet it seems many people have trouble figuring out the best approach. "After I diet, the pounds just come right back" is a common theme.*

So why aren't Canadian women more successful in the fight against flab? Because the best way to lose weight and keep it off for good is not by doing something drastic, but by making little changes you can live with. That's why we came up with the **Swap & Drop** *concept: to show you that when you trade in one unhealthy meal or snack for a better one, it really does add up over time to a happier, healthier and—big bonus—SLIMMER you. For example, I now know that if, once a week, I swap my afternoon snack at Tim Hortons from the raisin bran muffin for the trail mix cookie, I'll save myself about 10,000 calories over a year—which adds up to almost three pounds.*

Best Health *is the Canadian healthy-lifestyle resource that's all about balance, not extremes. That's what* **Swap & Drop** *is all about, too. Here's to weight-loss success that lasts!*

Bonnie

Bonnie Munday

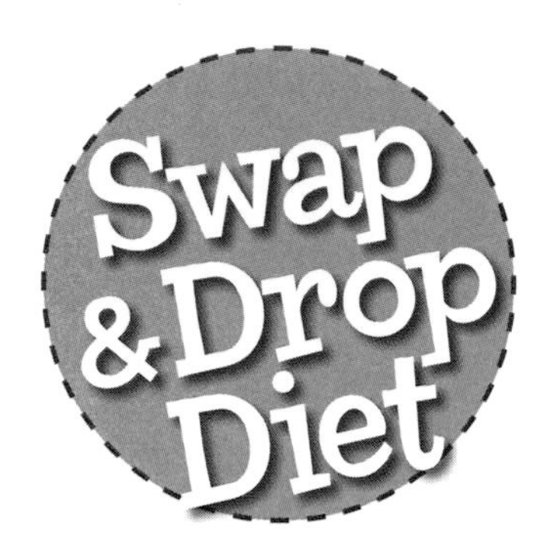

What is the Best Health **Swap & Drop** diet?

It's a uniquely Canadian plan for getting slim and staying slim by making small food and lifestyle changes, one week at a time. No risks, no fads, no craziness–just easy weight loss.

Swap & Drop by the numbers

The meals and menus you'll find in **Swap & Drop** have been designed to offer maximum nutrition with few calories—you shouldn't cut back on vitamins, minerals and fibre just because you want to lose weight. Scientific studies have also shown that diets with decent amounts of healthy fats are actually more successful than diets that restrict fat to an absurd minimum. And on **Swap & Drop**, you won't have to weigh every gram or calculate every calorie—we've already done it for you.

Our meal plans are designed to meet the following daily guidelines:

- Calories: from 1,300 to 1,600
- Calories from fat: 30 to 35 percent
- Saturated fats: no more than 10 percent of calories
- Fibre: at least 25 grams
- Calcium: about 1,000 milligrams
- Fruits and vegetables: seven to eight servings a day

:) KEEPING TRACK OF WEIGHT LOSS

Dieters want to see change on the scale. Weigh yourself daily or weekly—the choice is yours—and keep a log of your weight.

But remember, logging pounds on the scale is only one way to measure progress. If you're losing fat and adding muscle, for instance, your weight may remain the same, but you'll look and feel a lot better (as will your waistline). So keep an eye on your belt and reflection, too.

It's not easy to find a truly motivating diet plan—one that makes you excited to start your weight-loss journey. That's why the editors of Best Health magazine created **Swap & Drop**—a sensible, balanced and very Canadian approach to slimming down. **Swap & Drop** cuts through the hype surrounding trendy, ineffective diets, and empowers you to make simple changes that will not only shrink your waistline but lead to overall better health.

At the heart of **Swap & Drop** is an innovative 12-week plan that takes you step-by-step and swap-by-swap to a better body. We'll show you how to tweak your eating and lifestyle habits for steady, sustainable weight loss, and how to keep it off once it's gone. It'll work wonders for your confidence and energy, too!

Each week introduces a new healthy diet habit to learn and practice. No foods are forbidden—as long as you eat appropriate amounts. **Swap & Drop** recommends eating about 1,300 calories a day on this plan, although you can add roughly 300 more calories daily if you have a bigger frame or are very active.

Most diets ask you to throw out your old habits overnight and instantly adopt a new way of eating. That's far from sustainable. Instead, **Swap & Drop** makes losing weight as straightforward and stress-free as possible. So don't worry about being overwhelmed. We're here for you, every swap of the way!

PART 1

A 12-week step-by-step, swap-by-swap plan ■ Part 1 of **Swap & Drop** (page 16) delineates our well-balanced approach, which tackles one weight-loss issue at a time and gets it right before moving on to the next.

We start by adjusting your portions in week one, then revamping your breakfast in week two, before taking on lunch, dinner, snacks and so on. We also provide vital coping strategies to deal with some of the most difficult diet saboteurs, such as stress, restaurant meals, holidays, weekends and even the dreaded Canadian winter.

The secret to weight loss isn't restricting specific food groups—it's about controlling portion size and making the best choices for your needs. **Swap & Drop** advises readers to forget about points, carbs, protein grams or any other diet math. Instead, use our innovative Portion Checker—with actual-size photos of healthy food portions, based on Health Canada's Food Guide—and you'll know just how much constitutes the correct portion of all major food groups.

PART 2

A 12-week meal planner with over 100 healthy, delicious recipes ■ It can be hard to change your eating habits when you're so busy you hardly have a moment to yourself. The **Swap & Drop** diet makes it easy for you to get in the healthy-eating groove: Just follow our

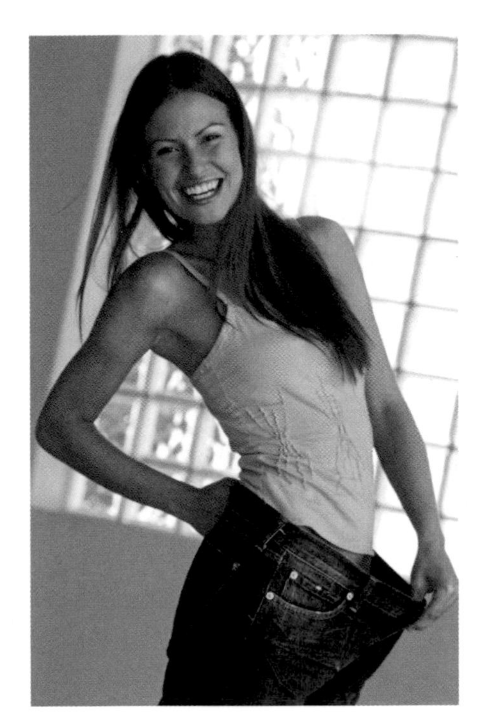

complete 12-week meal planner (page 96). You'll be able to enjoy three delicious meals—plus snacks—every day, without dedicating time to planning. No special diet foods, scales, supplements or expensive meal substitutes will ever be required.

Not only that, but we include over 100 mouthwatering recipes that the whole family will love—no need to cook separate meals! Plus, **Swap & Drop** includes many alternative and vegetarian recipes, for whenever you want to switch it up or go meat-free.

PART 3

Eating in, dining out and grabbing a meal on the go ■ "Sure, it's easy to eat well at home," you might say. "But what about those of us who can't always control where we eat?" Never fear—**Swap & Drop** is all about facing real-life situations and adapting them to your diet needs. To help with that, we rounded up major restaurants and fast-food chains from across Canada and singled out the best items on their menus, so you can eat out without worrying about gaining weight. **Swap & Drop** followers are encouraged to dine out twice a week—it's even in the meal planner!

Making some or all of the swaps in this section will really add up. In fact, we've already done the math, so you can see just how much weight you stand to lose. We'll also show readers how easy it is to do a healthy makeover of some of Canada's favourite dishes and snacks in this section (page 182).

PART 4

Walk it off in just minutes a day

■ Weight loss isn't just about eating right—it's also about getting moving. In **Swap & Drop**, we show you how to go from sedentary to active as easily as possible. You can do it while following the meal plan, or wait until you've mastered the 12-week program before you get started—you'll lose weight either way. But if you really want to shed pounds fast, you can easily get started on the **Swap & Drop** 12-week walking plan (page 210), even if you're not used to doing regular exercise.

It's not easy to cram time at the gym into an already overloaded schedule. That's why walking is the perfect active everyday movement: It restores the optimum balance between calories consumed and calories burned, without becoming a hassle. Plus, **Swap & Drop** also contains several key exercise workouts that will help you build strength, tone your body and burn belly fat.

With our easy-to-follow approach to transforming eating habits and improving health, **Swap & Drop** is the weight-loss plan that will get you started on a lifelong path to a leaner you. So what are you waiting for? Get swapping! ■

GET AN ATTITUDE ADJUSTMENT

Because we're so busy, we think of exercising as just one more thing to cram into our hectic day. That's why it feels like a chore.

To lose weight and keep it off for good, spread movement throughout your life. You can accomplish this by wiping the word "exercise" out of your vocabulary and replacing it with the word "activity." Forget about minutes and kilometres, and focus on individual steps. In Swap & Drop Part 4, our walking plan will not only help you lose more pounds, but it will stave off your food cravings, boost your energy levels and improve your mood. To begin, turn to page 210.

4 STRATEGIES to win the war on weight

1. **Make one change at a time. You can't become a new person overnight—lasting change requires a more balanced approach.**
2. **The secret to weight loss is understanding portion sizes, not doing math. If you don't want to count calories for the rest of your life, don't diet that way.**
3. **All foods are allowed. Let your meals be a source of healthy pleasure and never skimp on flavour.**
4. **Eating for a healthy weight is the same as eating for health. Think of Swap & Drop as a way of life, and this will be the last time you have to go on a diet.**

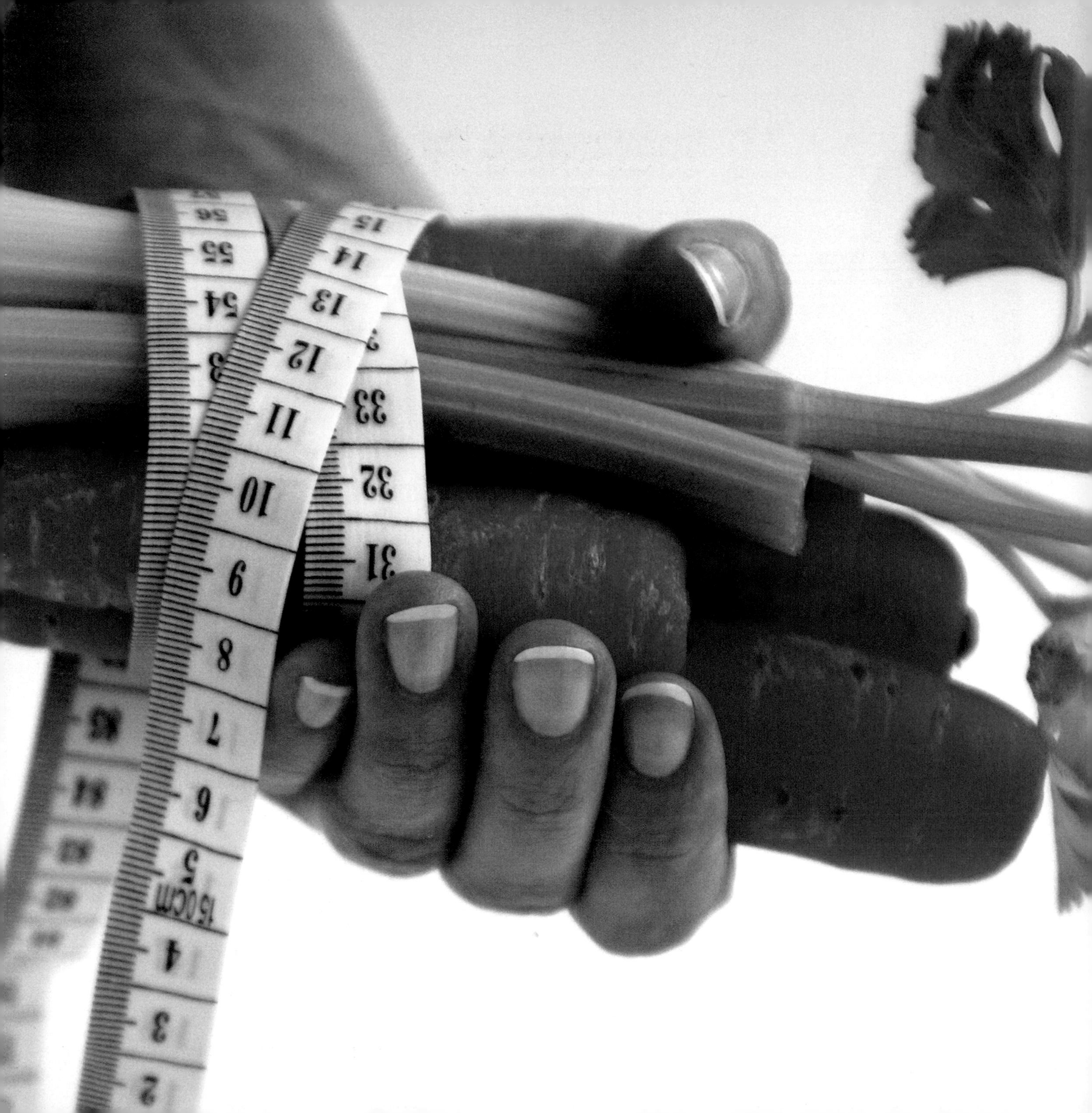

1

The **Swap & Drop** Diet Your 12-week step-by-step, swap-by-swap plan

Are you worried that a healthier relationship to food might not be fun? One of my favourite aspects of **Swap & Drop** *is that you're reminded to eat only what you like. If it doesn't taste great, don't eat it!*

You're in control, and I encourage you to really listen to your body as you go. Pay attention to how you feel after making new choices. I love the description of a lunch that refreshes and revives (page 36)–who wouldn't want that?

If you've already been eating fairly well, and don't understand why you're overweight (assuming you've ruled out medical causes with your doctor), you might be suffering from "too much of a good thing" syndrome. Eating more calories than you burn will lead to weight gain, even if you're eating nothing but rice cakes. Understanding the power of portion sizes will go a long way toward helping you achieve your goals, as will developing the fantastic, super-easy habit of filling half your plate with veggies.

As a doctor and a life coach, I approach change from both a medical and motivational perspective. It's one thing for me to tell you what you need to do, but until you understand that change in a context that's meaningful and relevant to you, it won't happen.

As you'll read in Swap 4 (page 42), it's essential to observe the unique associations you have with food. In Swap 9 (page 72), you'll be encouraged to observe the chains of behaviour that move a food from the store to your lips. I used to relax at home with a movie and a big slab of cake, and then wonder why my clothes didn't fit. These days I keep cake out of my shopping cart and chill with my favourite veggies and dip or a modestly portioned, as-healthy-as-possible sweet treat. I'm just as content with these, and as a bonus I look good in my favourite outfit.

It's important to learn and understand how to eat, but it's these real-life concepts that will really make your fabulous new habits stick.

– Dr. Susan Biali, M.D.

WEEK ▸ ONE

Right-size your portions

Small switches in portion size can make pounds disappear

Canadians eat more food than we need and it has a lot to do with portion sizes. Studies show that if people are served more food, they'll eat it, regardless of their hunger level. Throughout your first week on the **Swap & Drop,** you'll learn to right-size your portions. You'll be surprised by how quickly the weight will come off.

"My doctor told me to stop having intimate dinners for four unless there are three other people present."

— *Orson Welles, filmmaker*

EATING MORE, ENJOYING LESS

We may be eating more, but that doesn't mean we like it. In a 2006 U.S. survey, only 42 percent of respondents who self-identified as overweight also said they enjoyed eating—down from 56 percent in 1989.

You've opened this book for one simple reason: You want to lose weight. Maybe a little, maybe a lot. Maybe you'd like to improve the reflection looking back at you from the mirror. Maybe you're hoping to fit more easily into your pre-baby jeans. Or perhaps you simply want to be healthier and feel better.

Whatever your goal, the **Swap & Drop** diet will help you lose weight–and keep it off. That may sound like a big promise. But there's really no mystery to dieting, despite the bewildering number of diet plans out there. They can all work. Only one thing matters in the weight-loss game: Eat fewer calories than you burn. All diets restrict calories, and that's why you lose weight.

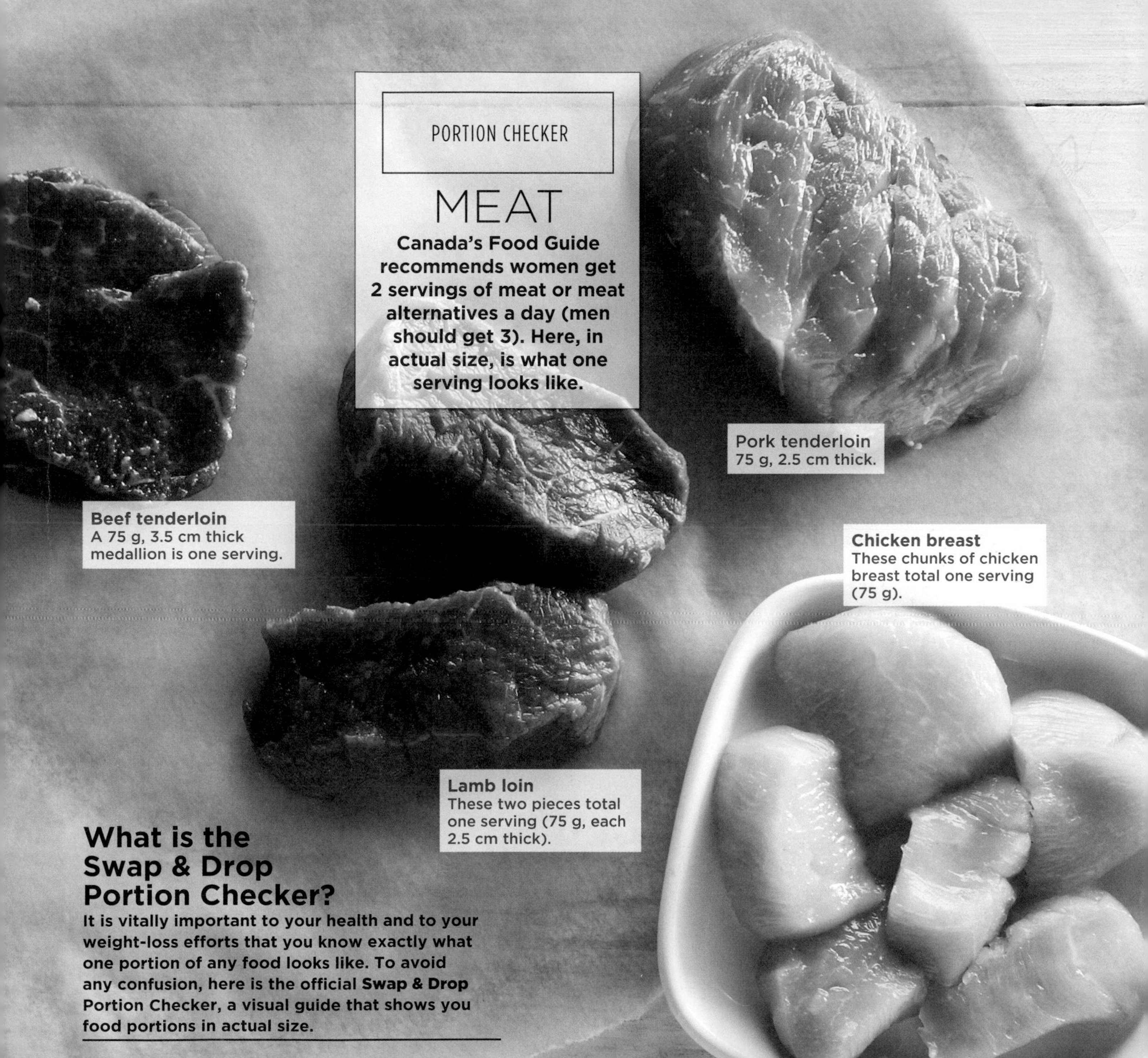

What is the Swap & Drop Portion Checker?

It is vitally important to your health and to your weight-loss efforts that you know exactly what one portion of any food looks like. To avoid any confusion, here is the official Swap & Drop Portion Checker, a visual guide that shows you food portions in actual size.

5 Tips for a healthy pasta dinner

- Choose whole-grain noodles whenever possible.
- Choose a tomato or veggie sauce, and skip the cream.
- Go easy on the parmesan—a pinch should do it!
- Prepare a salad and eat it before digging into the pasta.
- Cook any side veggies or sauce in a little extra-virgin olive oil—no butter, please!

BIRDS OF A FEATHER

You know the saying about how people start to look like their dogs? Turns out the same may be true when it comes to human friends. One major study that followed people for more than 30 years found that a person's risk of obesity increased 57 percent if they had a friend who became obese, and 37 percent if their spouse became obese.

Scientific studies comparing popular diet plans reveal that the biggest variable in weight loss isn't the diet type, but the dedication of the dieter. Those who found a program they liked enough to stick with it not only lost the most weight, but kept it off–no matter what program they were on. And of course, people who did a fad program for three months and then reverted back to their old habits regained the weight.

That's why we designed **Swap & Drop** the way we did: to teach you lifelong healthy eating habits by sensibly swapping out bad choices for good ones. Don't waste your time chasing after the latest diet trends. In the end, eating fewer calories, each and every day, is the only way to lose weight for good–and we're here to make that a little easier. A dieter's golden rules should be to eat reasonable amounts of food and add in some calorie-burning exercise. Follow those simple guidelines, and the pounds will melt away.

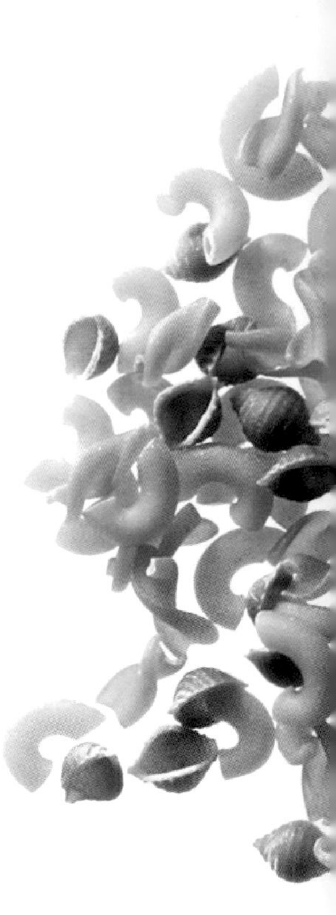

Blowing up portion sizes

The single biggest problem Canadians face in the battle of the bulge isn't what they eat, it's how much. We now annually gobble up 140 pounds more food per person, on average, than we did in 1990. How is that possible? Take a look at lunch: With so many of us opting for fast-food offerings like bacon-covered cheeseburgers, jumbo drinks and fries, it's no wonder we're gaining all this weight.

In the first week, you'll make just one change to your diet: Overhauling your portion size. To make it as easy as possible, we've provided a visual guide to right-sizing the food portions you put on your plate–just take a look at all the pages in Swap 1. In each case, we've counted the calories, so all you have to do is learn to recognize and eat reasonable portion sizes. This measured approach makes it easy to experiment, allowing you to incorporate the foods that you enjoy while still cutting calories.

The 50-percent trick

We know what you're thinking: Getting used to smaller portion sizes is easier said than done. If the portions you've been eating are significantly larger than the ones shown on these pages (or if your fruit and vegetable intake is considerably smaller), then it might be a shock to realize how much you need to change habits.

Relax! There's no need to go hungry, now or at any time on the **Swap & Drop** diet. **(continued on page 24)**

PORTION CHECKER

PASTA

Half a cup of cooked pasta is one serving, according to Canada's Food Guide, and adults should get between 6 and 8 servings of grains daily. Here's what one serving looks like before cooking (shown in actual size).

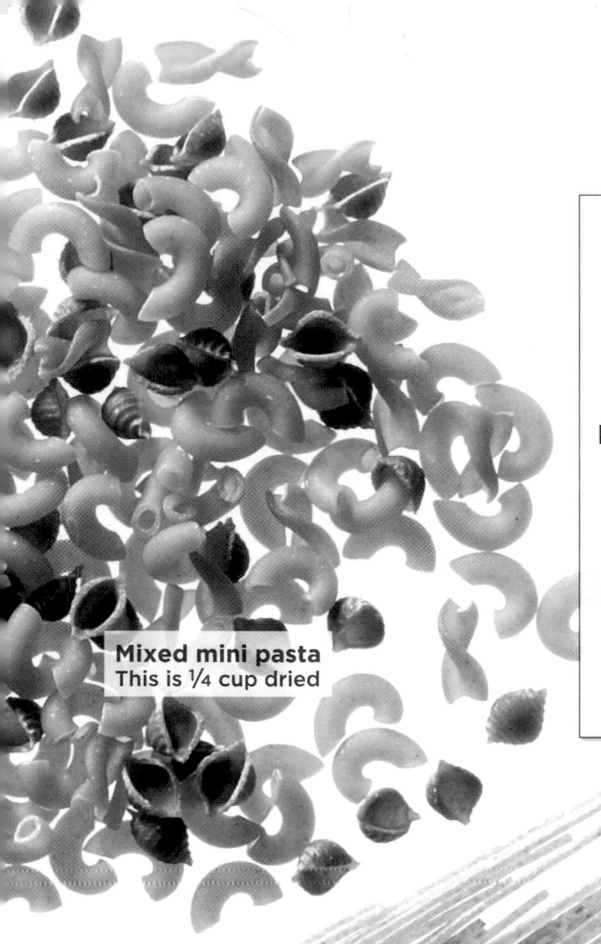

Mixed mini pasta
This is 1/4 cup dried

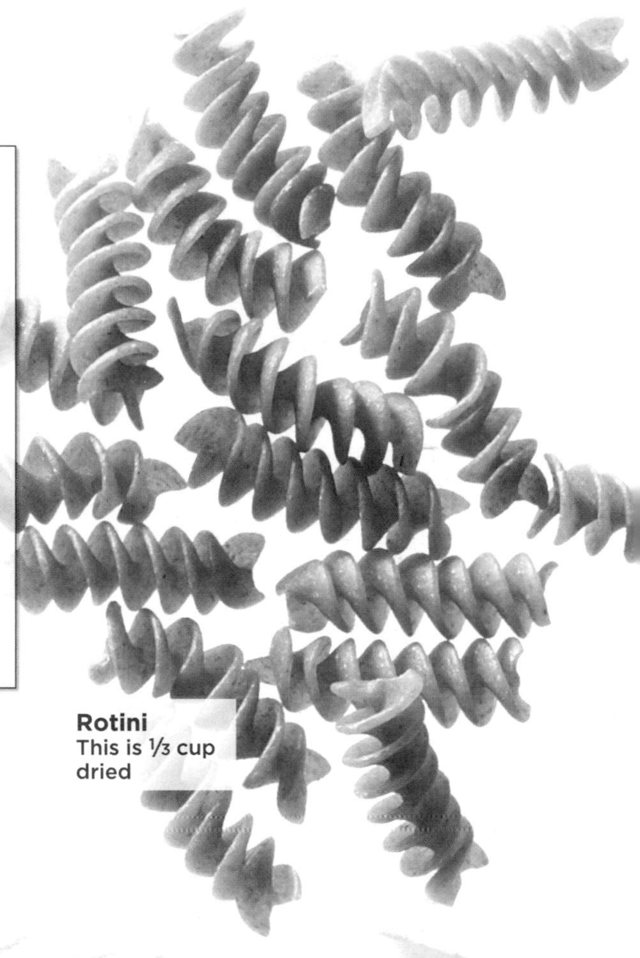

Rotini
This is 1/3 cup dried

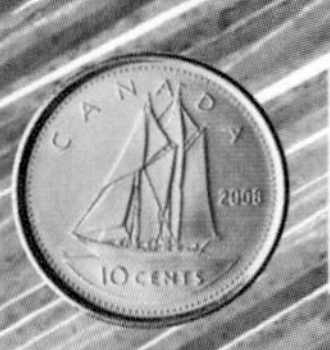

Spaghettini
When held in the hand, this bunch has a diameter no bigger than that of a dime!

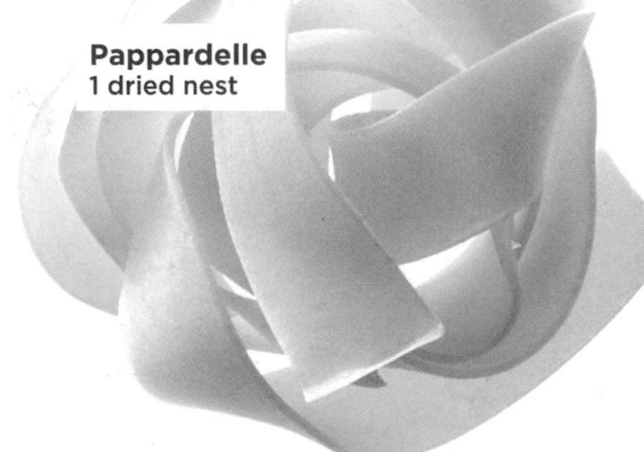

Pappardelle
1 dried nest

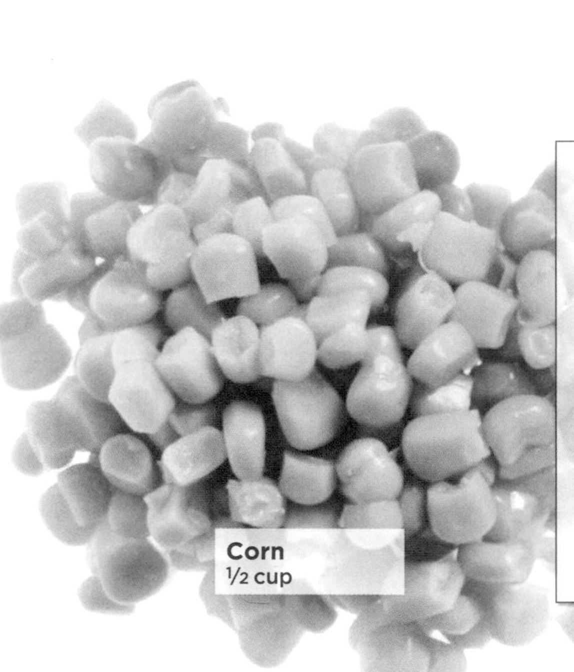

Corn
½ cup

PORTION CHECKER

VEGETABLES

Are you getting enough? Women need 7 to 8 servings of fruit and vegetables a day, according to Canada's Food Guide (men need 8 to 10). Here's what one serving looks like of a few different types.

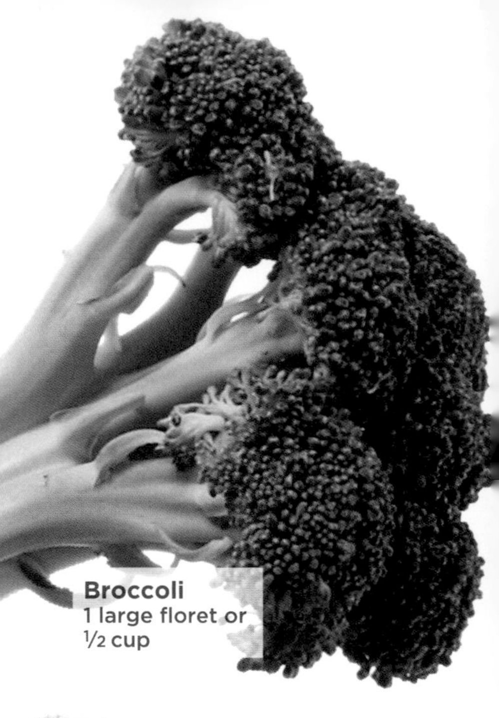

Broccoli
1 large floret or ½ cup

FILLING UP ON VEGGIES

When you go to serve yourself, start with the freshest thing on the menu: vegetables. Fill half your plate with non-starchy veggies right off the bat. Most, not including corn and potatoes, fill you up on very few calories—far fewer than whatever other food your plate contains. Fill another quarter of your plate with a healthy carbohydrate, such as brown rice, and top it off with a lean protein.

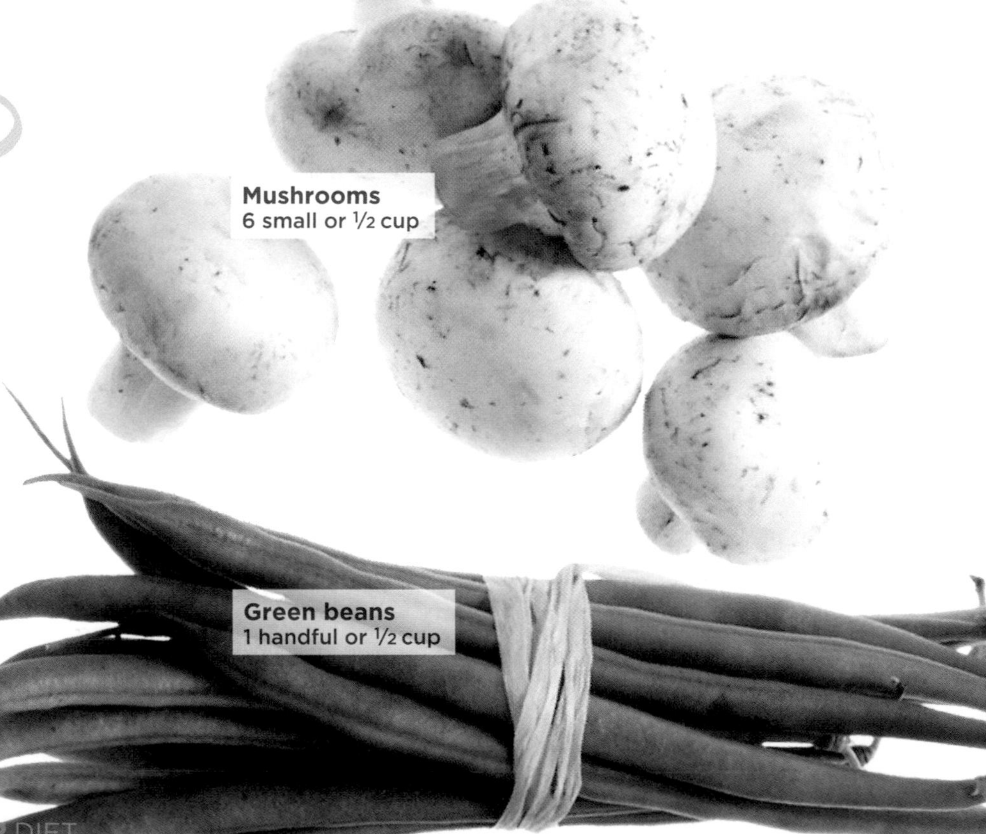

Mushrooms
6 small or ½ cup

Green beans
1 handful or ½ cup

How many veggies?

While many of us need to pare down our meat and cheese consumption, we usually need more veggies than we already get. Aim for at least 8 servings a day. That doesn't have to mean salad; add spinach and mushrooms to an omelette, or bring pre-cut celery sticks to the office.

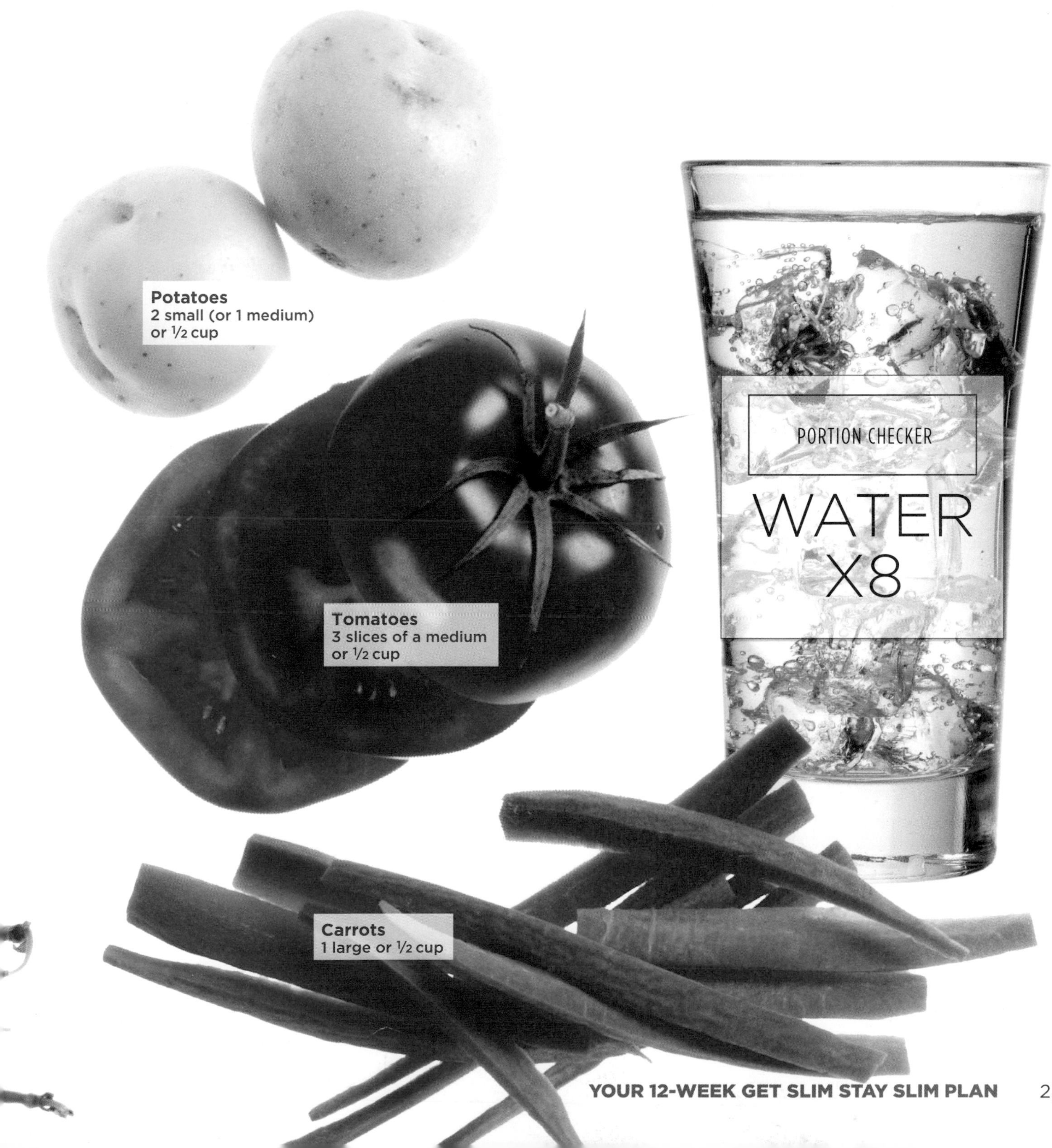

Potatoes
2 small (or 1 medium)
or ½ cup

Tomatoes
3 slices of a medium
or ½ cup

PORTION CHECKER

WATER X8

Carrots
1 large or ½ cup

(continued from page 20) Sure, you might feel as if you should eat more the first time you follow our tips. But soon you'll learn to recognize how hungry you really are–and it's probably less than you think.

This week, ease into healthier portion sizes by using the 50-percent trick at dinnertime: Serve yourself half of what you eat normally. After you're done, take a few minutes to relax and savour the meal. If you're still hungry, help yourself to half of what's left over (meaning, a quarter of what you normally serve yourself). Otherwise, get up and clear the table.

Eating slowly helps you eat less because it allows your body time to realize it's full (for more on this, see Swap 5, page 48). It actually takes your body about 20 minutes to register fullness. If you've been overeating, that means you don't even realize until it's too late. You shouldn't feel sluggish after meals. Instead, you should feel energized and ready to get on with your day.

Visualize this

Finding the "right" way to eat can be difficult and complicated in a world of conflicting nutritional advice and disingenuous claims. In response to all this craziness, American food writer Michael Pollan had this simple advice: "Eat food. Not too much. Mostly plants."

We completely agree, but determining how much is too much can be hard. If you've already tried the 50-percent trick described above, and you're still unsure what you should be eating, carry this book with you everywhere this week. Compare servings to the images on these pages. These visual guides provide a quick and easy way to keep on track. But sometimes you'll be faced with food not shown here, or you may accidentally leave your guide at home. Don't panic: Just remember these handy comparisons.

- **Starches and grains:** 1 serving should be about the size of a tennis ball–and that includes cereal in the morning, a baked potato, dinner roll, bowl of rice or noodles.
- **Cheese:** a small palmful
- **Lunch meat** (for sandwiches): size and thickness of 2-3 CDs
- **Seafood** (shrimp, scallops, crab): size of a baseball
- **Chicken, turkey, beef, veal or salmon**: deck of cards
- **Whitefish/non-fatty fish**: chequebook
- **Most dairy**: 1 cup, or about enough to fill a small coffee cup.

(continued on page 28)

Are you !#*@%?& kidding me?

PORTION DISTORTION In North America, we're eating as much as 25 percent more food per person than we did 40 years ago.

Photographic proof

Taking photos of meals before digging in may help you become more conscious of portion sizes:

- Use your cellphone to take a quick snapshot of what you are about to eat, then store it.
- Refer to the photo later when you write down what you ate and how much in a food diary.
- Looking at the photos might change your mind about over-indulging. Use the erase button to delete the photos—use your judgment to cut the extra calories.

PORTION CHECKER

CHEESE

Wondering what the right portion might be? Here's your visual guide to what 100 calories looks like.

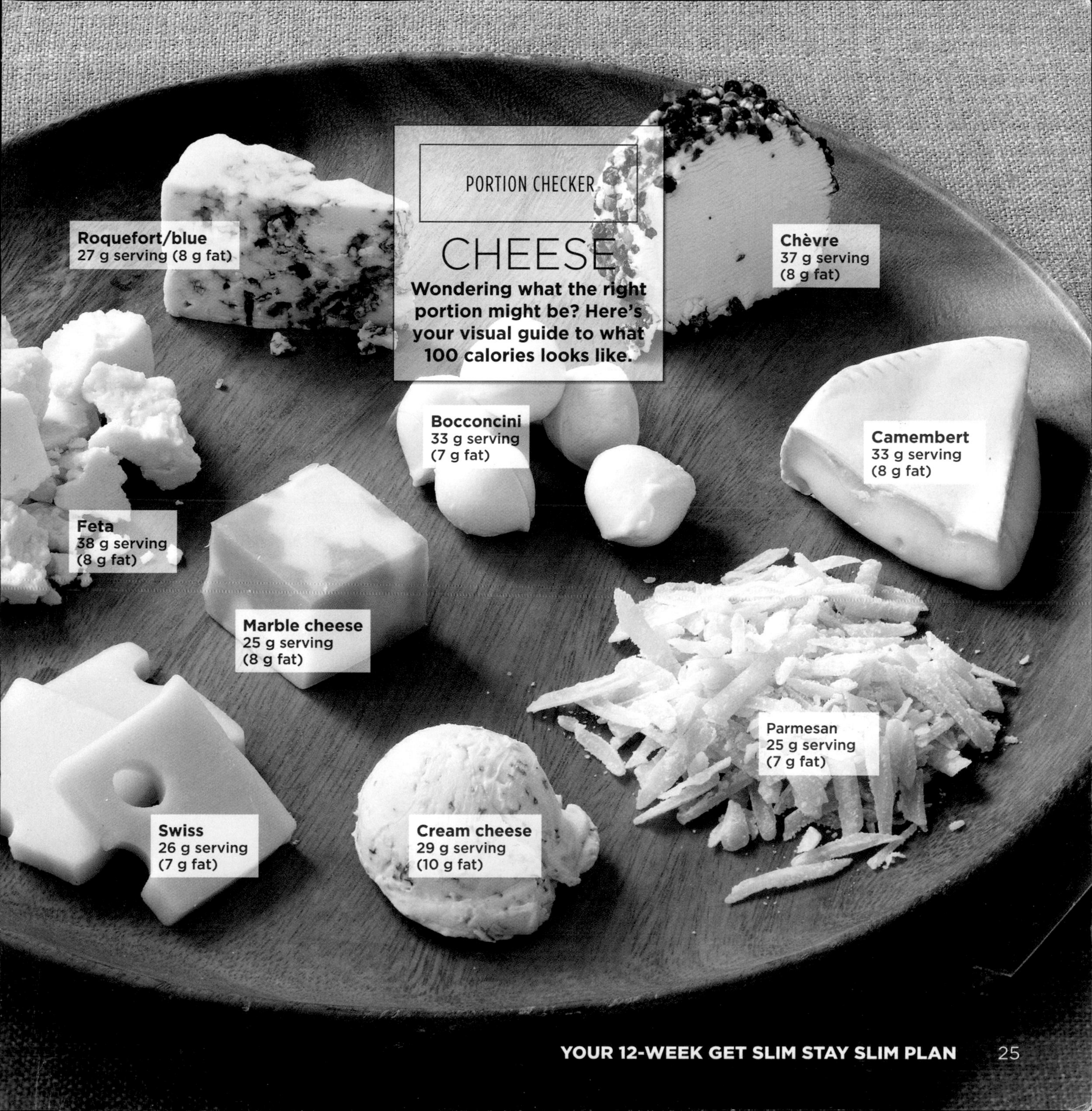

Roquefort/blue
27 g serving (8 g fat)

Chèvre
37 g serving
(8 g fat)

Bocconcini
33 g serving
(7 g fat)

Camembert
33 g serving
(8 g fat)

Feta
38 g serving
(8 g fat)

Marble cheese
25 g serving
(8 g fat)

Parmesan
25 g serving
(7 g fat)

Swiss
26 g serving
(7 g fat)

Cream cheese
29 g serving
(10 g fat)

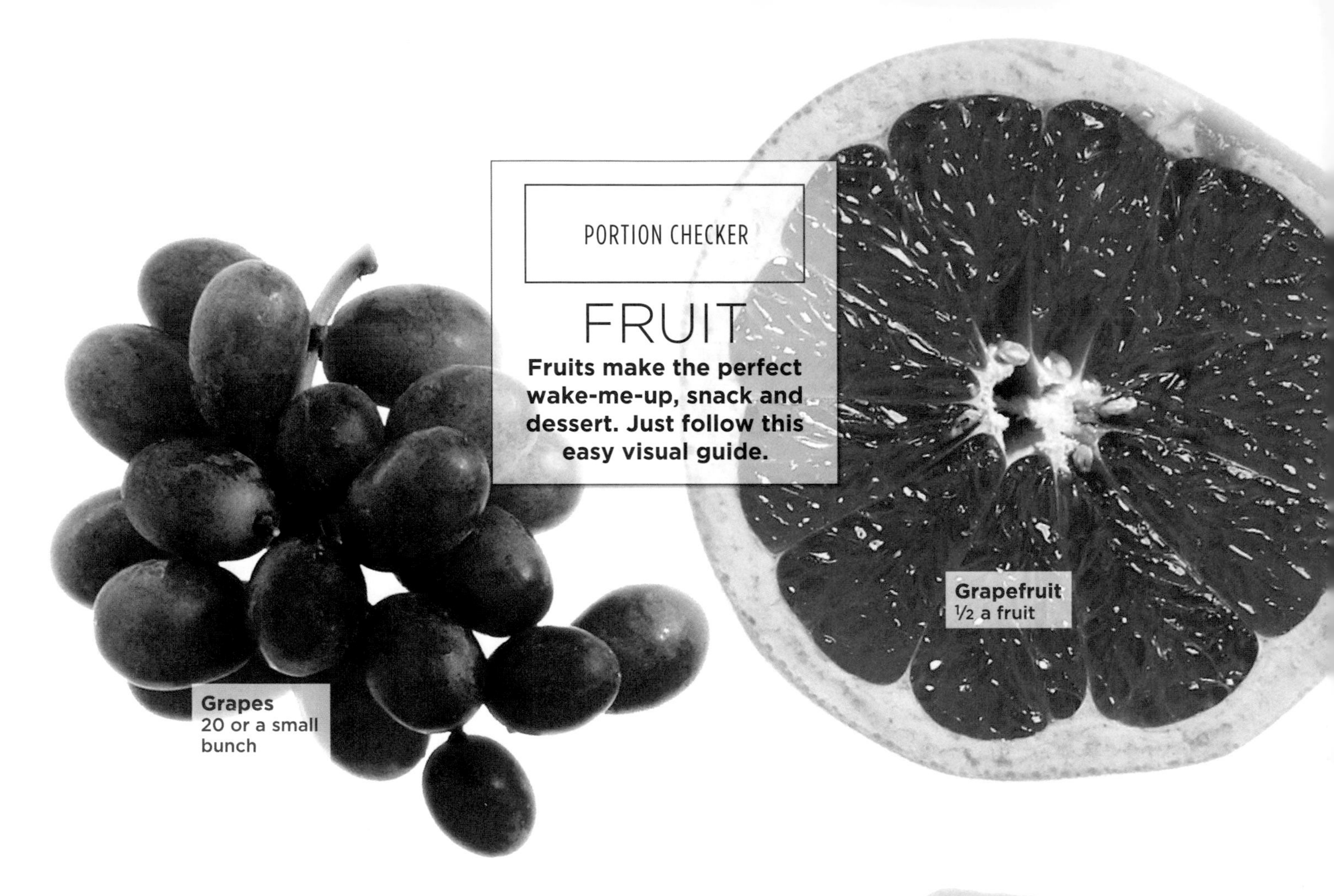

PORTION CHECKER

FRUIT

Fruits make the perfect wake-me-up, snack and dessert. Just follow this easy visual guide.

START YOUR DAY ON A FRUITY NOTE

The morning is a great time to eat fresh fruit: It's sweet, refreshing and not too heavy. You might find crunching on an apple helps you wake up (almost) as well as a cup of joe—and it's better for your teeth, too!

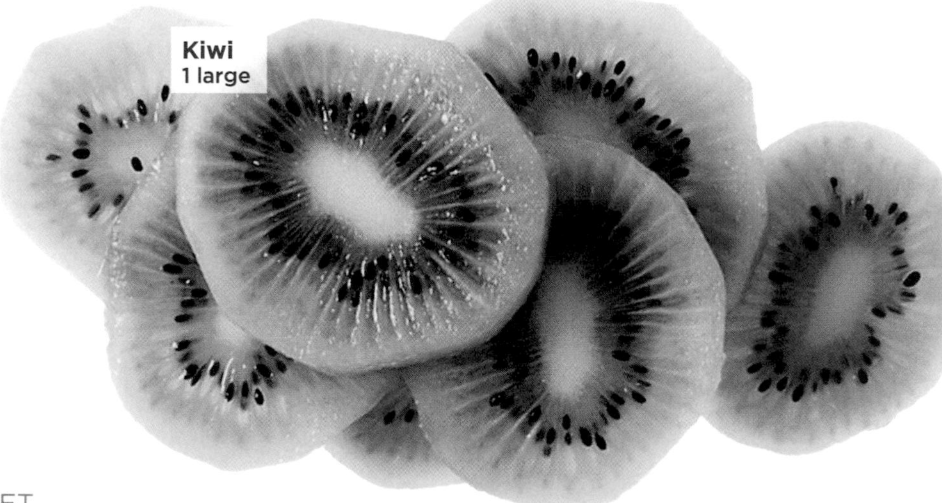

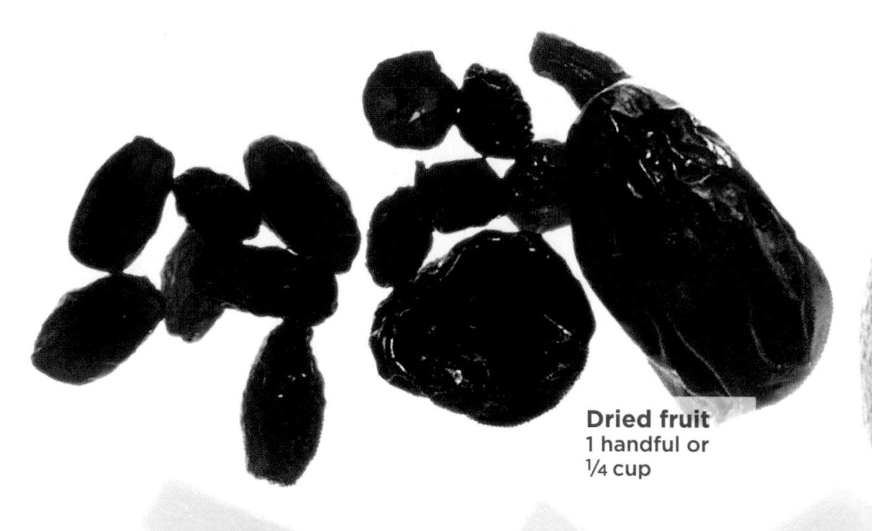

Dried fruit
1 handful or
¼ cup

Orange
1 medium

Pineapple
2.5 cm-thick
slice or ½ cup

Honeydew melon
½ cup

(continued from page 24)

Keeping restaurant meals under control

Canadians dine out frequently, with many of us eating at restaurants and cafés multiple times a week. That's understandable: Sometimes it can feel as if planning and preparing dinner is just one more stress you don't need. Besides, eating out can be fun! However, the restaurant habit can spell peril for people trying to lose weight: Restaurant portions have steadily inflated for the past several years, often including more than 20 percent more food than meals cooked at home.

What meal do you typically eat out? Breakfast, lunch, dinner—or all of the above? If you dine out this week, ask your server if half portions are available. If not, ask that you be served only half the meal, and that the other half be packed in a take-out container for you to bring home. At cafés and lunch counters, go for *just* the sandwich, without the bag of chips or creamy soup, no matter how cheap a combo may be.

It's harder to resist temptation when you're not the one in the kitchen. But just remember: It's your money and your order, and there's no reason you have to tailor your intake to suit a restaurant. Huge portion sizes are about giving you bang for your buck, after all—and in this case, the best value is just eating half. But we'll deal with dining out at length in Swap 7 (beginning on page 60) as well as in Part 3, where you'll find the best choices to order when eating out at Canada's major restaurant chains.

Downsize your dishes

Portion sizes aren't the only things that have grown bigger in recent years—the sizes of the plates and bowls on which those portions are being served have grown, too. If you have a tendency to pile your plate high and finish it all, try switching to smaller dinnerware.

Use a bread plate instead of a dinner plate for your entrée. Ditch the giant pasta bowls and use a smaller cereal bowl to serve spaghetti. If the plates you already have won't do, buy an inexpensive set of downsized plates and bowls for everyday use. Another clever way to make a little less food seem like more: Try using a salad fork instead of a regular fork at your next meal and change to a smaller spoon for your soup and cereal. You can do it! ■

For more on learning how to tell when you're full, turn to Swap 4 (page 42).

EAT, SWAP, LOVE

The **Swap & Drop** isn't a plan you follow until your weight improves; it's a new way of living that will make you feel so good that you won't ever want to go back to eating the way you did before.

SHOPPING

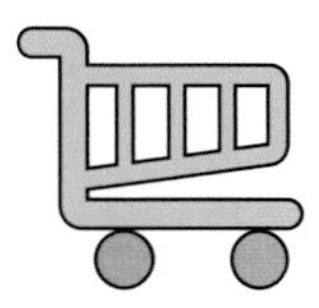

Supermarket portion control

If you buy huge amounts of dairy or meat, you may feel pressure to eat it all before it goes bad. Try buying smaller amounts more often or, if a sale on meat is just too seductive, give in to it, but when you get home, divide it into individual portions and freeze it right away for later use.

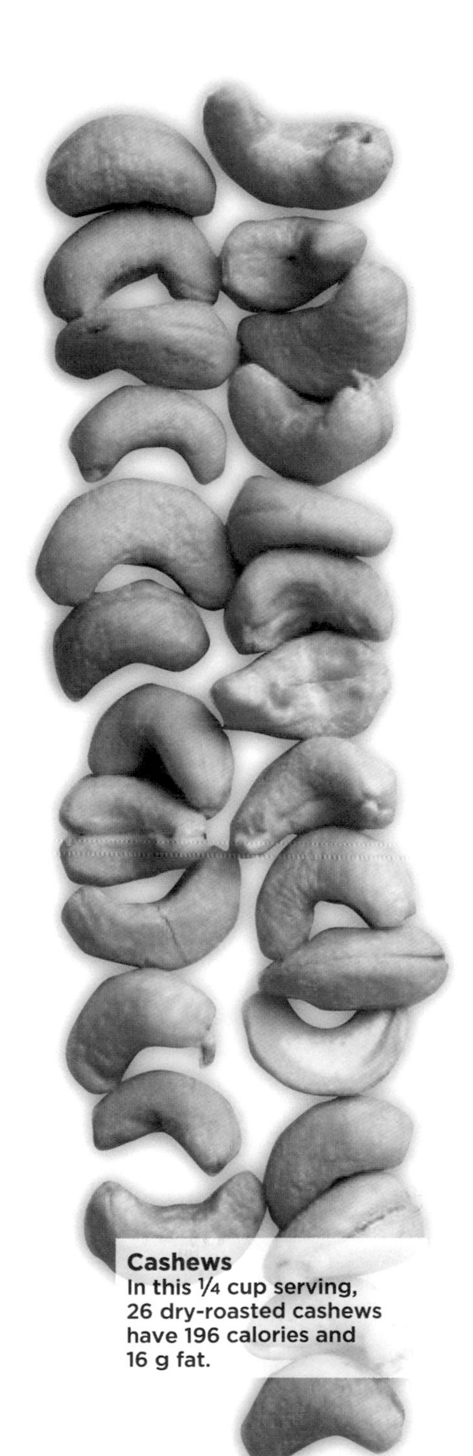

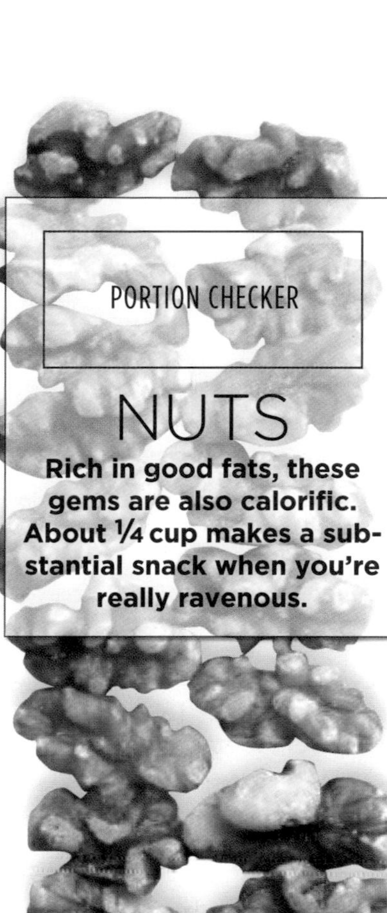

PORTION CHECKER

NUTS

Rich in good fats, these gems are also calorific. About 1/4 cup makes a substantial snack when you're really ravenous.

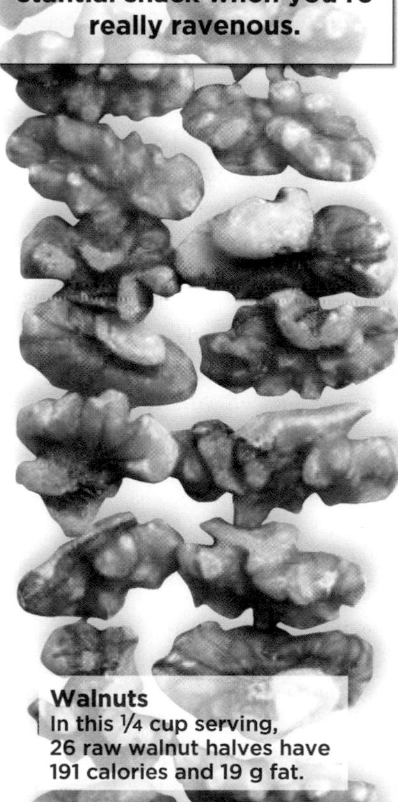

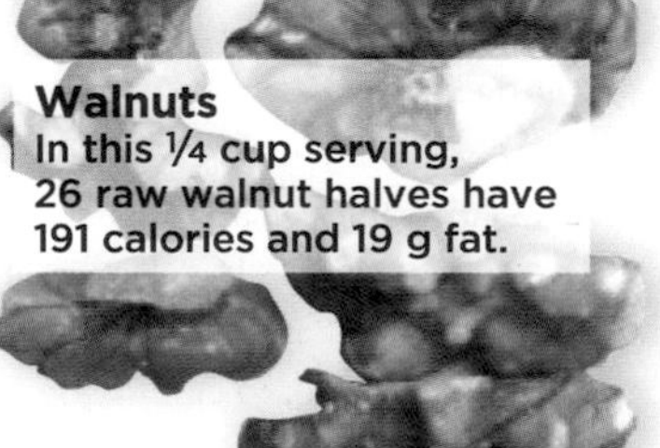

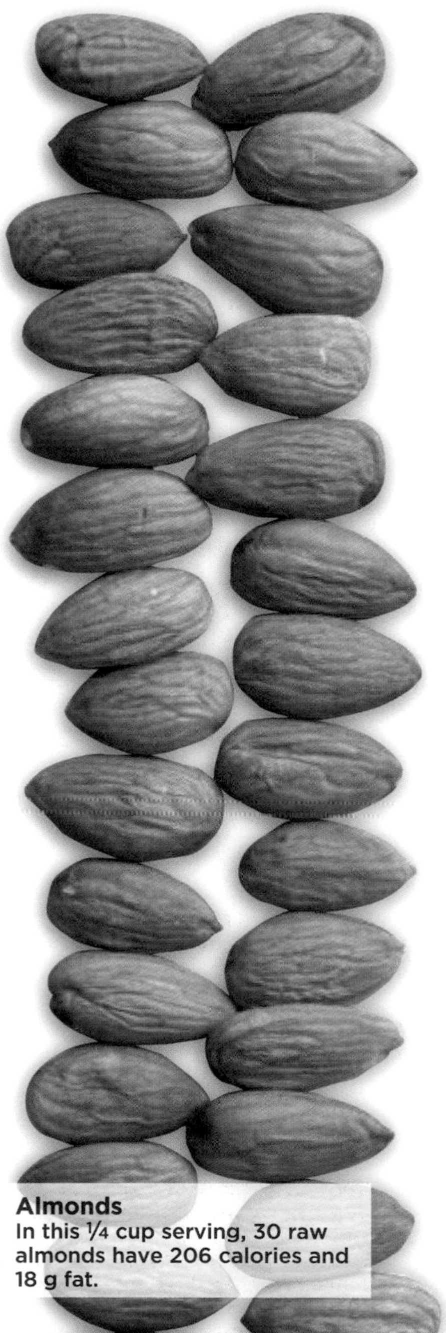

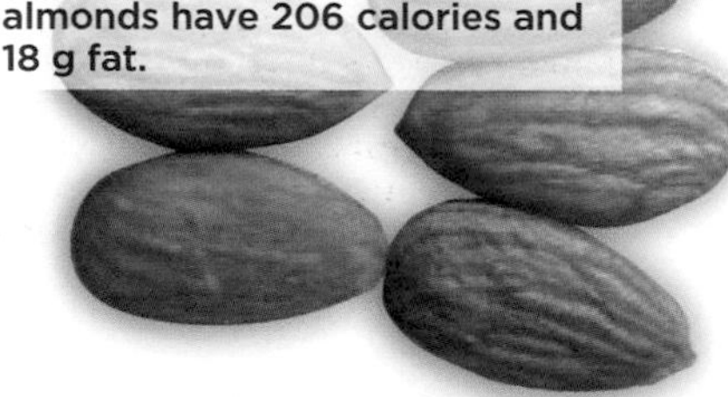

Cashews
In this 1/4 cup serving, 26 dry-roasted cashews have 196 calories and 16 g fat.

Walnuts
In this 1/4 cup serving, 26 raw walnut halves have 191 calories and 19 g fat.

Almonds
In this 1/4 cup serving, 30 raw almonds have 206 calories and 18 g fat.

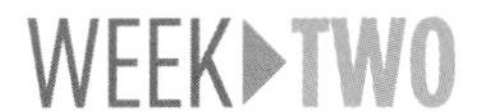

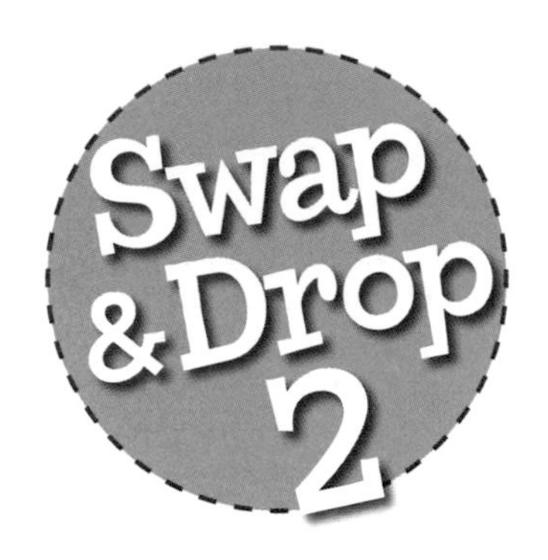

Eat a proper breakfast

Have it every morning—even if you're not hungry

There's a reason it's called the most important meal of the day: People who eat breakfast are significantly less likely to be obese than those who don't. The key is to choose energy-enhancing, health-invigorating foods. That's the focus of your second week on the **Swap & Drop** diet.

"Eat breakfast like a king, lunch like a prince, and dinner like a pauper."

— *Adelle Davis, nutritionist*

START YOUR DAY SUNNY SIDE UP

Studies prove that eggs make you feel full longer than many other foods, lowering calories eaten the rest of the day. A single egg has 6 grams of high quality protein, 14 essential nutrients (such as zinc, iron and vitamins A, D, E and B12) and contains only 85 calories.

For some people, the thought of food is repulsive early in the morning. Others just never feel they have the time. Plenty of dieters forgo the first meal of the day, figuring they'll end up eating fewer calories that way–when in fact, it works the other way around. People who skip breakfast often end up consuming more calories during the day, whereas those who start the morning with a healthy meal end up consuming fewer calories overall.

Why breakfast is key

If you usually skip the morning meal, you may need a little convincing. But there's plenty of evidence to back this up: Researchers at Vanderbilt University recruited dieters who typically missed breakfast, and put all women on a 1,200-calories-a-day diet. One group divided calories between lunch and dinner. The second group ate those two meals plus breakfast. Twelve weeks later, the breakfast eaters had lost 17 pounds; the women who didn't eat breakfast had shed 13.

"Wait a minute," you might say. "Weren't both groups consuming the same number of calories?" Only in theory, the researchers concluded. The women who ate breakfast were better able to stick to the 1,200-calorie diet, while those who went hungry until lunch were more tempted to cheat a little.

If you pass up breakfast, this study shows, you're likely to eat more, not less, than if you start the day with a meal. The longer you go without eating, the hungrier you get. And the hungrier you get, the more likely you are to reach for an

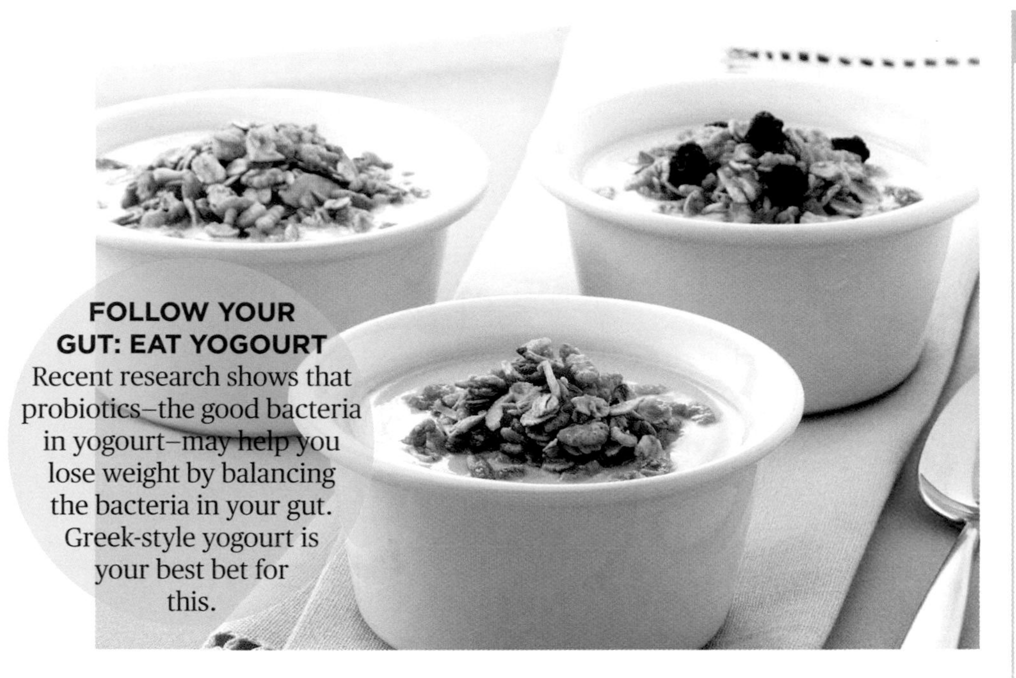

FOLLOW YOUR GUT: EAT YOGOURT
Recent research shows that probiotics–the good bacteria in yogourt–may help you lose weight by balancing the bacteria in your gut. Greek-style yogourt is your best bet for this.

unhealthy snack. When you greet the day with breakfast, you begin by taming the hungry beast inside and make it easier to keep cravings in check.

Hunger is closely related to blood sugar, which is to the human body what gasoline is to a car: its primary source of fuel. Eating a good breakfast makes sure there is plenty of blood sugar in your bloodstream available for your body to convert into energy. When blood sugar dips, your body responds with food cravings–and for many people, those cravings are for sugar, since sweet foods convert quickly into blood sugar. But this wreaks havoc on your body's chemistry, particularly your insulin levels, leading to unhealthy eating. Long story short: You want generally stable blood sugar and insulin levels for both your optimum weight and overall health.

The way to achieve that is to eat small amounts frequently. A healthy breakfast not only sets you up for good eating patterns throughout the rest of the day, but immediately takes care of the lower blood sugar level that you have after a night's sleep.

One other good reason why **Swap & Drop** advocates breakfast: It's an easy success. Of the three meals, a healthy, sensible breakfast is the simplest to pull off, and it will help you stay on track with your diet for the rest of the day.

Psychologists say that levels of two brain chemicals that give us a sense of control–cortisol and adrenaline–peak right after we get up. The confidence they

GETTING AHEAD

Don't let a hectic morning rush sabotage your dieting effort. Putting breakfast together doesn't have to require more time than it takes to put cereal in a bowl, scatter a little fruit over it, and pour the milk. If you're really in a hurry:

- **Set the table for breakfast before going to bed. You'll save time, and the table will be a reminder when you get up.**
- **Take care of a few morning chores the night before. Instead of deciding what to wear after you get up, for example, select your outfit before bedtime.**
- **Prepare a fruit salad on Sunday so that you can quickly spoon some up every morning of the week.**
- **Set the alarm clock earlier so you'll be guaranteed a little more time to eat and get organized.**

:) SIP A CUP OF GREEN TEA WITH YOUR BREAKFAST

In addition to its heart-protective benefits, green tea may also have some weight-loss benefits, with one study finding that it appears to raise the rate at which you burn calories and increase the speed at which your body uses fat.

provide may make it easier to stick to our good intentions, such as a healthier diet. These chemicals ebb later in the morning, making it tougher to say no to the doughnuts someone brings into the office—especially if you're starving because you skipped breakfast.

Here's another compelling argument: Since 1993, researchers at the University of Colorado and the University of Pittsburgh have been gathering data on dieters who lost 30 pounds or more and kept the weight off. This unique project, called the National Weight Control Registry, was designed to find out what it takes to shed pounds permanently.

And guess what? Four out of five participants in the registry—people who have managed to lose and keep off a significant amount of weight—say they eat breakfast every day.

Swap & Drop breakfast 101

Every day this week, help yourself to whichever **Swap & Drop** breakfast strikes your fancy (recipes start on page 104). Most of these recipes are 300 calories or less. That's enough energy to power your morning and still give you a headstart on losing weight.

What's more, each breakfast includes at least one food that's high in fibre. There are several good reasons for this. The biggest shortfall in most people's diets is fibre, experts say. We should get about 25 to 30 grams a day to be our healthiest; most people average a mere 15.

Fibre's an important defence against several common health problems. It's also a key player in a healthy weight-loss diet. Because it's filling, fibre makes a meal feel more satisfying with fewer calories. One form, called soluble fibre, absorbs water to form gels that slow digestion; foods that are high in this kind of fibre stay with you longer than those without, keeping you from getting hungry.

By slowing down digestion, fibre also helps keep blood sugar steady, which cuts cravings and evens out insulin levels. This has several benefits, including signaling to your body to cut down on the amount of fat it is storing.

In fact, to test the hunger-taming effects of high-fibre foods, scientists at Australia's University of Sydney compared two seemingly similar breakfasts: a bowl of bran flakes, which are high in fibre, and a bowl of cornflakes, which are not. Volunteers in the bran group reported feeling less hungry later in the morning than those who ate cornflakes.

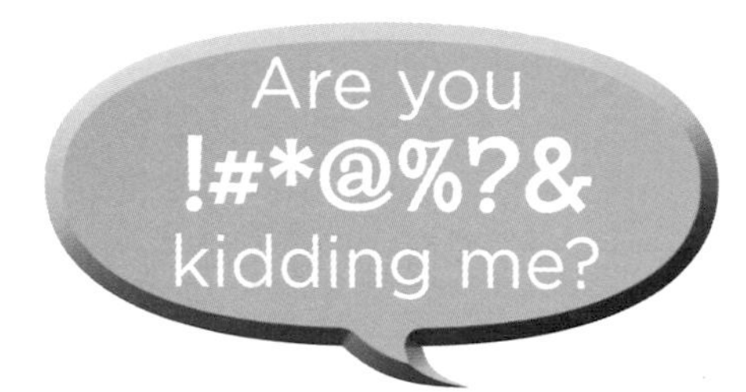

Just one cup of cranberry juice cocktail contains a hefty 140 calories, while a cup of apple juice weighs in at 116 calories. Millilitre for millilitre, that's more than most soft drinks!

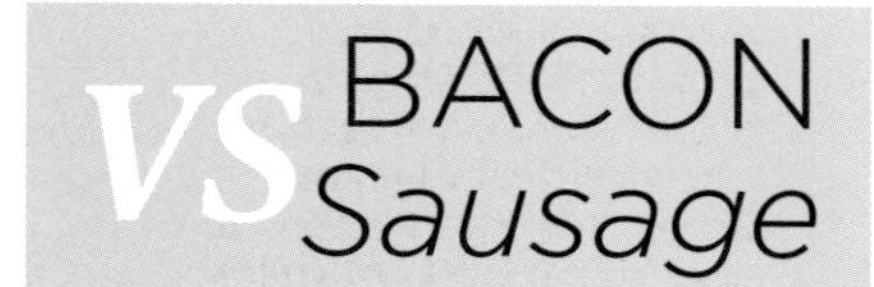

A SLICE OF CRISP BACON has fewer calories than a typical sausage. Your best bet is a slice of lean back bacon with the rind and fat cut off, rather than fatty, streaky bacon.

SWAP & DROP

SWAP THIS		FOR THAT
Bagels may look innocuous, but surprise, surprise: These ultra-dense baked goods often have more than 300 calories!	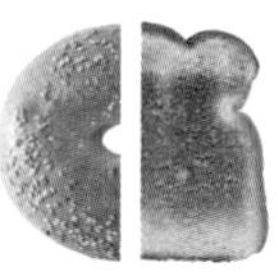 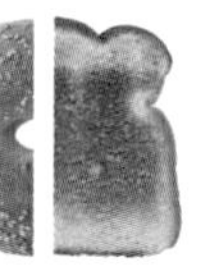	**Whole-wheat toast** is a much less calorific choice: One slice usually has around 70 calories.
Eggs are a healthy source of protein, but go easy on the yolks: No one absolutely needs to eat two.	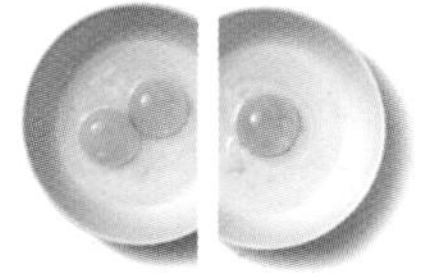	**Use two whites and one yolk.** You'll save about 60 calories and 5 grams of fat.
Black tea with milk and sugar may be a comforting start to your day, but it also adds unnecessary calories.	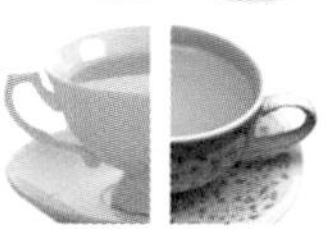	**Green tea** is virtually calorie-free and packed with antioxidants.

In a similar experiment, researchers at the New York Obesity Research Center at St. Luke's-Roosevelt Hospital pitted a sugary, low-fibre breakfast cereal against oatmeal, which is among the highest-fibre cereals you can have. When volunteers ate the sweetened flakes, they tended to eat as much at lunch as if they'd had nothing but a glass of water at breakfast. When they sat down to a bowl of oatmeal, they felt fuller for longer and ate as much as 40 percent less for lunch.

Swap juice for fruit

Fruit, like whole grains, is a terrific source of fibre. Your breakfast should include at least one serving of it—but when we say fruit, we mean fruit you can actually chew.

Fruit juices are surprisingly high in calories, especially if they've been sweetened. What's more, most fruit juices don't have nearly as much fibre as the fruit from which they're made. Compare three of the most popular:

Orange juice (1 cup)	One orange
Calories: 100	Calories: 64
Vitamin C: 80 mg	Vitamin C: 80 mg
Fibre: 0.4 g	Fibre: 3.3 g
Apple juice (1 cup)	**One apple**
Calories: 116	Calories: 81
Vitamin C: 2.2 mg	Vitamin C: 7 mg
Fibre: 0.2 g	Fibre: 4 g
Grapefruit juice (1 cup)	**Half a grapefruit**
Calories: 115	Calories: 60
Vitamin C: 67 mg	Vitamin C: 62 mg
Fibre: 0.2 g	Fibre: 1.3 g

Swap & Drop encourages you to help yourself to fruit not only at breakfast, but in between meals, too. We stop short of saying you can eat as much fruit as you want—most fruit contains a fair amount of sugar, which means it adds calories to your diet—but we've never met anyone who got fat eating too many mangoes. Certainly, if the choice is between a candy bar and a piece of fruit, reach for the fruit.

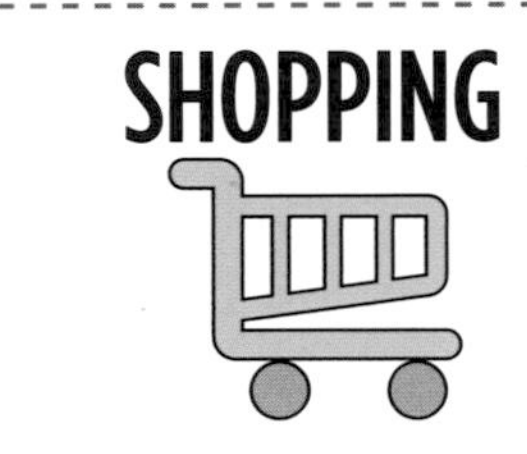

GOT MILK?

Studies indicate that dairy products may play a role in weight loss. A group of 323 girls in Hawaii lost both weight and abdominal girth when they consumed just 1.5 servings of dairy foods daily. One cup of milk or a small piece of cheese resulted in 9 mm less abdominal fat and a decrease of as much as 2.2 pounds of body weight.

4 GREAT REASONS TO MAKE HIGH-FIBRE SWAP & DROPS

Fibre, which is the indigestible part of plant-based food, gives whole grains, fruits and vegetables their snap, crunch and crispiness. And since your body can't digest fibre, it passes through without adding calories. Fibre is great for you because it:

1. **Sustains long-term weight loss.** In a study published in the *Journal of the American Medical Association*, scientists tracked the diets of 2,909 men and women over the course of 10 years. Those who chose high-fibre foods ended up weighing almost 10 pounds less, on average.

2. **Keeps cholesterol levels in check.** High-fibre foods have been shown to lower LDL or "bad" cholesterol. A study by University of Toronto researchers showed that a diet that gets more than one-third of calories from high-fibre foods can lower LDL cholesterol by 33 percent. Volunteers on a high-fibre diet saw their LDL drop within the first week.

3. **Prevents diabetes.** In two major studies conducted by researchers at the Harvard School of Public Health, people who ate the most fibre from whole grains had the lowest risk for type 2 diabetes. Eating high-fibre grains cut their risk for the disease by 30 percent.

4. **Reduces cancer risk.** Many studies show a lower risk of several kinds of cancer among people who include lots of fibre in their diets. By eating a healthier diet based on plant foods, most of us could cut our cancer risk by at least one-third, experts say.

324

That's how many calories you can burn in 60 minutes of walking the dog.

EAT BREAKFAST TWICE

Instead of having your usual lunch, make your midday meal another breakfast. Eating breakfast twice during the day isn't our idea—several big cereal companies have been touting it as a novel weight-loss method. Help yourself to a bowl of high-fibre flakes for breakfast and lunch, and you can have a full dinner and still shed pounds. It works, especially if high-calorie lunches are your downfall.

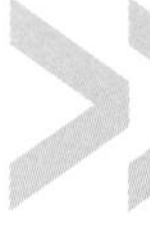

For tasty, healthy breakfast recipes, turn to page 104.

Swap coffee for dairy

Something else you'll notice about **Swap & Drop** breakfasts: Most of our meal plans include milk or yogourt. Non-fat or low-fat dairy products are a terrific low-calorie source of calcium, which you need for three key health reasons: It helps keep bones strong, reins in blood pressure, and recent studies suggest it may lower the risk of colon cancer.

Calcium also seems to change the efficiency of weight-loss. The evidence first showed up in a study designed to test whether men who added two cups of yogourt to their diet every day would lower their blood pressure. Their readings did drop, and they also lost weight–11 pounds a year, on average.

Another study showed that dieters who ate three to four servings of dairy products daily lost 70 percent more weight in six months than people on the same diet who were not eating dairy. And better still, those in the dairy group also lost more fat from around their middles.

The magic ingredient in dairy products seems to be calcium. One two-year study found that young women who ate a low-calcium diet gained weight, while women who got plenty of calcium in their diets maintained a steady weight or even lost a few pounds.

Why? Experts have found that getting too little calcium triggers the release of a hormone called calcitriol, which tells the body to store fat. When calcium levels are high, calcitriol levels remain low and the body burns fat instead of storing it. Calcium's not quite the whole story, however, since subjects who took a calcium supplement pill in the diet studies didn't lose quite as much weight as people who got the mineral in their meals. That finding suggests that something else in dairy products may help spur weight loss.

Don't be concerned if you can't digest dairy–you're certainly not alone. Many Canadians are lactose intolerant, which means they do not have enough of the enzyme lactase, which is crucial for the digestion of milk sugars.

But experts say that, even with low lactase, you may still be able to digest milk with no stomach discomfort, thanks to sugar-processing microbes we all carry in our intestines. If you're lactose intolerant

NO FAIL *get-slim* STRATEGY

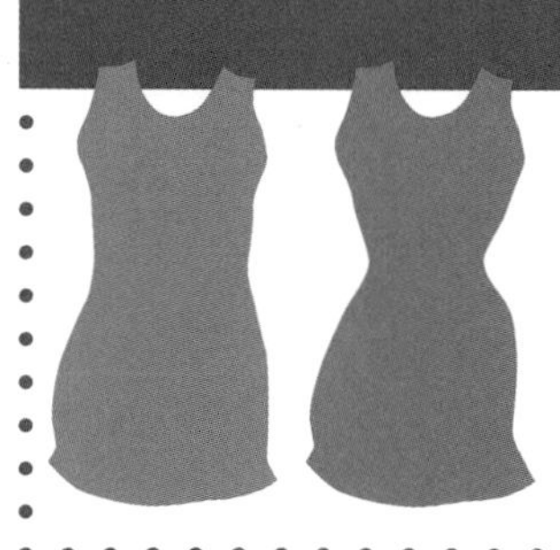

SLIM MILK

Still drinking whole milk? Time to lighten up, one swap at a time. Go from whole to 2%, then 1%, then skim. It won't take long before skim milk tastes as good as whole. Here's what you'll save in artery-clogging saturated fat and calories:

Type	Fat per cup	Calories
Whole (3.5%)	5.0 grams	149
Reduced fat (2%)	2.9 grams	122
Low fat (1%)	1.6 grams	102
Skim (0%)	0.3 grams	86

and want to find out if these microbes will help your body digest dairy on a small level, try gradually adding milk to your diet, rather than all at once. Start with a half cup a day. If you have an actual dairy allergy–which is different from lactose intolerance–you should still avoid dairy in any form.

Rise and shine!

Not only is breakfast important for your physical well-being, but a morning routine is also a great way to start the day on a happy note. You may not think of yourself as a morning person–but how much of that has to do with feeling rushed and stressed out, so soon after waking up?

This week, get your affairs in order before you hit the sheets every night, and set your alarm a little earlier than usual–say, 20 minutes. If you have a hard time getting out of bed the next morning, don't hit that snooze button. Instead, force yourself to walk over to the window and draw the curtains. Natural light is the ultimate wake-up call. Morning light can be hard to come by during long Canadian winters, but just performing this ritual will make you feel more awake.

Now use your extra time to prepare a healthy breakfast, drink a steaming mug of green tea and collect your thoughts. As we've already said, be sure to include plenty of fibre, at least one serving of fruit and a little dairy. Once you see how great this jumpstart makes you feel, you won't miss the tiny bit of lost sleep! After all, every morning is beautiful when you're well on your way to a healthier, slimmer you. ■

Although regular oatmeal is a great cereal choice in the morning, few of us have time to cook. Here are some of the best cereal options for Canadian dieters.

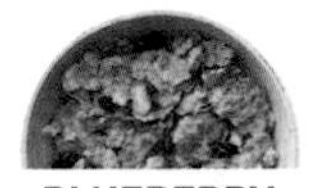

BLUEBERRY POMEGRANATE ANCIENT GRAINS
Post Great Grains This one has a delicious fruity taste, and the large-sized flakes give it great bite.

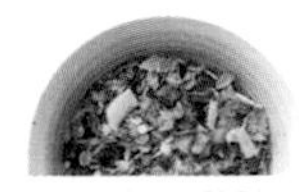

SUPER HIGH FIBRE MUESLI
Dorset Cereals The coconut slices are delicious, and this cereal has a nice, toasty taste. There's no added sugar, but it has plenty of sweet fruit.

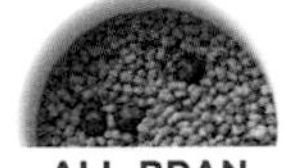

ALL-BRAN BRAN BUDS
Kellogg's This cereal has a substantial 11 g of fibre in a ⅓-cup serving. Add some fresh blueberries for an antioxidant punch.

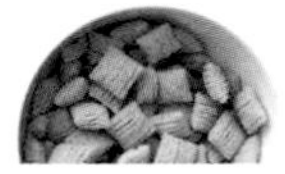

OATMEAL SQUARES
Quaker These are great if you love oats but can't be bothered making hot oatmeal. They're crispy, yet have a light-and-airy bite.

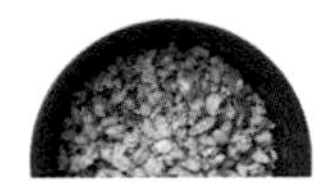

PUMPKIN FLAX PLUS GRANOLA
Nature's Path Organic The granola base is tasty, but what makes this cereal so good are the pumpkin "pepitas" and flaxseeds—both sources of omega-3s.

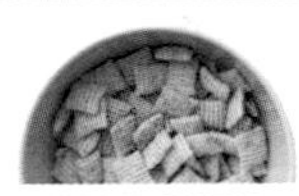

RICE CHEX
General Mills This gluten-free option has a light bite, yet stays crunchy in milk and has a good flavour. And though it has some added sugar, it doesn't taste very sweet.

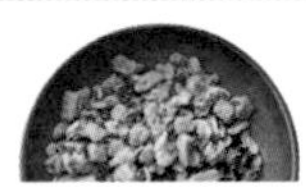

TOASTED BERRY CRISP CEREAL
Kashi Thanks in part to the soy bits, this has 9 g of protein in ¾ cup —about the same as a similar amount of black beans. The berry sweetness is nice, and this is *very* crunchy!

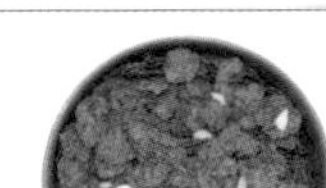

MULTIGRAIN FLAKES WITH ALMONDS
Compliments Balance Light and tasty at only 120 calories per ¾ cup serving (170 calories with ½ cup 1% milk), and the almond flakes provide a refreshing crunch.

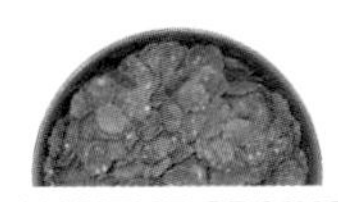

ANCIENT GRAINS
President's Choice Organics Made with organic kamut flour, wheat bran, barley flour and quinoa, among other ingredients, this crunchy, tasty cereal delivers 12 percent of the daily value of fibre. Its sweetness comes from organic honey.

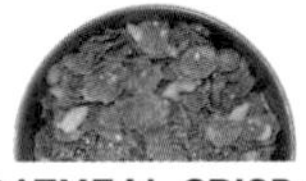

OATMEAL CRISP & ALMONDS
General Mills Although this cereal has added sugars, it also contains lots of vitamins, including 50 percent of your daily value of iron.

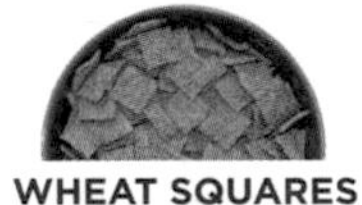

WHEAT SQUARES
President's Choice Organics A great-tasting cereal that's rich in protein at 6 g per 1¼ cup serving, supplying 24 percent of your daily fibre needs.

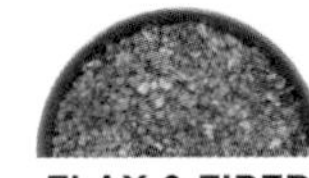

FLAX & FIBER GRANOLA CEREAL
Compliments Balance Crunchy and sweet, this cereal delivers 10 g of protein, or 20 percent of your daily recommended intake.

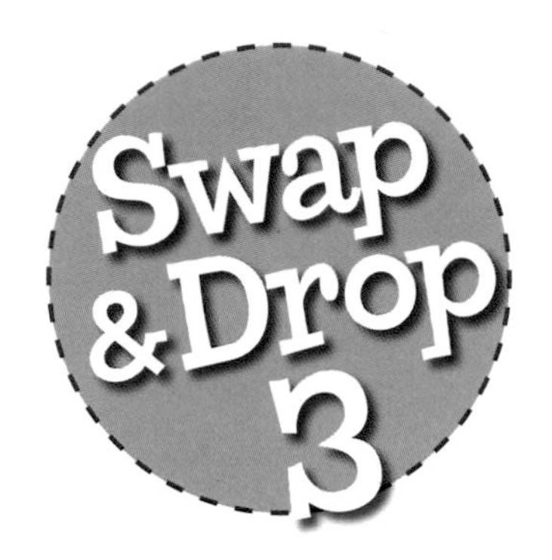

WEEK ▸ THREE

Reinvent lunch

Always plan your midday meal—especially if you have to brown-bag it!

For many of us, the lunch break has become just another extension of our already overburdened day–and since it's the meal we're least likely to eat at home, it can be extra challenging for dieters. This week, you'll learn how to make lunch a great-tasting, sensible meal that you can really enjoy.

"I haven't trusted polls since I read that 62 percent of women had affairs during their lunch hour. I've never met a woman who would give up lunch for sex."

— *Erma Bombeck, writer*

BEATING THE MIDAFTERNOON SLUMP

You know the feeling: It's 3 p.m., you ate lunch a couple hours ago and you are dying for a boost. A croissant may sound great right about now, but reach for cherry tomatoes and celery sticks instead. The crunch of the celery will wake you up, while the tomatoes provide a welcome flavour hit. Pack them with your main meal.

Don't let lunch blindside you: Decide in advance what and where you're going to eat. Right off the bat, that puts you in control. No more putting yourself at the mercy of the food court. No more scouring nearby restaurants or cafés for palatable low-calorie choices. No more desperately searching the lunch room's vending machines for anything that looks halfway healthy. It's time to start eating lunches that refresh and revive you.

The lunch swap

This week, while you keep up the good work at breakfast, help yourself to a healthy, delicious lunch, **Swap & Drop** style. **Swap & Drop** lunches contain about 350 calories. That includes everything–food and drinks. Compare that to the calories in most fast-food and deli meals, and you'll see why sticking to the **Swap & Drop** menu will speed your weight loss.

The meal plans you'll find in this book (starting page 96) include lunches you can make at home, lunches you can pack and even fast-food meals that will work for you. (Turn to page 40 to discover your lunch IQ.)

If you usually eat out

Make a list of the **Swap & Drop** lunches you'll be able to order at your favourite lunch spot or company cafeteria. Try to choose a place that really will do it your way, and keep portion sizes under control. When in doubt, eyeball the serving sizes in Swap 1 (page 18) for a rough idea of what a **Swap & Drop** portion should look like. Keep those handy visual equivalents in mind. Before you dig into lunch, make

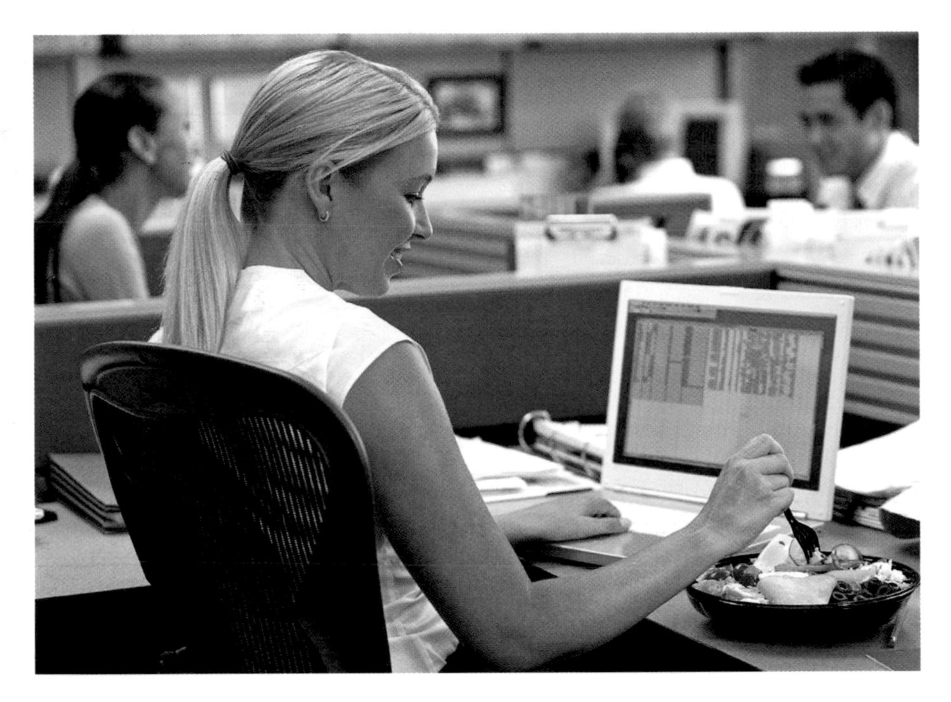

sure that what's on your plate matches up. At some lunch places, you may end up eating just half of what you're served and taking the rest home. Just think of it as two meals for the price of one.

If you usually eat at home

Choose the meals you think you'll like the best from the **Swap & Drop** lunch suggestions (starting page 108). You may find that something you wouldn't normally eat tastes great and really fills you up.

To stay motivated, consider writing each day's lunch menu on your blackboard or calendar the same way restaurants post their daily specials. When you begin to feel hungry as lunchtime approaches, you'll know exactly what's coming.

If you feel ravenous by midafternoon, you can have a snack and have your usual dinner later.

If you plan to brown-bag it

Make a shopping list and buy what you'll need at the beginning of the week. (Don't forget to pick up microwave-safe containers if you don't have them already.)
If your early mornings are crazy, do as much preparation as you can the night before: until you get in the swing of packing your lunch, it's easy to rush out the door empty-handed. Write "Got Lunch?" on a note and stick it on the refrigerator or front door to make sure you won't forget. If you don't have a refrigerator at work to store your lunch, try a refreezable ice pack or freeze a small plastic water bottle

3 Tips for a healthy lunch break

- Have a snack mid-morning, so you're not ravenous by noon.
- If you have the time, go outside and take a walk around the block—it'll clear your head and add a little activity to your day.
- Don't feel guilty about snacking again after lunch. Just opt for a healthy piece of fruit.

GO WHOLE

Always buy bread with the word "whole" in it: 20 grams of additional fibre per day may reduce the risk of heart disease by some 26 percent. Whole-grain breads are a great source of fibre.

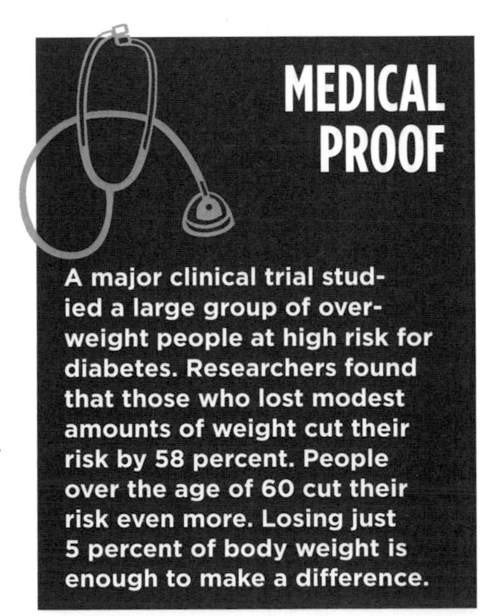

MEDICAL PROOF

A major clinical trial studied a large group of overweight people at high risk for diabetes. Researchers found that those who lost modest amounts of weight cut their risk by 58 percent. People over the age of 60 cut their risk even more. Losing just 5 percent of body weight is enough to make a difference.

Steer clear of processed foods

When it comes to making healthy (yet delicious) food choices, you only need to remember one thing: Eat *real* food. If you choose real food, you will not only see a big difference in your waistline, but you'll feel like a new person, too. Processed foods often contain an unnatural mix of fats, simple sugars, too many calories and not enough nutritional value. Look at the labels on foods and go for choices that use as few ingredients as possible.

THINK AHEAD

When preparing dinner at night, make enough that you'll have leftovers the next day. If you don't like eating repeats, this is still useful for preparing sandwiches: Leftover chicken or beef you roasted yourself is far healthier (and lower in sodium) than prepackaged deli meats.

to use as your lunch chiller, and then as a drink once it thaws. An insulated lunch box or bag (there are a lot of attractive ones to choose from these days) would be a wise investment.

Keep it simple

Many people prefer not having to decide what they're going to eat when they are hungry, but not everyone wants to sit down to the same thing every day. By trying out several **Swap & Drop** lunch options, you'll find the ones that work best for you. All that really matters is arriving at a plan for lunch that you can stick with.

Swap & Drop lunches 101

You may be surprised by some of the choices you find on the lunch menu, such as avocado, peanut butter, cheese and nuts. None of these would make it into a low-fat diet, but we included them in the **Swap & Drop** diet for a very good reason: The latest evidence demonstrates that you don't have to cut way back on fat to lose weight. Recent data shows that most people shed pounds more successfully on diets containing moderate amounts of fat than they do on very low-fat regimens.

Surprised? For years nutritionists told us to cut back on fat; too much fat on the menu makes people gain weight, they said. Gram for gram, fat contains twice as many calories as protein or carbohydrates, they pointed out. Just as bad, it puts our hearts and arteries at risk by increasing cholesterol.

We listened. Over the past decades, the total percentage of calories from fat in the Canadian diet has fallen considerably. But now, in a stunning reversal, the experts are offering very different advice: Some fats are actually good for our hearts. What's more, rather than helping you lose weight, slashing fats may actually make it harder to maintain a healthy weight. Very low-fat diets could even be unhealthy.

Good fat, bad fat

The truth is, experts have long known that there are various kinds of fat. The two main categories are saturated fat and unsaturated fat. Saturated fat comes mostly from animals, either in the form of meat or from cheese, milk and other dairy. Unsaturated fat comes mainly from plants and fish. Some of the biggest sources in our diets are vegetable oils such as corn, safflower, olive, peanut and canola.

When it comes to heart disease, the culprit is saturated fat. Because of its chemical makeup, saturated fat causes the

SWAP & DROP

SWAP THIS	FOR THAT
Switch from cream soups Most cream-based soups have about 140 to 200 calories per cup.	**Try a soothing broth** Most chicken or vegetable broths come in under 50 calories per cup.
Be salad savvy A Caesar salad with all the typical ingredients can clock in anywhere from 200 to a whopping 600 calories.	**A garden salad** uses lots of additional veggies. Add a low-cal dressing on the side, and you have a meal at about 115 calories.
Drop the pop A 500 mL Pepsi or Coke contains about 200 calories.	**Drink club soda** Club soda is refreshing and inexpensive, and has 0 calories.

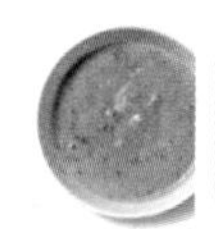
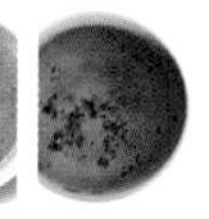
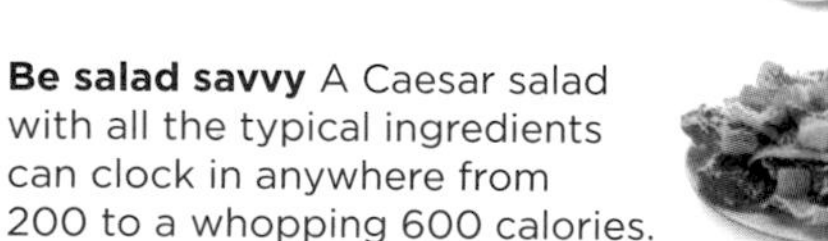
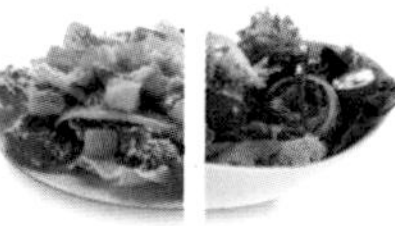
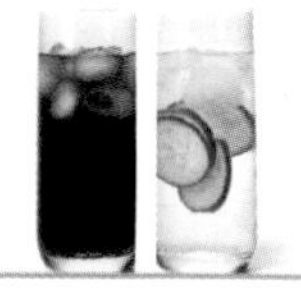

body to churn out extra LDL cholesterol, which is the harmful, artery-clogging kind.

Unsaturated fat, in contrast, has been shown to lower LDL and raise HDL cholesterol, the friendly form that removes dangerous cholesterol from the body. Remarkably, getting plenty of unsaturated fat actually protects your arteries from hardening. Studies around the world have found the same thing: The less saturated and more unsaturated fat people eat, the lower their risk of heart disease.

Some particular unsaturated fats called omega-3 fatty acids are not only great for your heart and arteries, but battle inflammation throughout your body and help prevent several major diseases. Omega-3s can even help lift mild depression, making you feel more energetic. They are abundant in salmon, mackerel, tuna and flaxseed oil. Because these are foods most people don't eat frequently, they are increasingly being taken in supplement form. Who knew doctors would one day be recommending a kind of fat pill?

Carbohydrates: Not so simple

When we cut back on fat, we replaced it with carbohydrates, mostly the simple kind found in white rice or bread. That's bad news: A high-carb, low-fat diet increases levels of triglycerides, a form of fat in the blood linked to a greater danger of heart disease. Second, a diet low in fat and high in simple carbohydrates may make it harder, rather than easier, to lose weight. The surge in blood sugar caused by simple carbs triggers a surge in insulin from the pancreas. One of insulin's jobs is to move blood sugar into muscles, where it provides fuel for movement. But another of its roles is to prompt the body to store excess energy as fat. If blood sugar and insulin levels continually spike and then drop, it can spell trouble.

The resulting rollercoaster makes people hungry more often, and the surges of insulin prime the body to store fat. Cutting back on total fat and filling up on simple carbohydrates hasn't made us thinner. Instead, we're fatter than ever.

Are you !#*@%?& kidding me?

Salad may seem like the best option at fast-food restaurants, but watch out: At McDonald's, for example, the Southwest Salad with Crispy Chicken has 430 calories—more than a Bacon Cheeseburger!

LIKE A FINE WINE

Leftovers don't have to be a letdown. Many dishes actually taste better the next day after their flavours have had time to develop, making them ideal lunchtime fare. Try the Curried Red Lentil Soup (page 145), Rice Salad with Ginger Soy Dressing (page 149) or Couscous Salad with Chickpeas (page 150).

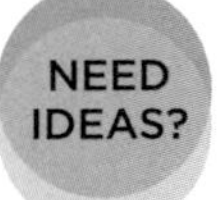

Stuck eating the same thing every day? Try some of these sandwich fillings:

- *Roast beef, tomato and sprouts*
- *Canned tuna, cucumber and a thin slice of light Swiss cheese*
- *Veggie paté, roasted red pepper and goat cheese*

NO FAIL get-slim SWAP

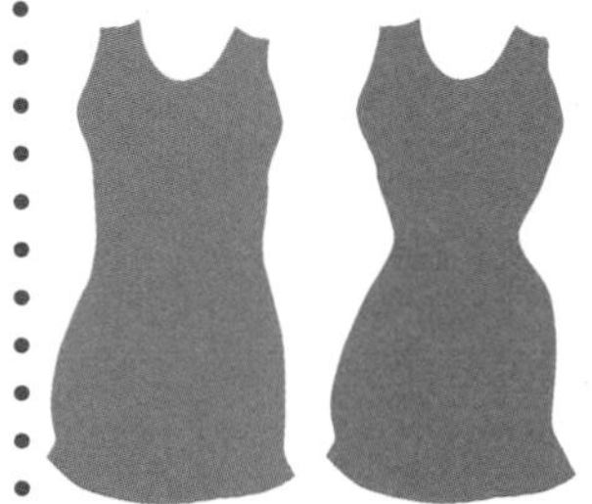

SWAP SHELLED NUTS FOR NUTS IN THE SHELL

Don't always buy shelled nuts—they make it easy to eat too much. Besides, their nutrient values drop during processing and they tend to be salted. A little elbow grease with the nutcracker not only helps to limit portions, it also burns calories, provides the freshest nut and gives the most nutritional bang for your buck. So stock up on peanuts, walnuts, pecans, almonds and pistachios, and get cracking!

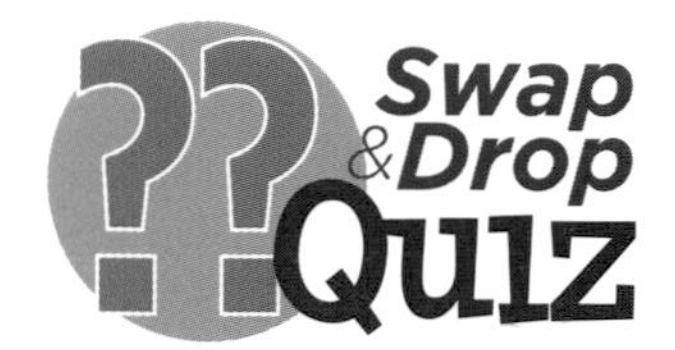

What's your lunching IQ? Complete these nine questions by circling the number to the right of the appropriate answer.

1. Last week, how often did you know in the morning what you'd have for lunch?

Never	1
A few days	2
Most days	3
Every day	4

2. How often did you know at least *where* you would have lunch?

Never	1
A few days	2
Most days	3
Every day	4

3. How often did you grab whatever happened to be handy?

Most days	1
Several days	2
Rarely or never	3

4. Which phrase best describes the choices available to you at lunch?

Very little choice	1
Some choice—same three or four things	2
Ample choice—varied and interesting	3

5. How would you rate your typical lunch?

Not very healthy	1
Healthy enough	2
Very healthy	3

6. How many servings of vegetables did you typically eat at lunch? (French fries don't count.)

None	1
1	2
2 or more	3

7. What was your usual choice for a sandwich bread?

White or French roll	1
Whole-wheat, rye or other dark brown bread	2
Seven-grain or other whole-grain bread	3

8. How often did you eat lunch at home this past week or bring lunch to work?

Never	1
1-2 times	2
3-4 times	3
5-7 times	4

9. What was your usual beverage at lunch?

Regular pop	1
Sweetened fruit drink	2
Milk, diet pop or water	3

Add up the numbers you've circled in the right-hand column.

A score of 24-30: You're already well on your way to eating a good lunch.

A score of 19-23: A few simple strategy changes and you'd be on your way to enjoying lunches **Swap & Drop**-style.

A score of 9-18: Okay, you've got serious work to do. By improving your lunches, you can take a giant step toward trimming calories and slimming your waistline. Put checks beside questions that scored a 1 or 2. Then look for the corresponding answers in the key below for tips that will help you this coming week.

1, 2, 3. If you have no idea where you'll have lunch—or what you'll choose—you're at risk of grabbing whatever's handy when lunchtime rolls around. That could spell trouble for your diet. Study the tips in this Swap to master lunch by planning ahead.

Of course, not all of us always know ahead of time where we'll eat lunch. If that sounds like you, then it's time to keep a very close watch on portion sizes, wherever lunch hour finds you.

4. When your choices are limited, your best option may be to pack it in—lunch, that is. You'll find several tasty packable lunches in the **Swap & Drop** meal planner (page 96). If you're pressed for time in the morning, put your lunch together the night before.

5. Is your lunch falling short on good nutrition? If your typical lunch rarely includes a green vegetable, it needs work. If the lunch spots available don't offer much choice, your best bet is to bring your own meal.

6. What, no vegetables? You're missing out on one of the best health and diet foods around. Follow the **Swap & Drop** menu this week, and you'll get at least one serving at lunch, usually two.

7. Breaking the white-bread habit can be tough, but you'll get more nutrients—and feel fuller for longer—when you eat breads that are made from whole wheat or rye flour. You'll get even more fibre, plus healthful vitamins and minerals, from breads that contain whole grains like oats.

8. Don't dismiss the idea of brown-bagging your lunch. This week, give it a try for a day or two. There's no better way to control exactly what and how much you eat. Many people find that packing a lunch relieves them of the pressure of having to choose a healthy meal when they're already hungry. (Not to mention how much money you'll save.)

9. Sugary pop and fruit-based beverages pack a load of calories. Some experts place much of the blame for our growing weight problems on their popularity: The sugar and corn syrup in soft drinks and juices now supply a hefty percent of our total calories.

That's an awful lot of calories from foods that don't supply much else in the way of nutrition. Switch to a sugar-free beverage or help yourself to a glass of plain or sparkling water, and you'll shave 150 calories from your diet just like that.

Low-fat milk is another smart choice, since it's loaded with protein and calcium. Calcium is essential for healthy bones, and there's evidence that it also helps speed weight loss.

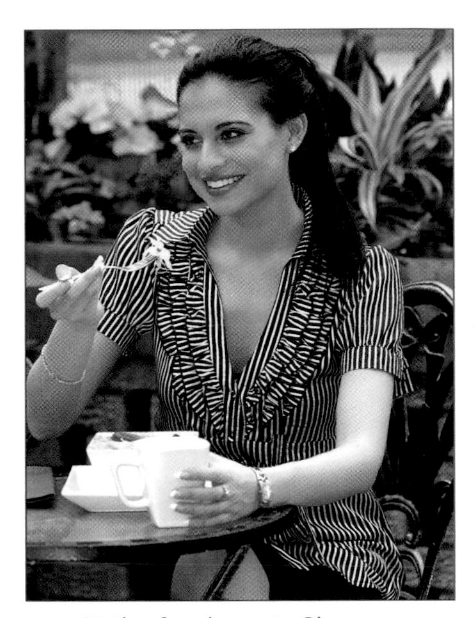

At the food court: Choose a salad either as a main course or side dish, with low-cal dressing on the side to help fill you up.

Eat fat, get slim

A diet with moderate amounts of fat is simply more satisfying than a harsh low-fat regimen. And it's the only kind of diet that really works over the long term. Another reason may be that people consuming moderate amounts of fat are less likely to overdo simple carbohydrates and will find it easier to keep hunger in check.

Replace saturated fat with unsaturated fat wherever you can. Switch from butter to olive or canola oil, for instance, and eat less meat and more fish. Keep portion sizes and calories under control, and steer toward more complex carbohydrates like those in whole-grain breads and cereals.

The perfect diet food

Every meal on the **Swap & Drop** lunch plan includes at least one serving of vegetables, often two. No other food fills you up on fewer calories with more nutrients. Vegetables are rich in fibre and disease-fighting antioxidants. They're mostly complex carbohydrates, the kind that keep blood sugar levels off the rollercoaster.

And as any chef will tell you, nothing brightens up a plate like dark leafy greens, yellow peppers or carrot slices. On the **Swap & Drop** lunch menu, you'll find plenty of clever ways to add a serving or two of vegetables to your favourite sandwiches and soups to make them not only more filling, but more flavourful–without piling on calories. ■

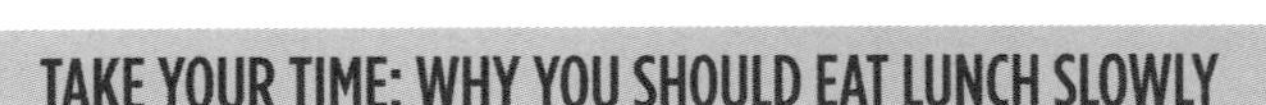

TAKE YOUR TIME: WHY YOU SHOULD EAT LUNCH SLOWLY

Researchers at the University of Rhode Island supplied two groups of women with huge plates of pasta, instructing one group to eat quickly and the other to eat slowly. Those who ate slowly ended up consuming significantly fewer calories, largely because they were more attuned to their appetites and were able to stop when they were full. They also reported enjoying their meals more (no surprise there!). So take it easy during lunch, even if you're rushed.

For Swap & Drop lunch recipes, turn to page 108.

Eat less meat, more veg

Want to whip up a quick and easy side salad to go with your lunch? Try these two:

- **Quick-cooking whole-wheat couscous with cherry tomatoes, diced cucumber and an oil and red wine vinegar dressing**
- **Baby spinach with orange segments, dried cranberries and toasted sunflower seeds, tossed with oil and balsamic**

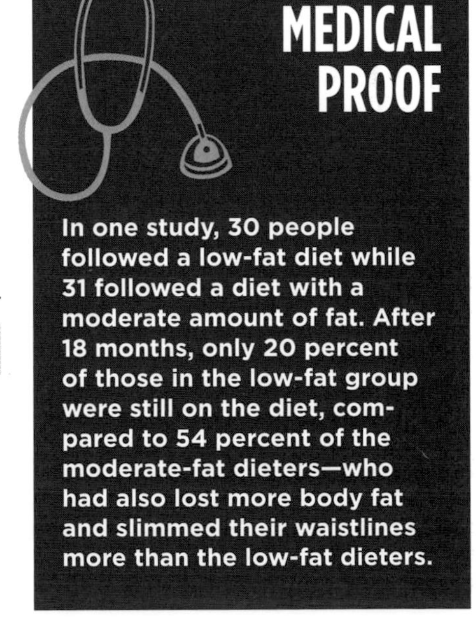

MEDICAL PROOF

In one study, 30 people followed a low-fat diet while 31 followed a diet with a moderate amount of fat. After 18 months, only 20 percent of those in the low-fat group were still on the diet, compared to 54 percent of the moderate-fat dieters—who had also lost more body fat and slimmed their waistlines more than the low-fat dieters.

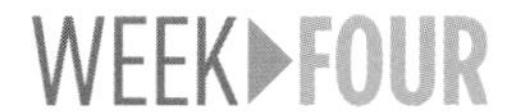

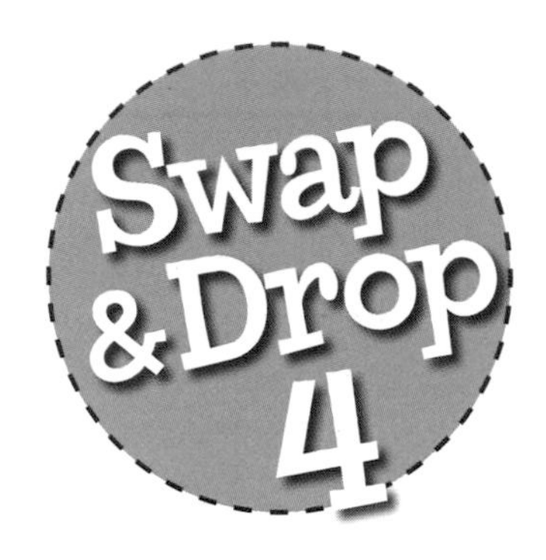

Learn to snack well

Never get so hungry that you'll devour just about anything—smart snacking is key to diet success

“I want to get a vending machine with fun-sized candy bars, and the glass in front will be a magnifying glass. You'll be mad, but it will be too late.”

— Mitch Hedberg, comedian

SNACKING AND WEIGHT LOSS

Worried that snacking will make it harder to lose weight? Surprisingly, several large studies have found no link at all between how many snacks people eat and how much they weigh. Even people who snack before bedtime—once considered a big diet taboo—don't seem to be any more likely to be overweight than people who skip late snacks.

A whole chapter on snacks–in a diet book? Of course! Anyone who wants to lose weight and keep it off needs a great snacking strategy to take the edge off hunger between meals. This week, you'll learn just how easy it is to fit nutritious, low-calorie nibbles into your day.

Eating something between meals can be one of a dieter's smartest strategies. When asked, people are most likely to describe “hunger” as the single biggest fear they face in dieting. That's not surprising, and this week we want you to pay close attention to hunger cues. And instead of resisting them, we want you to give in–the **Swap & Drop** way. Here's why.

Hunger is an extremely powerful force. Getting enough fuel for our bodies is essential to survival. It is a matter of life and death, literally, so the body has a variety of internal signals to tell it when its energy stores are dipping low. Some come from the belly. Some originate in the brain.

The longer we go without eating, the more powerful those signals become. It doesn't take long before they're so urgent that almost all we can think about is food. As your hunger intensifies, your willpower weakens. If you get hungry enough, you'll reach for anything.

That's where smart snacking comes in. Help yourself to something sensible when you feel hungry, and you'll help ensure that hunger doesn't rise up and devour your determination.

Eating more often than just three times a day might actually have advantages over that traditional pattern when it comes to health. In a study at St. Michael's Hospital at the University of Toronto, researchers tested two nutritionally identical diets where one group of volunteers ate their allotted food in three square meals, and the others ate the same amounts of the same food but divided it among 17 snacks. The frequent snackers saw their choles-

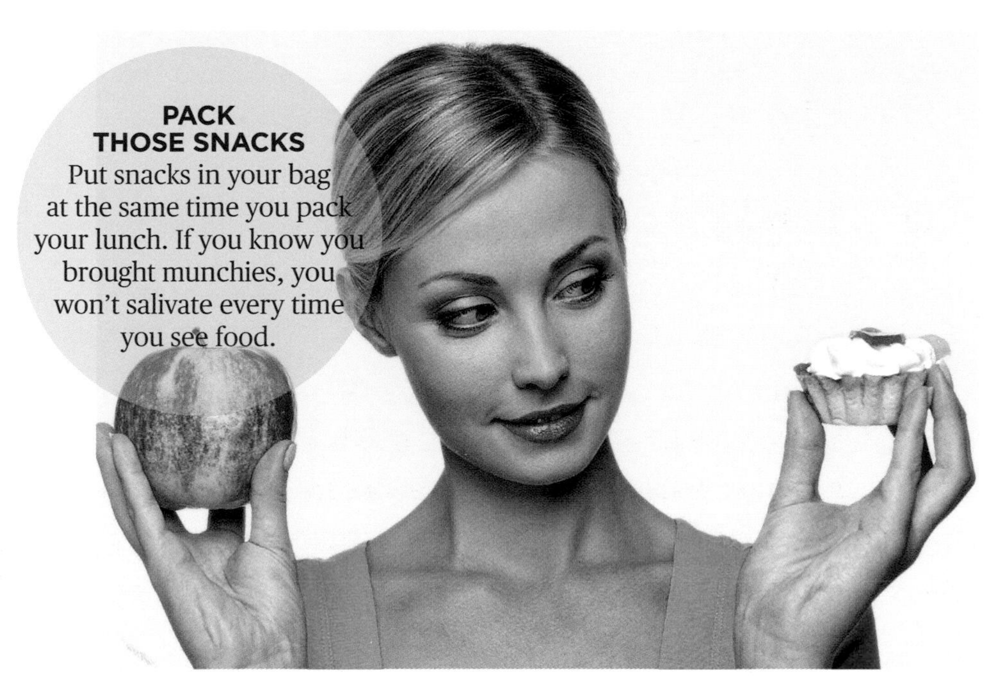

PACK THOSE SNACKS
Put snacks in your bag at the same time you pack your lunch. If you know you brought munchies, you won't salivate every time you see food.

terol levels drop more than those who ate three meals. Eating smaller amounts more frequently, the experts concluded, kept blood sugar and insulin levels down, which in turn reduced the body's output of cholesterol. Plus, holding blood sugar and insulin levels steady can keep hunger in check.

For many, eating 17 snacks a day might be going a bit overboard, but having several during the day is vital to weight loss. A majority of successful dieters in one study reported that they ate five times a day: three small main meals and two snacks.

This week, help yourself to a snack. But before you do, we're going to ask you to do one simple thing: Make sure you're really hungry.

Learn to spot hunger cues

In **Swap & Drop**, we've grouped snacks and desserts together. One of our reasons is that the same foods often serve both purposes–frozen yogourt, fruit, a piece of chocolate, an oatmeal cookie–depending on when we eat them. Another reason is that most of us think of snacks and desserts as optional foods, a treat that's not part of our basic diet. Help yourself to sensible portions of snacks and desserts–but only eat them to satisfy genuine hunger.

Isn't that the reason most of us eat in the first place? Surprisingly, no. Weight-loss experts say we typically eat for reasons that have nothing to do with genuine physical hunger. We take a tub of buttered popcorn or a box of chocolate-covered raisins to our seat at the movies simply

For more yummy snack and dessert recipes, turn to the recipes on page 122.

8 SNACKING STRATEGIES to control hunger

1. **Instead of buying snacks at a movie, hockey game or other event, chew a stick of sugar-free gum.**
2. **At parties, stand as far away as you can from the bowls of chips, dips and other munchies.**
3. **On car trips, plan ahead by bringing a few Swap & Drop snacks. If you have a tendency to munch in the car, bring just a single serving, not the whole box. Put the rest in the trunk.**
4. **Buy snacks in small packs. If you buy the jumbo size to save money, divide it into single-serving bags or containers as soon as you get home.**
5. **Put the healthiest snacks where you'll see them when you open a kitchen cabinet or the refrigerator.**
6. **Don't snack in your office. (And definitely don't keep bags of chips or pretzels in your desk drawer.) Go somewhere else—the kitchen, cafeteria, lounge or outside. That way you won't associate your office with food.**
7. **At home, enjoy your snacks in the kitchen—and nowhere else.**
8. **Don't eat to relax. Relax, then eat. Stress is such a big factor in diet that we've devoted a whole swap to stress-busting tips (starting page 78).**

because that's what we've always done. We eat because one of our colleagues just brought a homemade coffee cake to the office, and who can resist?

The experts call these reasons for eating "environmental cues": Something in your surroundings gives you the urge to eat. You may have just finished a big, filling meal, but a sight or smell will trigger memories of past occasions, prompting you to eat—so you're likely to simply help yourself, often without thinking.

Emotional eating

Many of us eat for emotional reasons, too. After all, food can be comforting. Getting together over a meal with friends or family can be a pleasant way to relax after a long day. And there's no need to make it overly complicated: Food simply tastes good.

When we eat something delicious, the experience triggers the release of feel-good endorphins in the brain. Certain foods may have their own mood-enhancing effects: Carbohydrates are thought to increase the absorption of an amino acid called tryptophan, which in turn boosts levels of serotonin, another brain chemical associated with mental well-being.

There are other reasons why eating is linked to emotions. If your parents comforted you or rewarded you with food, for instance, you may tend to reach for something to eat when you're feeling low or want to congratulate yourself for a job well-done. You may get into the habit of eating when you're bored or lonely.

If you eat when you're not genuinely hungry, you'll almost certainly consume more calories than your body needs. There are healthier ways to deal with stress, boredom or loneliness. To find out if environmental or emotional cues are controlling when and how much you eat, you need to pay attention to what genuine hunger feels like.

Knowing when you're genuinely hungry

Try this simple experiment. If you typically have either a mid-morning or mid-afternoon snack, skip it and push the next meal about an hour later than usual. Then pay attention to how you feel. After you've gone four or five hours without eating anything, your body will begin to send out physical hunger cues. Some of these

Are you !#*@%?& kidding me?

MANY FAST-FOOD CHAINS include "snack-size" items on their menus, hoping to pull you in with the small size and super-low price—but these snacks also pack a surprising amount of calories: At KFC, the Colonel Snacker sandwich is 260 calories, and McDonald's Pesto Crispy McMini Sandwich is 330 calories. For that many calories, you could instead have two or three healthy homemade snacks to keep you going.

SWAP & DROP

SWAP THIS		FOR THAT
Most store-bought muffins are your enemy: A store-bought blueberry muffin has a whopping 444 calories.	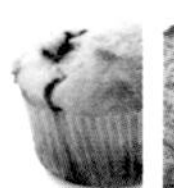 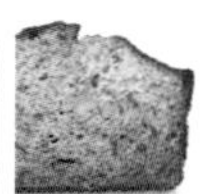	**Homemade banana bread** has far fewer: One slice has 225 calories, if you skip chocolate chips.
Sugar cones are a cute and tasty way to eat ice cream, but they add even more calories to an already indulgent treat.	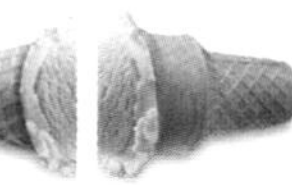	**A plain wafer-type cone,** plus frozen yogourt instead of ice cream, will save you 175 calories.
Potato chips are dangerously addictive—and even just a 28 g bag can have 150 calories and 10 g of fat.	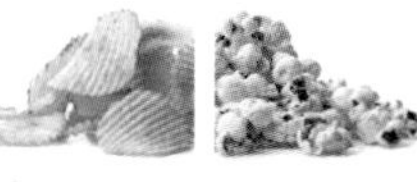	**Air-popped popcorn** has only 31 calories and 0 g of fat per cup. Sprinkle with a little salt.
Strawberry ice cream is a classic treat, and a classic calorie bomb—500 per cup!	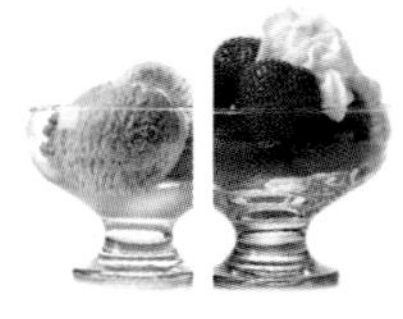	**A cup of strawberries and whipped cream** is much fresher and lighter—86 calories together.

come from a part of the brain called the hypothalamus. When blood sugar levels fall, the hypothalamus senses an impending energy crisis and begins to issue "feed me" orders by way of the central nervous system. Your stomach growls. Your thoughts zero in on food. You may find yourself getting cranky.

This physical hunger is different from the emotional or environmental kind, and it is not the same as a food craving. Food cravings target specific foods. You may crave chocolate when you're feeling lonely. You may find yourself craving a hamburger when you're on a car trip. Cravings are almost always responses to emotional or environmental cues.

Physical hunger isn't so specific. When your body needs more energy in the form of food, you don't focus on the taste of a particular food. What you want is any food to fill you up.

Essential questions

As part of your hunger test this week, try another experiment. When you finally sit down to eat, make a point of slowing down and paying close attention to how you feel as you eat. Notice what it feels like as your hungry sensations give way to a feeling of satisfaction.

During the rest of this week, each time you feel the urge to grab a snack between meals, pause for as long as it takes to ask yourself these two simple questions: Am I really hungry? Can I wait until my next meal to eat?

If the answers are a resounding "Yes!" and "No!" help yourself to a snack. But if your answer is a lukewarm "Well, maybe,"

GOT CALCIUM?

Not only does calcium build strong bones, there's research that shows it also helps the body burn fat. Some favourite calcium-rich snacks, in 100-calorie portions, include:

- Low- or non-fat yogourt, plain or artificially sweetened (1 cup)
- Yogourt smoothie: In a blender, mix ½ cup low-fat plain yogourt, ½ cup skim, low-fat or soy milk and 1 cup frozen, unsweetened strawberries (or other fruit) until mixture is smooth
- Low-fat or skim milk (1 cup)
- Skim or low-fat milk flavoured with sugar-free syrup (1 cup)
- Reduced-fat cheese (see Swap 1, page 18, for portion sizes)
- Skim or low-fat latte (medium size)
- Hot cocoa made with skim or low-fat milk (1 cup)
- Calcium-fortified orange juice (1 cup)
- Juice pop made with calcium-fortified juice (1 cup)
- Sugar-free pudding made with skim or low-fat milk (1 cup)

BAKED VS *Fried*

MANY BRANDS of crackers and potato chips boast that they're "baked, not fried." The implication, of course, is fewer calories. But the calorie difference isn't always that great. The baked brands still use some fat, and their calorie count is often close to that of the fried products. So don't buy something simply because the label says "baked." Look for brands that supply at least 1 g of fibre and less than 3 g of fat per single serving.

Savoury snacks

Here are a dozen fresh and delicious alternatives to the usual chips. Each is just 100 calories—the perfect amount for a snack. Remember: On Swap & Drop, we want you to enjoy food!

- Soup (minestrone, vegetable, tomato, chicken noodle), 1 cup
- Edamame (soybeans ready to eat from the shell), 100 g
- V-8 juice, 1 cup
- Three-bean salad, 1 cup
- Hard-boiled egg, 1
- String cheese, low fat, 1 piece
- Hard cheese, 20 g
- Peanut butter, 1 tbsp
- Corn tortilla topped with grated, reduced-fat cheese, 2 tbsp
- Hummus, 2 tbsp, and ½ pita, cut into wedges
- English muffin pizza: half muffin spread with 1 tbsp pasta sauce and 2 tbsp grated cheese, baked at 350°F (175°C) until cheese bubbles.
- Sugar snap peas, 1 cup (crunchy and good, and only 40 calories!)

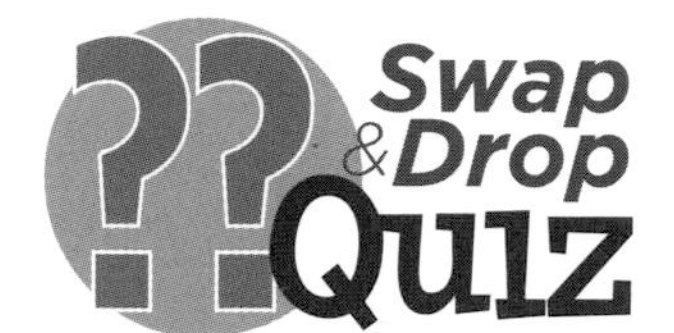

The hungry "I." What drives your snacking—emotions, environment or just plain old hunger? Check only the shapes with the statements that apply to you.

- ● When I go see a movie, I almost always get popcorn, candy or some other treat.
- ■ When I'm very busy, I sometimes don't even notice that I'm hungry.
- ◆ On stressful days, I often find it relaxing to eat something.
- ● If I'm bored and there's food around, I'll eat it.
- ■ It's no big deal for me to say no to treats if I'm not really hungry.
- ◆ There are certain foods I really crave, like chocolate or salty snacks.
- ■ I like the feeling of being really hungry when I sit down to a meal.
- ● I have a tendency to clean my plate even if I'm not really that hungry.
- ◆ If I'm feeling a little down or blue, eating something can really help.
- ● If there's a plate full of cookies or chips in front of me, I won't be able to resist taking some.
- ● I have to be careful about having junk food around the house. If it's there, I'll eat it.
- ■ My way of dealing with stress is to get up and do something.
- ■ As long as I know I'll be sitting down to a meal soon, I can deal with feeling hungry.
- ● Dinner just doesn't feel like dinner without dessert.
- ◆ I definitely don't like the feeling of being hungry.

Score: Tally up the number of coloured shapes you checked according to colour.

■ green ______________

● **red** ______________

◆ yellow ______________

What your score means:

■ If you checked mostly green boxes, at least you're not snacking because you're bored or stressed. This week, choose from among the recommended **Swap & Drop** snacks (recipes start on page 122), and you'll keep calories under control.

● If you checked mostly red circles, you tend to be an "on cue" snacker: You reach for a snack not necessarily because you're hungry, but because of cues in the environment around you. Recognizing them—and asking yourself if you're really hungry—could help you avoid gobbling up calories you don't want or need.

◆ If you checked mostly yellow diamonds, you tend to be an emotional snacker. You have the urge to eat something when you're feeling anxious, sad, lonely or stressed out. Many people do. Recognizing what real hunger feels like and finding ways other than eating to deal with your emotions will help you control calories and eat more healthfully. Turn to Swap 10 (page 78) for help dealing with stress.

If your score was divided evenly among greens, reds and yellows, you're on your way to becoming a smart snacker! But you still need to be aware of eating only when you're hungry. The tips in this chapter will guide you the rest of the way.

---

take five–get up and change what you're doing. Some options:

- Take a quick stroll.
- Drink a tall glass of water.
- Complete a chore that needs doing–dusting, tidying up, sweeping.
- Wash your face or hands.
- Brush your teeth.
- Practice a relaxation technique like deep breathing.

Food cravings typically disappear as quickly as they come. But if after five minutes or so you're still hungry, then by all means, it's time for a snack.

Swap & Drop snacks 101

Every snack on the **Swap & Drop** diet contains about 100 calories–enough to ease hunger pangs and still keep you within your calorie guidelines. We've chosen snacks that offer plenty of flavour. It may be a no-brainer, but it's worth repeating: If something doesn't taste good, don't eat it. Why waste calories on a fat-free cracker that tastes like sawdust when you can help yourself to a handful of rich-tasting nuts or a piece of pita with sizzling salsa?

Beyond good taste, a snack worth its calories should also be satisfying in other ways. If it's 32°C in the shade, you want

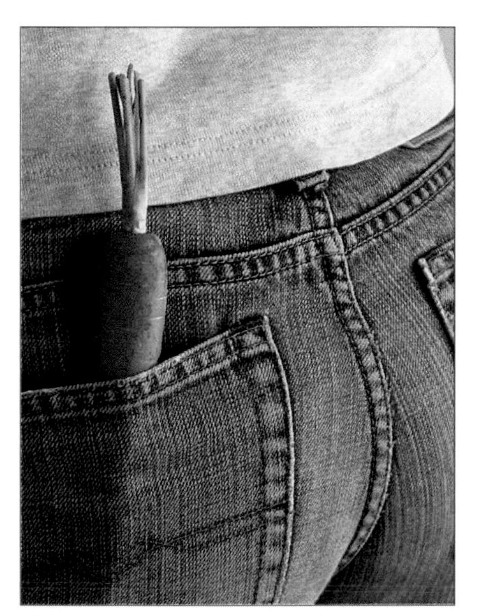

Carry a carrot in your back pocket—why not? Carrots are portable, crunchy and delicious!

something cool and refreshing, like a raspberry sorbet. If you're just in from shoveling snow, hot chocolate might be the pick. Naturally, a snack should also satisfy your hunger long enough to tide you over until the next meal. Research shows that snacks that take up a lot of volume per calorie–popcorn or fruit-and-yogourt smoothies, for instance–tend to make people feel fuller on fewer calories.

Snacks that pack a lot of nutrition also turn out to be more satisfying and filling than those with a lot of empty calories. Remember the nuts we mentioned earlier? One recent study found that snacking on nuts might actually help people keep their weight down. The reason: Nuts are loaded with protein, vitamins, and, yes, fat. With all of that nutritional content, it doesn't take very many of them to satisfy your appetite.

Choosing a nutritious snack is important for another reason: When you're on a low-calorie diet, it's just good sense to make those calories count. On **Swap & Drop**, snacks should make up about 15 percent of your total calorie intake. We've also included some less nutritious favourites just because, well, they're tasty. After all, it's not about avoiding candy and cookies forever–it's about eating them less often, in reasonable portions, and learning to enjoy them more.

Salty, crunchy—healthy?

No chips are really ideal snack foods—they tend to be too high in salt and fat (and too low in other nutrients) to make the grade. But you can buy these healthier-than-usual options:

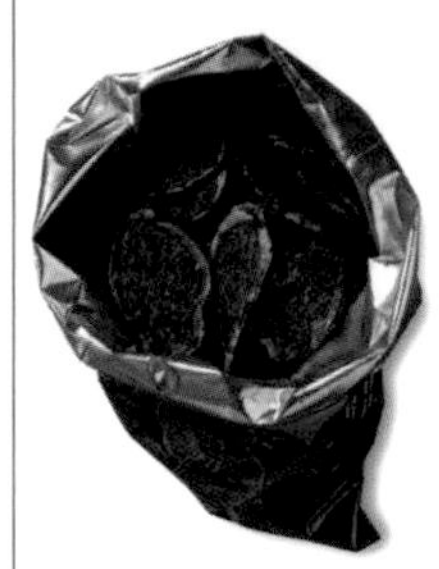

TERRA BLUES POTATO CHIPS These thick, satisfying chips are made from blue potatoes.
A 50 g serving has 230 calories.

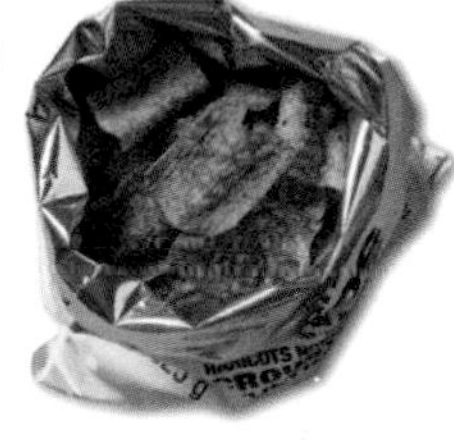

PC MULTIGRAIN CHIPS These whole-grain chips have great crunch.
A 50 g serving has 240 calories.

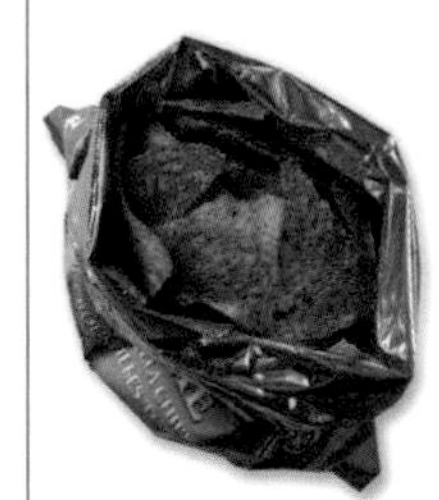

GUILTLESS GOURMET CHILI LIME TORTILLA CHIPS These baked organic corn chips are nice and spicy.
A 50 g serving has 210 calories.

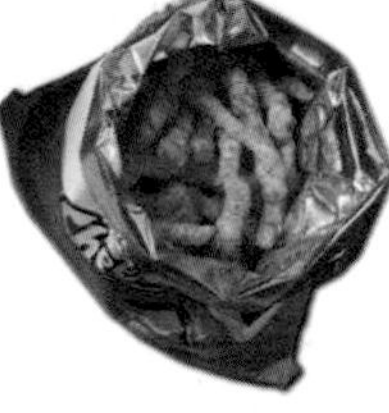

BAKED! CHEETOS CRUNCHY These may have a neon-bright colour, but they're also yummy.
A 50 g serving has 230 calories.

NO FAIL get-slim STRATEGY

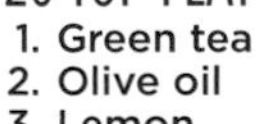

20 TOP FLAT TUMMY FOODS

1. Green tea
2. Olive oil
3. Lemon
4. Chicken
5. Cinnamon
6. Green chai tea
7. Cucumber
8. Bran
9. Low-fat yogourt
10. Legumes
11. Turmeric
12. Quinoa
13. Pears
14. Dark chocolate
15. Berries
16. Leeks
17. Salmon
18. Miso
19. Eggs
20. Greens (spinach, broccoli, etc.)

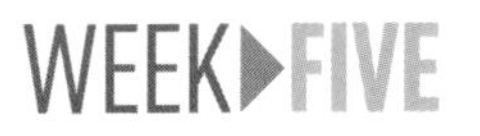

Eat nutritious, delicious dinners

One of the best ways to eat less is to eat slower, so try to make dinnertime a special occasion

Dinner is the time we relax and reward ourselves—often with an overload of calories, carbs and fat. This week, we'll show you how to make dinner a daily celebration. You'll learn to slow down, savour the flavours and enjoy the company. And when you start doing so, you'll find that you naturally eat less.

> A man seldom thinks with more earnestness of anything than he does of his dinner.
>
> — *Samuel Johnson, author*

IS THERE A RIGHT TIME TO EAT?

You might have heard that eating late at night will cause you to gain weight, but what really matters is how long you go between meals. If you wait too long to have dinner, you may be tempted to wolf it down when you finally do eat. No matter when you dine, fit some small, healthy snacks in between.

Dinners are typically the biggest meal of the day and the source of the most calories. That's why taking charge of dinner can have the biggest weight-loss payoff. By being sensible about portions and using the photos in Swap 1 (page 18) as guides, you'll discover that you can still enjoy delicious dinners while the pounds just melt away.

Slow down. Relax. Enjoy.

Of all the meals of the day, dinner is the one that most reflects our family histories and special tastes. When you sit down to dinner this week, no matter what's on the table, slow down and really taste the meal. Too often these days we're doing a mad dash from here to there, gobbling down meals without really taking the time to taste what's in front of us. And eating too quickly is one reason so many of us find ourselves struggling with weight.

This week, give dinner your full attention. Set aside enough time that you don't feel rushed. You may not be able to treat yourself to a leisurely dinner every night, but if you can make sure you enjoy an unhurried dinner at least three times during the coming week, you'll begin to see why savouring a meal is one of the simplest and smartest dieting strategies around.

Here's why: Research shows that, just as a body sends hunger signals, it also communicates when it's had enough food.

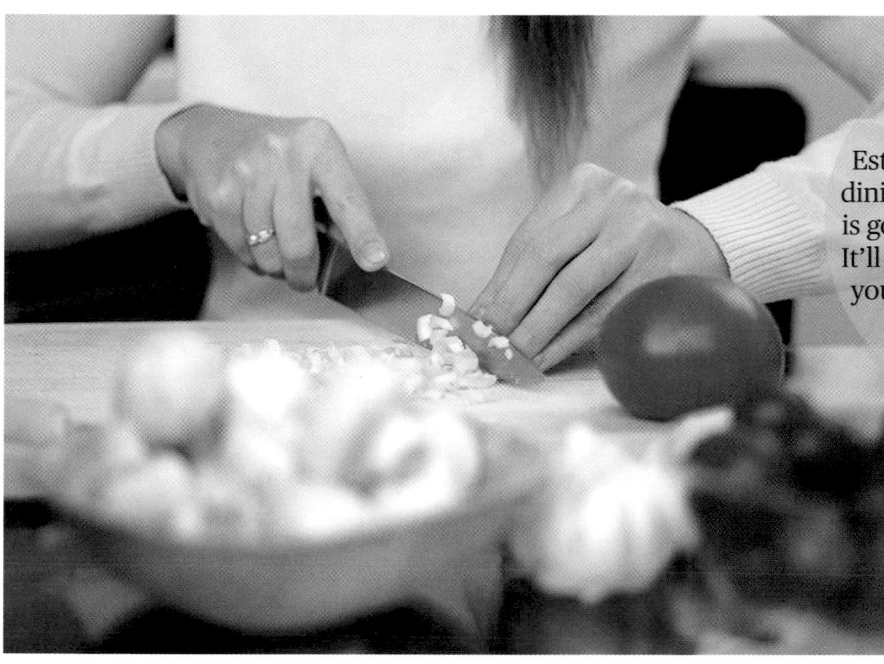

WHY WE LOVE ROUTINES
Establishing a routine—like dining together every night—is good for the whole family: It'll help you to control what you eat, and give your kids a sense of comfort and security.

Those cues, called satiety signals, are the body's way of balancing calories we consume with calories we burn. They work effectively as long as we take the time to notice them.

If you've ever stood up from a holiday feast feeling as stuffed as the turkey, you know that it's easy to eat more than you really need—sometimes a lot more. Studies show that it takes up to 20 minutes after food reaches your stomach for satiety signals to kick in—and you can eat a lot in 20 minutes.

That's the problem with fast food, and fast eating in general. If you scarf down food in a big hurry, you don't even give your body the time to tell you, "Hey, enough already!"

Making the change

We know, we know: Given how busy life is for many of us, taking time for dinner isn't always easy. Even so, give it a try. Make it a goal to have everyone in your house sit down for a meal together. It's worth the effort, not only for the food, but also for the chance to spend time with your family. If you're used to an eat-and-run approach, you can rediscover dinner's pleasures—and make yourself a smarter eater—with these seven simple changes:

1. Arrange your schedule so you have at least 30 quiet minutes for dinner.

2. When you have dinner at home, always have it in your dining area. That way you won't associate food with other parts of the house—the couch in front of the television, for instance.

8

The number of hours of sleep you need to lose weight.

Insomnia, or even chronically depriving yourself of an hour or two of sleep, may keep you from reaching your weight loss goal. Some researchers suspect that overtired people unwittingly compensate for their lack of energy by eating more. Research suggests that staying up late also prompts your body to store more calories. Losing sleep can also make people more susceptible to stress, and thus more likely to overeat. Whatever the reason, weight-loss experts recommend trying to get eight hours of sleep every night.

:) HAPPINESS IS A LONG MEAL

Nothing would be more tiresome than eating and drinking if God had not made them a pleasure as well as a necessity.
—Voltaire

More Healthy Swaps

- sandwiches → **soups**
- sour cream → **2% Greek yogourt**
- coffee → **herbal tea**
- mashed potatoes → **mashed cauliflower**
- cookies → **fresh fruit**
- milk chocolate → **dark chocolate**
- pasta → **quinoa, brown rice or bulgur**
- salt → **herbs**

3. If the menu allows, divide your meal into courses–for instance, main course and vegetables, salad and dessert. Choose the order that works best for you.
4. Make the meal the focus of dinnertime. Turn off the television. Put away the newspaper. Let your voice mail pick up your calls. A little dinner music is fine, as long as it doesn't distract you from the meal.
5. Serve a 250 mL glass of water with dinner. Between each bite, put down your fork and take a small sip of water. Sipping water forces you to slow down. Water with dinner also makes a meal more filling without adding any calories. Many people find that it helps them clear their palates and more fully experience the flavours in a meal.
6. Pay attention to how the food tastes. Take small bites and let them linger in your mouth long enough so that the full flavour is released.
7. Between courses, take a minute or two to relax, chat and savour what you've just eaten. It may sound paradoxical, but lingering over dinner could help you drop pounds and maintain a healthy weight.

Knowing when enough is enough

Paying attention to satiety signals is just one more way to make sure that you keep portion sizes–the key to **Swap & Drop** success–under control. Most of us underestimate how many calories we're really consuming.

Consider, for example, a study from researchers at the United States National Cancer Institute in Maryland. In the study, men underreported daily calorie intake by 12 to 14 percent; women, by 16 to 20 percent! They honestly didn't know how much they were eating. The implication: Merely getting better at knowing proper portion sizes could cut daily calorie intake substantially.

Some dieters discover that once they learn to stop eating when they're no longer hungry, they automatically eat reasonable portions. The art of knowing when you're satisfied takes time to learn, however, and it doesn't work for everyone. So practice memorizing the portion sizes from Swap 1 (starting page 18).

SWAP & DROP

SWAP THIS		FOR THAT
Cream of tomato soup has 140 calories and 9 g of fat.	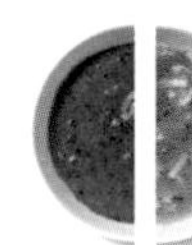 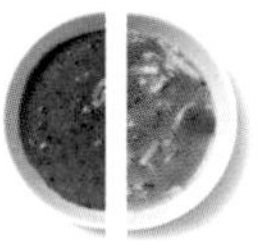	**Chicken noodle soup** only has 110 calories and 2 g of fat. Dress it up with fresh herbs.
Alfredo sauce sure is delicious, but since it's made with cream and parmesan, it also has 180 calories per ½ cup.	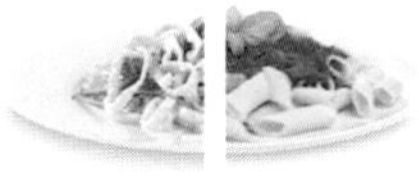	**Red sauce** will save you 100 calories—and give you antioxidants from those vibrant tomatoes.
White wine has heart-healthy benefits, but a 150 mL glass of Pinot Grigio has 120 calories.	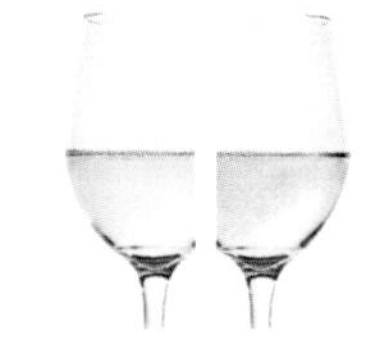	**A wine spritzer** cuts those calories in half: Combine equal parts wine and soda water.
A slice of chocolate fudge cake sure is luxurious—too luxurious at 490 calories.	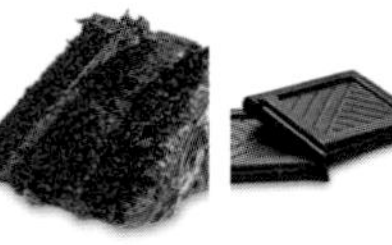	**Two pieces of dark chocolate** will satisfy your cravings for only 106 calories.

Swap & Drop dinners 101

Most of the dinners in the **Swap & Drop** meal plan (page 96) contain between 400 and 460 calories. By following **Swap & Drop** breakfast, lunch, snack and dinner recommendations, you'll tally between 1,300 and 1,600 calories a day. As we promised before, that's a level that will guarantee you lose weight at a reasonable, healthy pace.

How can **Swap & Drop** dinners be so thrifty with calories? By including at least two servings of vegetables. Vegetables are extra low in calories–a half-cup of spinach contains only 27, for instance, and the same amount of sliced carrots just 30. Therefore, you can think of them as "free" foods, calorie-wise, and help yourself to as much as you want.

One exception is vegetables that are fried, creamed or sautéed in butter or oil. In these cases, you do need to pay attention to serving sizes. Millilitre for millilitre, the fats in butter, cream and cooking oil have more than twice as many calories as either protein or carbohydrates. So even small amounts can drive up the calorie total fast. A teaspoon of butter, for instance, packs 34 calories. A teaspoon of cooking oil contains 40.

While the **Swap & Drop** dinner menus are relatively low in fat, we've been careful to include some fats, especially the unsaturated kinds that can improve cholesterol levels. Fat adds flavour and enjoyment to food. As you've learned already, diets with a moderate amount of fat offer much more variety and flexibility than strict low-fat diets.

In fact, research has shown that diets that include moderate amounts of fat actually work best–they're easier to stick to, and meals feel more satisfying. As long as you keep portion sizes under control, you can eat any kind of food you enjoy, even if it contains fat.

Of course, it is wise to eliminate fatty foods that you don't really like or want. It's smart, too, to replace saturated fat with unsaturated fat. You can do this easily by using olive oil or canola oil instead of butter, for instance, and choosing a low-fat mayonnaise made with canola oil. But don't get hung up on fat grams. Managing portion sizes is a much smarter way to keep calories under control.

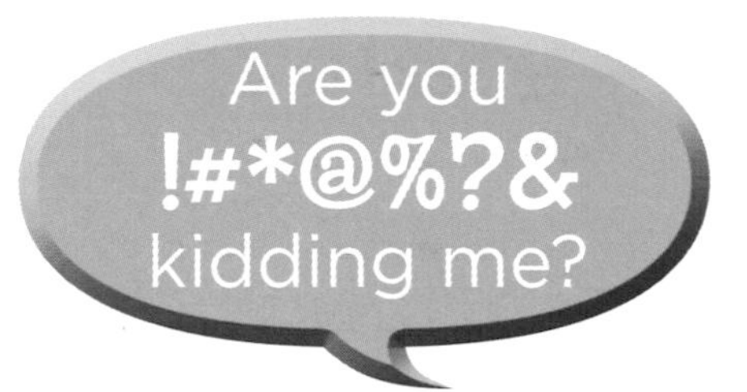

In developing countries, fats make up 10 percent of daily calories. In North America today, daily fat intake is about 35 to 40 percent! This is the equivalent of approximately 90 g of pure fat a day, and more than six to eight times what we need.

SALT OF THE EARTH

Canadians are major salt-lovers: A 2009 international study found that sodium levels in many restaurant-chain meals and prepared foods are higher in Canada than anywhere else!

Mealtimes are even more fun when everyone helps cook—enlist your family as sous-chefs!

EATING ALONE

In 2005, Statistics Canada reported that, in the past two decades, Canadians had become significantly more likely to eat at least one meal alone every day–a change that also correlated to less time spent with family.

Chew on this

Pick up some packs of sugar-free gum and place them everywhere: your kitchen, desk, car and purse or briefcase. When you're tempted to reach for a sweet, grab a piece of gum instead. You may find that the act of chewing relieves your cravings. Also, try chewing a stick while you're cooking meals—there's no way you can sample your wares while you're blowing bubbles.

SETTLING IN

Having difficulty getting used to a change of diet? Give yourself a little time, especially if you're used to eating foods that are high in salt, fat and sugar–those foods create a kind of addiction, so it can be hard to give them up. Just keep on following **Swap & Drop**'s diet plan, and you'll create some mouthwatering associations with healthier food.

SHOPPING

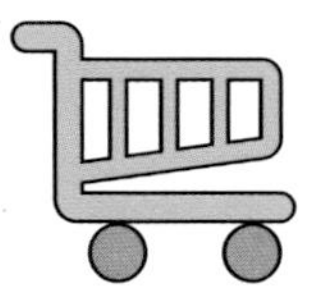

Shop on the edges of the grocery store and avoid impulse buys

Never go to the grocery store without a plan. (Just knowing you'll want dinner later isn't enough!) Make a comprehensive list and eat a snack before you head out—that'll prevent you from succumbing to sales on diet-unfriendly foods. And the more you shop in the outer aisles, the more calories you'll save. Essential foodstuffs are usually displayed around the perimeter, with pre-made meals and processed items in the centre aisles.

About high-protein and "low-GI" diets

For over a decade, there's been nonstop buzz over carb-cutting, protein-loading diets. It's easy to see why they've proved so popular–any diet that encourages you to live on steak is going to attract attention.

But approach these diets with caution. It's not that these regimens don't help people lose weight–they can. A study by Arizona State University scientists showed that young women who ate a meal high in protein burned more calories during the next several hours than women who ate a high-carbohydrate, low-fat meal.

The reason, researchers surmised, was that protein requires more energy to digest than carbohydrates do. That extra energy showed up in slightly elevated body temperatures for the women consuming the most high-protein meals.

Another study found that volunteers were more satisfied after eating a meal with 29 percent of its calories from protein, than after a meal with only 9 percent of its calories from protein. They also burned more calories digesting the higher-protein meal.

Before you get too excited, though, keep this in mind: You'll burn a lot more calories by taking a 15-minute walk after dinner than you will consuming extra protein. And while it's true that high-protein foods seem to satisfy hunger well, complex carbohydrates do the same, often with fewer calories.

High-protein diets may also pose long-term risks if you don't choose your foods wisely. Many foods high in protein, like most meats, are also high in saturated fat, which can be rough on your arteries.

Probably more important when you're controlling calories is the fact that overloading your diet with protein raises the risk that you'll come up short on other nutrients, such as the essential vitamins, minerals and fibre in vegetables.

If you follow weight-loss trends, you've probably also heard of the low-glycemic-index diet as well. The glycemic index (GI) is a measurement of how fast your digestive system can convert certain foods into blood sugar. The approach is simple:

NO FAIL *get-slim* SWAP

WHERE'S THE FISH?

Switch from beef to to fish once a week. A 75 g serving of broiled steak has 230 calories and 14 g of fat. Compare that to the same-size serving of broiled cod, at just 80 calories and 1 g of fat. Make this change once a week and slash 7,800 calories a year—easy!

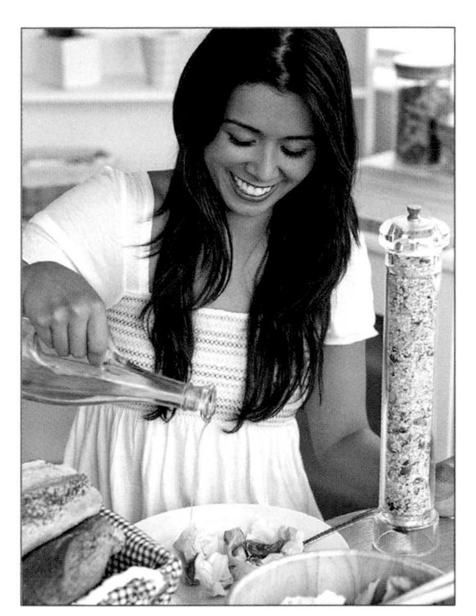

Making your own vinaigrettes using extra-virgin olive oil and balsamic or red wine vinegar will save you money and calories.

Foods that convert quickly into blood sugar (in other words, high-GI foods, primarily dietary sugars and simple carbohydrates) are bad for you; slow-to-digest, low-GI foods are good for you.

There's some validity to this premise as well, and most high-protein diets are also low-GI, since protein is very low-GI food. One recent study showed that people on low-GI diets burned 80 calories more per day than dieters on a regular low-fat diet. Plus, they reported feeling more energetic and less depressed and hungry.

The problem here is that it is extremely hard to monitor the glycemic index for all the foods you eat. You could spend all your time consulting the GI index, instead of just learning to recognize healthy foods and reasonable portions. A long-term eating program shouldn't be mathematically complicated. Also problematic is that the glycemic index of a food can change based on what is being eaten with it. Who wants to work that out everytime they sit down for a meal? It's hard to stay on a diet that requires so much effort to maintain.

The bottom line is there are kernels of truth in many popular weight-loss trends. But why put all your weight-loss hopes in one narrow scientific theory, when your goal is to lose weight and maintain it—while staying healthy as well?

The **Swap & Drop** diet, by pairing plenty of protein with good fats and complex carbs, is sensible, easy to track, and provides all the protein and low-GI food you need to garner their benefits. And there's evidence that this triple combo of nutrients keeps people feeling so much better that they don't want to overeat!

This week, the most important thing is to enjoy long, leisurely suppers. So don't sweat over nutritional math: Relax! ■

BEWARE!

North Americans spend more than $25 billion each year on commercial weight-loss programs

Beware of any diet regime driven by an obvious profit motive—fad diets just don't work in the long term. Be wary of so-called "fat blockers" and "starch blockers" that claim to absorb fat and block starch digestion. These claims have not been proven. Also be wary of herbal weight-loss products—many of these are loaded with stimulants that can provoke cardiac arrhythmias and other serious side effects.

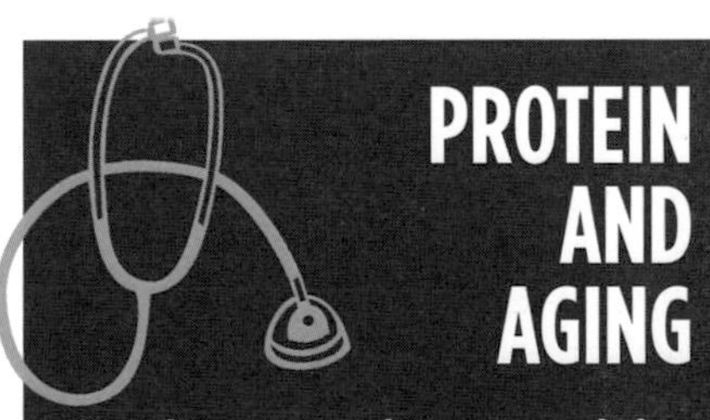

PROTEIN AND AGING

One instance when you might benefit from a higher protein diet is if you're an older woman. A 2011 study published in the *Journal of Gerontology* found that, because older women are at risk of losing muscle mass along with fat during diets, muscle-preserving protein will help them get more fit. If that's you, go for lean proteins such as fish.

GETTING YOUR AFFAIRS IN ORDER

Last-minute meal-planning is always tricky, but especially so when you're trying to lose weight. It's hard to make decisions when you're hungry! Try planning dinners at the beginning of the week, or use our handy meal planner (page 96).

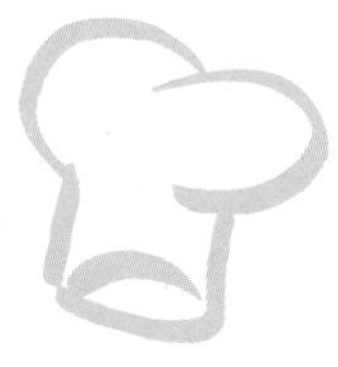

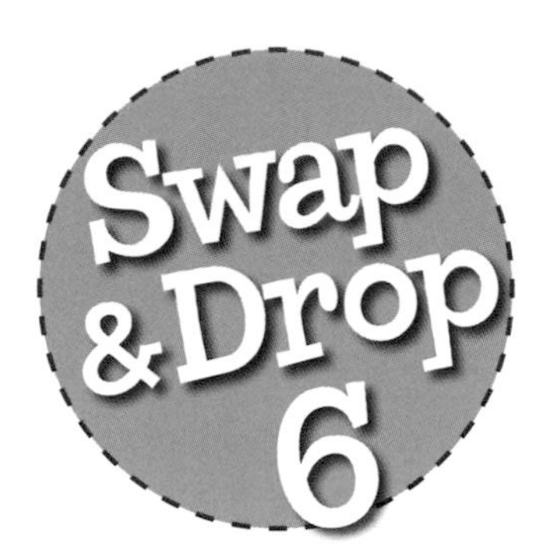

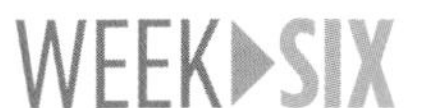

Dine out twice a week

It's time to relax and let someone else do the cooking. Just make sure they do it the **Swap & Drop** way

> We should look for someone to eat and drink with before looking for something to eat and drink.
>
> — *Epicurus, Ancient Greek philosopher*

Now that you've mastered eating healthy at home, it's time to take the next step: Dining out. This week, you'll learn that even though a chef may rule her kitchen, you rule your table. Order exactly what your meal plan calls for and assume responsibility for the food you're served.

Even though you're watching what you eat, that's no reason to deny yourself the pleasure of eating out. Yes, the serving sizes can be enormous, and many restaurant chefs seem to think "cooking light" means one cup of butter in the sauce instead of two. But if you approach dining out with confidence and common sense, you can have a great meal while sticking with your plan.

This week, dine out at least twice. Order exactly what your diet calls for, and get the waiter and chef to deliver a more personalized meal. Remember, there's no need to fear a restaurant's menu: You shouldn't go somewhere unless you like their offerings, but you are also paying to get what you want. Be polite but firm. There's no reason you can't make every night out a **Swap & Drop** evening.

A Swap & Drop date

Dining out has become one of the great national pastimes. In fact, Canadians spend close to $40 billion per year doing it. But there is a downside to dining out: Experts say restaurant food typically contains 22 percent more fat than food consumed at home–and, at many eateries, portion sizes have spiraled out of control.

Portion increases happened so gradually that most people didn't realize exactly how big those entrées had become until an American organization called the Center for Science in the Public Interest (CSPI) rounded up meals from the kinds of restaurants that many of us dine in regularly. What they found made headlines: Portion sizes and fat content at many well-known restaurants had become so bloated that many meals bordered on health hazards.

GO AHEAD—SPOIL YOUR APPETITE

If you and your family are planning to eat out tonight, you may feel as if you need to "save up" your hunger in order to really enjoy it. After all, this is a special occasion! But it's much healthier to approach this as you would any meal: Eat a healthy snack a couple hours before, so you aren't too ravenous by dinnertime.

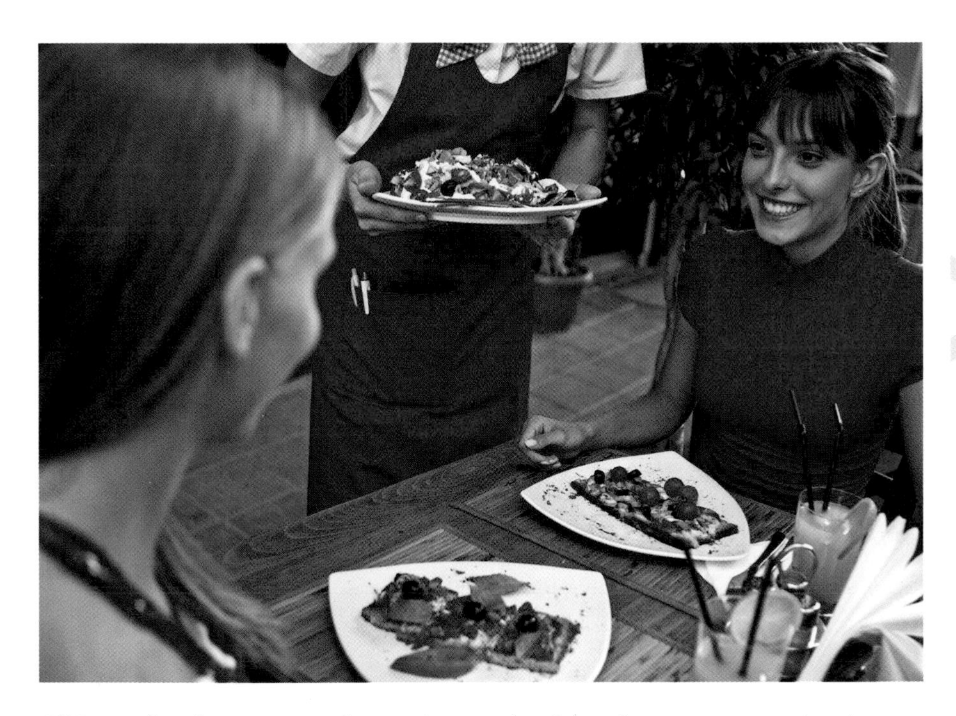

CSPI even found some cases where a single entrée exceeded what you should eat in a whole day on the **Swap & Drop** diet. At some Chinese restaurants, for instance, a single order of kung pao chicken packed 1,400 calories.

If you dine out a lot–and many of us do–numbers like those can be discouraging. But even though the chef rules the kitchen, remember that you rule the table. You're the one footing the bill, after all. You choose what to eat, how much of it you want and how quickly you want to eat it. In some restaurants, you can even give the chef specific directions for how you want your meal prepared.

Many of the strategies you'll use to take charge in restaurants are the same ones you've already been practicing: planning ahead, keeping an eye on portion sizes and monitoring hunger and fullness signals. This week, keep those ideas in mind when you take yourself out to dinner.

Do your menu homework

If you're considering a restaurant you've never tried before, look up its menu online or stop by to make sure you'll be able to order the meal you want–many establishments display their menus outside. You won't be able to learn much about portion sizes, of course, but at least you'll know whether the menu includes some decent options. You could even pick the safest bets before you go in. That way you won't have to look at the menu and be tempted by steak smothered in hollandaise sauce or deep-fried cheese blintzes.

For a guide to ordering at popular Canadian chain restaurants, turn to page 190.

5 Questions to ask before ordering

- Does it come with a cheese or nut topping?
- What cooking oils are used?
- Can it be prepared to order—say, if I want olive oil used instead of butter?
- Are half portions available?
- Can I make substitutions?

Turning Japanese

Are you worried that going to the same old restaurants you've always frequented will make you tempted to order something you shouldn't? Try a new cuisine—and if possible, choose Japanese. A lot of Japanese food is low-calorie and **Swap & Drop** friendly. Think green tea, sashimi (raw fish), miso soup and edamame (steamed soy beans). Just skip deep-fried offerings like tempura and gyoza.

ORDERING PIZZA

A pizza party might sound like a diet disaster—but it doesn't have to be! Opt for a thin crust if possible, and forget the meat—load up on veggie toppings. Order half the cheese (or none at all). Start with a salad, eat two pizza slices and wrap up the rest for later. For a guide to ordering pizza at popular restaurants, turn to page 190.

FIRST THINGS FIRST

It may seem counterintuitive, but always order a starter–say, a fresh green salad. It'll help you temper your hunger when you get to the main course.

If you dine out frequently, keep your own personal list of diet-friendly restaurants in your area–places where you know you'll be able to get a great-tasting, low-calorie meal.

There are some kinds of restaurants you should avoid altogether...unless you have an iron will. All-you-can-eat joints, buffet-style restaurants and even sprawling salad bars pose a hazard; salad bars can be great for dieters, but many are stocked with calorie-rich dishes like creamy pasta salads. Better to go somewhere where you can get a simple garden salad with dressing on the side. As for fried-chicken and barbecue joints, most of what's on their menus is so high in calories and fat, you'll bust your calorie budget before you satisfy your hunger.

Fast-food restaurants have made some progress in offering healthier alternatives to their usual fare, such as grilled chicken sandwiches and salads. But even those can be loaded with hidden calories. Menus change all the time, as chains constantly seek offerings that sell better. And even as they test healthier fare, fast-food restaurants keep adding bigger, unhealthier items as well, or loading up salad with fried chicken and creamy dressing. So while fast-food restaurants offer convenience and familiarity, you'll need to be extra careful when eating at them. Remember, you're shooting for at least two servings of vegetables; at your local burger joint, you'll be lucky to get a piece of lettuce and thin slice of tomato.

Even at pricier restaurants, you need to be specific about your desires or you'll end up with piles of high-calorie food on your plate. Take control from the start, and don't let the restaurants dictate your dining experience. Then check out page 190, where you'll find swaps for some of Canada's most popular restaurant chains.

Take control of the table

Be the director of your dining experience right from the start, and you really *can* have it your way. Here are four guidelines that will put you in charge:

1. **Ask and you shall receive.** The waitstaff should know how a dish is made, what the ingredients are and how big the portion size is, so don't be afraid to ask. If the burrito looks good except for the fact that it's smothered in sour cream, ask them to hold the cream. If you'd like the grilled chicken breast without the skin, say so. If the vegetable side dishes are usually prepared with gobs of butter, request yours lightly sautéed in olive oil or steamed. At pizza joints, ask the kitchen to make yours with no cheese and an extra topping of vegetables.

Decoding menus

Some restaurant's menus are overwhelmed by trendy terms you might never use in your own kitchen. So how do you know which items to order? Follow this handy guide.

WORDS TO AVOID

- Fried/deep-fried
- Au gratin
- Braised
- Buttered
- Creamed
- A la mode
- Hollandaise, cheese or cream sauce
- In gravy
- Pan-fried or -roasted

WORDS TO LOOK FOR

- Baked
- Broiled
- Grilled
- Poached
- Roasted
- Steamed
- In its own juice
- Garden-fresh
- Raw

2. Order one course at a time. One of the pleasures of dining out is taking your time–or at least it should be. Unfortunately, waiters often snatch up one course and rush in with the next before you've had time to put your fork down. Most restaurants want to turn tables around as quickly as they can, so more customers can be served in one evening. But don't worry: Just relax and take the time you need, within reason.

If you're worried about being rushed, order just one course at a time. Start with an appetizer. Once you're done, look back at the menu. Allot at least 20 minutes per course–the time your body needs to send satiety signals. (Better restaurants assume you'll take a couple hours, anyway.) Feeling full? You're under no obligation to keep ordering.

3. Draw the line. Ask whether the kitchen can prepare half portions. Some even offer half portions on the menu. If the dish you order turns out to be too big, ask the waiter to pack up half so you can take it home. Don't depend on your willpower to eat only half of what's in front of you. If you already know that the dishes at a particular restaurant are outsized, ask that half be brought to the table and that the other half be brought at the end of your meal in a take-out container.

4. Rule the table. When you're dining out, you're in charge–not only of what you eat, but of what's on the table. Lots of restaurants start you off with a basket of dinner rolls. If you're hungry when the rolls arrive, you'll automatically gobble up mediocre white bread smeared with butter and loaded with calories without even giving it a second thought. Tell the waiter, "No bread, thanks."

If you're famished when you sit down, order something more sensible to take the edge off your hunger before you do anything else, such as a side salad, vegetable side dish or glass of spicy tomato juice. At the same time, ask for a glass of water. Heck, ask for a whole pitcher. Then you won't have to keep the busboy busy filling

Are you !#*@%?& kidding me?

A lot of Italian restaurants splash extra-virgin olive oil over everything. We think of it as a healthy fat, and it is, but it *is* still oil—only one tablespoon has a whopping 119 calories! Better ask the chef to go easy.

NEED IDEAS? *If you've checked out a restaurant's website and you're still not sure whether you should visit, check out customer reviews on websites like yelp.ca. You'll learn whether the service and ambience are worth the money.*

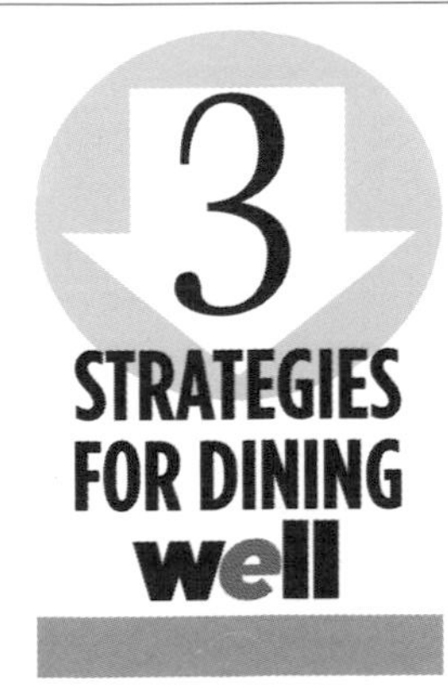

1 **Don't feel pressure to order everything right away. Start by ordering a healthy appetizer and hold onto your menu. That way, your eyes won't be bigger than your stomach—ordering gradually means following your appetite.**

2 **Instead of ordering pop or even diet pop, order a sparkling water with a slice of lemon. It'll still feel special, while adding virtually no calories to your meal.**

3 **Split some dishes with your tablemates, or go out for cuisines such as Chinese and Indian, which are well-suited to ordering several dishes for the table to share. This is a fun way to get some variety in your meal without feeling pressure to clean your plate.**

THE PROS AND CONS OF TAPAS

At a tapas restaurant, you order a variety of small dishes to share instead of one big item each. This Spanish custom may seem tricky—how will you keep track of portions? But each serving is small, and if you eat them gradually, you'll give your body time to let you know it's satisfied. If you eat slowly, order wisely and pay attention to hunger cues, this is a great option for a fun night out.

FULL DISCLOSURE

Restaurant servers can have stressful jobs, but that doesn't mean they should give you attitude if you ask for a substitution. If your server is less than understanding, consider coming out and telling him or her that you're watching your weight, and asking what items he or she would suggest. There's nothing to be ashamed of, and sometimes being direct will get servers to help you make a good choice.

:) Studies have shown that more Canadians demand nutritious, low-calorie food in comparison to Americans, who tend to focus on speed. That's a good reason to feel patriotic!

your glass. Remember to drink plenty of water with your meal.

And don't forget who's boss. If something arrives at the table that you don't want, politely decline.

Manage the menu

Order wisely, and you can put together a meal that's long on flavour and short on calories. Here are five things to consider when you open the menu:

1. **Be colourful.** Meat and cream sauces are usually beige. Choose the most colourful dishes on the menu, and chances are you'll order the healthiest, lowest-calorie selections–the ones packed with veggies. Spicy red salsas, deep purple beets, green salads, yellow corn, and bright orange and yellow sweet peppers turn your plate into an extra-tasty rainbow. Not only that, but many of the substances that provide fruits and vegetables with their colours are also antioxidants–potent disease-fighters that have been shown to lower heart disease and cancer risk.

2. **Order appetizers and sides.** Consider forgoing the entrée section of the menu and ordering only from the appetizers and side dishes. With today's oversized restaurant portions, an appetizer or side often makes a perfect meal by itself. Skip things like the deep-fried mozzarella sticks, and make sure your choices include at least two servings of vegetables.

3. **Dip into the sauce.** Ordering salad dressing on the side is one of the oldest diet tricks. Remember that you can order other sauces on the side, too, from gravy to guacamole. Give yourself no more than a tablespoon.

Here's another tip: Instead of pouring on the sauce or salad dressing, every time you take a bite, dip the tines of your fork in the dressing, then spear a bite-size portion. You'll make a little bit of a good thing go a long way.

4. **Create your own smorgasbord.** If you're dining out with friends who share your concern about overdoing it, agree to order and share entrées. If there are four of you, order two or three main dishes. You'll get a chance to sample a wider variety of items and keep portions down to size.

NO FAIL *get-slim* SWAP

JUST SAY "NO" TO THE HOUSE DRESSING

Swapping out salad dressings at restaurants is easy—it could save you a ton of calories. And beware of so-called "house dressing": That name could mean anything, and it could contain high-calorie ingredients such as parmesan or cream. Ask that your salad come with a simple oil and vinegar dressing, served on the side. Every chef should know how to whip one up.

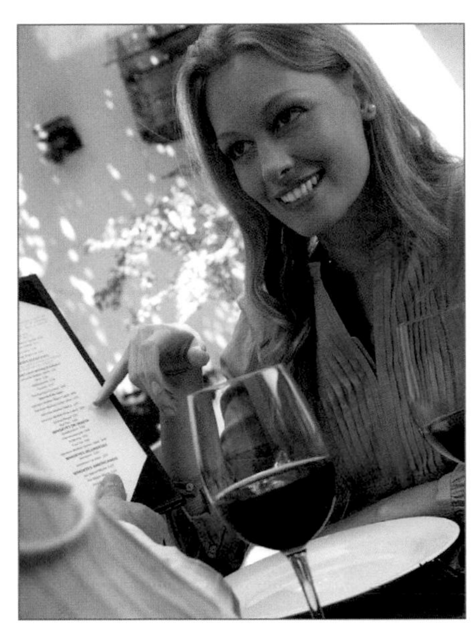

■ Don't feel that you have to order a full-sized entrée—many appetizers and side dishes are big enough for a full meal.

Be careful, though: When offered a lot to choose from, some people end up eating a lot more. Decide in advance to sample only two or three forkfuls of each dish. With lots of dishes on the table, it's especially important to be aware of hunger and satiety signals. Sit back from time to time and think about whether you've had enough. If you have, put your fork down, raise a glass of water, and enjoy the conversation.

5. **Be a discerning foodie.** Remember the credo of smart dining: If it doesn't taste great, don't eat it. Sure you paid for it, but to finish something you don't like is a greater crime.

When you're dining out this week, be a tough critic. Pay attention to the first few bites. Decide whether it's good enough to finish, or whether you'd just as soon put those calories toward something else.

One glass will do

Before you raise your glass, remember one key word: moderation. Alcoholic beverages contain calories–about 90 calories in a 120 mL glass of wine and 150 in a 355 mL glass of regular beer (depending on the kind). Surveys show that the average adult who drinks gets 10 percent of total calories from alcohol, so if you must have a glass of wine or beer with dinner, go on and enjoy just one.

It can be easy to get carried away if the people you're with are ordering tons of food and drinks, but only order what *you* want. It's your money and your meal. ■

120

That's how many calories there are in a single dinner roll–so tell your server right away that you do not want the bread basket.

NEVER, EVER, EVER USE THE FAST FOOD DRIVE-THRU

A British medical study revealed that people who eat fast food more than twice a week have 10 pounds more body fat than those who do not. If you must resort to fast food for a lunch on the fly, go inside the restaurant, take your time eating and consult the **Swap & Drop** fast-food recommendations starting page 190.

SALMON VS *Chicken*

CAN'T DECIDE whether to order the salmon or the chicken? When it comes to calories, they're actually roughly equivalent healthy choices. But it's good to know salmon is high in heart-healthy omega-3s.

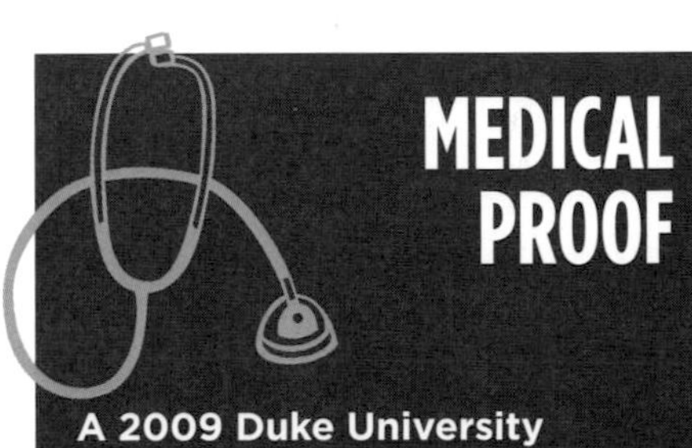

MEDICAL PROOF

A 2009 Duke University study found that when people ordered a side salad, they would also go ahead and order the least healthy thing on the menu. Sounds crazy, but researchers think it might be because people feel like eating salad is a free pass to load up on calories—which it definitely isn't.

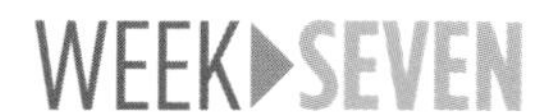

Be social, but eat smart

Getting together with family and friends is fun, but don't let socializing sabotage your diet efforts

This week, go out in all sorts of social settings–girls' night out, the movies or a family dinner–and practice flexing your control muscle. You'll also find out what to do when the people you rely on most feel threatened by your weight loss and even try to subtly derail your diet. Learn to stand up for yourself!

> Lots of people want to ride with you in the limo, but what you want is someone who will take the bus with you when the limo breaks down.
>
> — *Oprah Winfrey*

EATING WITH LARGE GROUPS

It's more difficult to stay motivated when surrounded by lots of people: One American study found that we tend to eat more when we eat with large groups. Whenever possible, share your table with just a few close friends, and spend more time talking.

Family and friends help determine your long-term dieting success, either through their support or lack thereof. Since they're the ones you spend time with on your days off, they can greatly affect how you eat when you're outside your normal routine. Weekends and holidays are full of new temptations, and the people closest to you may persuade you to eat more than you want.

This week, dive into your relaxation time with gusto–but try to focus less on food and more on active fun. The more confident you feel about adapting your diet to new social situations, the better your chances of success.

Control weekend temptations

If you distinguish between days when you follow a diet and days when you're on "vacation" from it, losing weight will feel like an unnatural chore. So when you're celebrating something special–say, your birthday or an anniversary–live it up. But strike a deal with yourself: In return for indulging a little, agree to skip snacks during the day or set aside 45 minutes for a calorie-burning activity. Keep track of what you eat in your food diary.

And remember, one indulgence doesn't mean you've failed. To gain one pound, you have to consume about 3,500 more calories than you burn–even the biggest holiday feast isn't likely to pack that many. The real danger is eating a little too much every day, or every weekend.

When food equals love

How do we celebrate Valentine's Day? With chocolate. How do we mark a wedding? With a feast. The simple act of offering someone food is a way to show af-

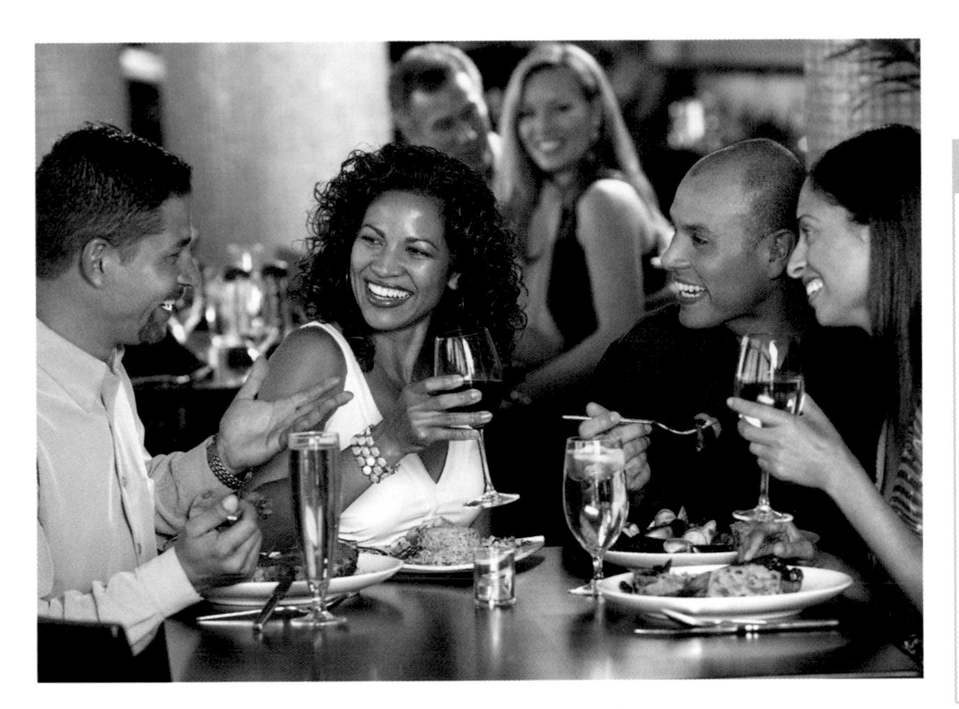

fection. There's nothing wrong with that. We just need to keep a clear view of why we're eating.

This week, if your loved ones pressure you to eat more than you should, look for alternatives. If your mother says, "Eat, eat," say, "No, thanks, Mom. I'm full right now–but let me help you clear the dishes so we can have a chance to talk." Remember that food is only part of what makes gatherings a pleasure. If you're engaged in conversation over the dinner table, no one will notice if you put your fork down.

Have a plan in place

Chances are you've already made at least a few plans for this weekend. Let's say you're taking a trip to your mother's house to celebrate her birthday with a big family potluck. Your schedule might look something like this:

Saturday
Breakfast: At home
Lunch: On the road
Dinner: Mom's house
Sunday
Breakfast: Mom's house
Lunch: Family potluck
Dinner: On the road

How can you handle this kind of irregular timetable? Here are a few ideas to get you started:

1. **Do it yourself.** The best way to control what you eat is to make it yourself. Pack a meal to eat on the road, and you'll save money and frustration. Then contribute a **Swap & Drop** dish (or two) to the family potluck. When eating other dishes, spend

What to do when....

Uh-oh—it's birthday-cake time at work. Passing up a colleague's cake looks as curmudgeonly as refusing to sing "Happy Birthday," but it's hard to celebrate the 300 calories—about half from fat—packed into a single slice of store-bought, super-sweet cake. Here are socially acceptable ways out:

- **Ask for a thin slice, and then eat only a small nibble, leaving the rest on your plate.**
- **If you can't resist, leave the icing on your plate and just eat the cake.**

SHOPPING

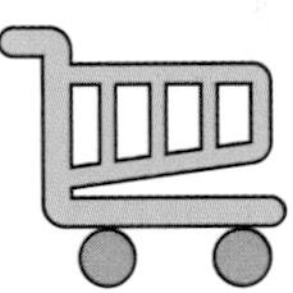

Never shop hungry—for the sake of your diet and your wallet!

Shopping marathons are like any other kind: You need constant, small boosts of energy to keep going, or you'll make choices you regret. Walking around a shopping centre can burn about 200 calories an hour! Avoid settling in at the food court; grab a small bag of nuts and a diet pop from a kiosk, and keep going.

Going out with family? For tips on how to order in Canada's most popular restaurants, turn to page 190.

:) THE REWARDS YOU DESERVE

When you reach one of your goals—like sticking to **Swap & Drop** through a long holiday weekend—give yourself a reward. For a little extra motivation, decide in advance what the reward will be, such as a new pair of shoes or a trip to the spa.

:(...AND THE KINDS YOU SHOULD AVOID

Never eat to reward yourself or feel better when you're blue. Emotional eating can make you feel bad. And what do you do then? Well, you eat some more. You can escape this cycle by becoming more aware of genuine hunger cues and distinguishing them from environmental and emotional triggers. After a stressful day, instead of reaching for the ice cream, give yourself five minutes of quiet time. Learn more stress-busting strategies in Swap 10, beginning on page 78.

your calories wisely and opt only for special homemade foods, not chips and dip.

2. **Pace yourself.** You may have to use every delaying tactic in the book during leisurely holiday feasts: Drink a sip of water between each bite. Put your fork down frequently. Sit back in your chair and enjoy the conversation for a few minutes without eating.

3. **Watch the alcohol.** Wine, punch and other calorific alcoholic beverages have a way of flowing freely at holiday meals. Don't let too much alcohol dissolve your best intentions. Limit yourself to one glass per meal, then opt for sparkling water.

4. **Get out and about.** Rally friends and relatives for hikes, bike rides, cross-country skiing, days at the pool or just frolicking with the dog. Burn 500 extra calories this weekend, and you can treat yourself to a piece of Mom's pie without worrying about upsetting your calorie balance.

5. **Take time for bedtime.** Catch up on sleep you may have missed during the week. Lack of sleep can erode your willpower, and obesity experts believe it can even cause you to gain weight. Get to bed a little early or allow yourself to sleep a little later than usual one morning.

6. **Fine-tune your expectations.** If your schedule is crowded with holiday parties, be realistic: Make it your goal to simply maintain your current weight. You can start shedding pounds again when the holidays are over. It's far better to take a little longer to reach your goal than to put yourself under unnecessary pressure.

Should you enlist your family and friends?

Behavioural scientists once assumed that the more social support dieters had, the better their odds of losing and keeping off weight. But studies on the subject have had mixed results: Some people do better when they have a strong social network, while others succeed on their own.

What is consistent among successful dieters is a sense of accountability for their weight loss. To find out whether you'd do better as a team player or flying solo, answer the questions in the quiz on page 64.

Your friends in need

Social support comes in many forms, and the first step is deciding what you need. Which of the following people do you think could help you?

- An activity partner
- Someone to talk to when I'm feeling discouraged about dieting
- Help in the kitchen

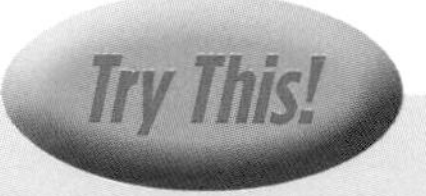

A great way to guarantee that you'll eat more slowly is to buy a stylish pair of chopsticks, then eat even non-Asian meals with them. This can slow you down because chopsticks pick up much less food with each bite than a fork. They also require more concentration if you're not used to using them.

- Someone who can answer specific diet questions
- Help around the house
- A lunch or dinner companion
- Others: ______________________
  ____

Now make a list of possible candidates to fill the positions you need help with. Keep in mind that support sometimes comes from unexpected places—a colleague who's also trying to slim down may be more helpful than a close friend who isn't. If you're looking for emotional support, identify someone you're willing to confide in, even if that means admitting weakness or failure.

Beware of saboteurs!

In a perfect world, family and friends would support you 100 percent—but sometimes the people closest to you can feel threatened by your efforts. Your spouse may interpret your decision to lose weight as a desire to be considered more attractive by other people. A friend who could also stand to lose a little weight may feel intimidated by your determination. Think about the people closest to you. Is there anyone who:

- Urges you to eat even when you say you're not hungry?
- Belittles your efforts to lose weight?
- Throws obstacles in the way of your activity goals?
- Seems resentful of or threatened by your recent weight loss?
- Expresses anger or surprise when you leave food on your plate?
- Undermines your efforts with negative messages? (He or she might do so with comments such as "You're going to gain it all back again during the holidays, anyway.")

If you answered yes to any of these questions, you may have a diet saboteur in your midst.

This week, ask that person for a heart-to-heart talk. Explain why losing weight is so important to you—and why their sincere support matters. And be specific:

- "I'd rather you didn't offer me seconds. When I say no, I feel like I'm hurting your feelings, but it's important to me that I cut back."
- "It would help me a lot if we kept snack food in the cupboard, rather than on the counter where I see it all the time. I have a tendency to eat when there's food out."
- "It really hurts my feelings when you say I never stick with things. I'm really trying and your encouragement means a lot to me."

When your lover surprises you with a box of chocolates, remember this quick lesson in love: He or she didn't bring them in hopes of watching you eat!

Before surrendering to the temptation of what's in the box, unwrap your lover. A concerted half-hour of sex can chew up 85 calories, and the longer you linger, the higher the calorie count. Afterwards, feel free to enjoy **a single piece** of chocolate —a Godiva truffle tucks a lot of sweetness into 105 calories.

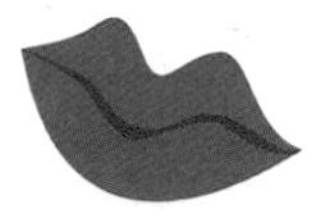

HOST A VEGETARIAN DINNER PARTY

There's far more to the vegetable world than salads. Check out Swap & Drop recipes (starting page 104) for inspiration, then invite a few friends over for a healthy and delicious vegetarian meal. It could help expand your culinary horizons!

BEWARE!

Don't drink too much—or fun could turn into fat

Think of this if you're having drinks with friends or co-workers: Juice, pop and other mixers ratchet up the calories in cocktails, but it's the alcohol itself that turns fun into fat. Undiluted alcohol contain 90 calories per 30 mL! Turn to our alcohol chart on page 65 for a more in-depth guide to the most calorific drinks.

BFF If going it alone isn't your thing, get a group of friends together who also want to slim down. It'll make you more likely to lose weight and keep it off. Researchers at the University of Pennsylvania recruited 166 people to participate in a weight-loss program, either alone or with three friends or family members. Among those who embarked on it with friends, 95 percent completed the program, compared to only 76 percent of those who dieted solo. Plus, after 10 months, 66 percent of the group dieters had maintained their weight loss, compared to only 24 percent of those dieting on their own.

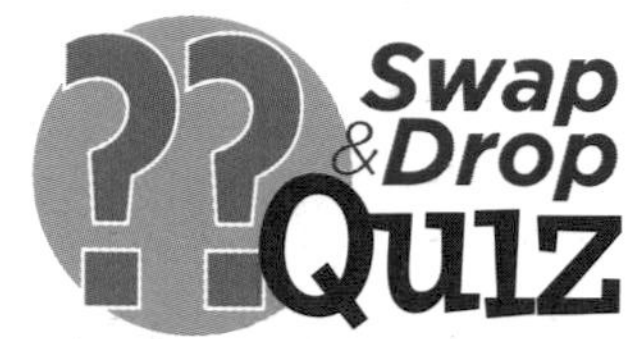

Team player or solo flier? Some people need the support of people around them. Others do best on their own. To find out what's best for you, answer the following:

1. **I'm comfortable talking to other people about my weight.**
   ▲ True ■ False
2. **If things aren't going well for me, I typically turn to family or close friends for advice.**
   ▲ True ■ False
3. **I'm embarrassed talking about my feelings with other people, even people close to me.**
   ■ True ▲ False
4. **Getting a little pat on the back now and then would help motivate me right now.**
   ▲ True ■ False
5. **When I set my mind to do something, I don't really need other people to push me.**
   ■ True ▲ False
6. **I have at least one person in my life with whom I can talk about almost anything.**
   ▲ True ■ False
7. **I tend to keep my personal feelings to myself.**
   ■ True ▲ False
8. **I suspect the people around me are part of the reason I've had trouble losing weight.**
   ■ True ▲ False
9. **I've always tended to tackle problems on my own.**
   ■ True ▲ False
10. **Sometimes I'm not really sure if the people around me have my best interests in mind.**
    ■ True ▲ False
11. **Just being able to talk things over with someone when I've got a problem can make things seem better.**
    ▲ True ■ False
12. **I'm very uneasy about letting people see my weaknesses.**
    ■ True ▲ False
13. **I've joined support groups in the past, and they really helped me.**
    ▲ True ■ False
14. **Frankly, I don't trust people to be honest with me or tell me what they're really thinking.**
    ■ True ▲ False

Score: Tally up the number of coloured shapes you checked—blue triangles or green squares:

▲ **Blue** ________

■ **Green** _______

▲ Blue answers indicate team players. The more blue triangles you checked, the more likely you are to rely on strong support from friends and family.

■ Green answers indicate solo fliers—people who typically go it alone. The more green boxes you checked, the more likely you are to depend on yourself above all.

Most of us are a little bit of both. Read the tips in this Swap for help strengthening your networks and learning to enjoy social gatherings, without feeling anxious about your weight.

Ask your spouse or friend to talk about his or her feelings. If a loved one feels threatened, make it clear that your love hasn't changed.

How to be your own best friend

Banish negative thoughts. Most of us have heard the little voice that whispers, "You just don't have what it takes." But that little voice doesn't know what's best for you! It's time to take charge and get happy.

Replace the naysaying with positive messages. Tell yourself, "One slip-up is no big deal," or "Keep up the good work."

Keep a journal. If that negative voice just won't let up, try carrying a small notebook around this week and surreptitiously jot down every negative thought. You may be surprised to find that writing them down makes you see how irrational they are. You'll also become aware of the situations that trigger negative thoughts and learn to avoid them.

Most importantly, learn to laugh at your foibles. If you take life–and yourself–too seriously, you could slip into the kind of all-or-nothing thinking that makes people give up before they've even given themselves a chance to succeed. Having a sense of humour goes a long way when you're trying to make big changes–and it'll make those holiday get-togethers a lot more fun. ■

Watch your consumption of empty calories

No foods are totally forbidden on the **Swap & Drop** diet, but it helps to avoid the empty calories in alcohol. Alcohol contains 7 calories per gram, compared with 4 calories per gram of protein or carbohydrate and 9 calories per gram of fat. Some wines provide small amounts of iron and potassium, and beer contains niacin, vitamins B6, chromium and phosphorus. But to benefit from the nutrients in these beverages, you would have to consume much more than the recommended limit of two drinks per day for a man or one for a woman. Each beverage listed below provide about 15 mL of ethanol, the usual definition of a drink. (Note that calorie amounts for beer and wine vary depending on the type.)

ITEM	ALCOHOL VOLUME	SERVING SIZE	CALORIES
MIXED DRINKS			
Bloody Caesar	12%	150 mL	156
Gin & Tonic	9%	220 mL	171
Manhattan	37%	60 mL	128
Martini	38%	75 mL	156
Piña Colada	12%	130 mL	262
Screwdriver	8%	200 mL	174
Tequila Sunrise	14%	160 mL	189
WINE			
Dry Wine	10-14%	120 mL	90
Wine Cooler	3.5-6%	355 mL	220
BEER			
Regular	3-5%	355 mL	150
Light	3-5%	355 mL	100

21

The percentage of total daily calories the average Canadian adult gets from beverages.

Are you !#*@%?& kidding me?

A British study confirmed what most waiters know—that people who have an alcoholic drink before dinner tend to eat more! The study found that men who drank a glass of beer 30 minutes before a meal ate more during the meal than men who consumed a nonalcoholic beverage. Those who drank alcohol also ate more fatty and salty foods and felt hungrier after the meal than men who didn't have alcohol. So when trying to lose weight, have alcohol with your meal rather than before.

NO FAIL get-slim STRATEGY

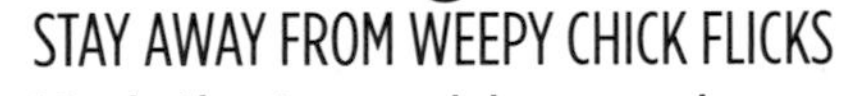

STAY AWAY FROM WEEPY CHICK FLICKS

Movie theatre snack bars are dangerous to your waistline, so take along a healthy snack and avoid tearjerkers. An Australian study found that women who watched a sad film were more likely to overindulge on chocolates than those who watched a travel movie. Another study from the University of Mississippi found that people munched nearly 30 percent more buttered popcorn when they watched *Love Story* compared to when they saw the comedy *Sweet Home Alabama*.

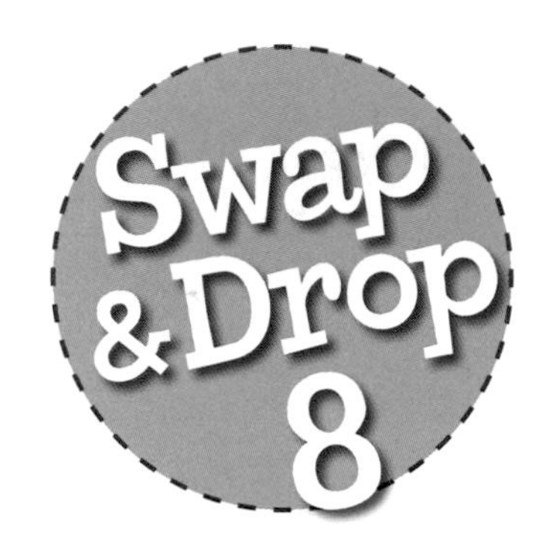

WEEK ▶ EIGHT

Stay motivated & engaged

Use this week to steel your resolve, keep your eyes on the prize and succeed in getting the body you want

"How long does getting thin take?"
— *Winnie the Pooh*

How much weight have you lost? Are you making reasonable progress toward your goal? What can you do when weight loss stalls? In week eight on the **Swap & Drop**, you'll assess how you're doing, give yourself a pat on the back or a kick in the pants–and find ways to get through any trouble spots.

After seven weeks on the **Swap & Drop** diet, spend this week reviewing your progress and solving any problems that you might be experiencing. To assess your progress, start by taking the "How motivated are you?" quiz, on page 70.

Succeeding your way

There is no single dieting approach that works for everyone. To help you overcome the challenges you face, let's go over those quiz questions from page 70 again.

1. **Disappointed in your results? Reassess your goals and renew your commitment.** Experts say a healthy weight-loss plan should shed an average of one to three pounds a week. So you may have lost from 8 to 24 pounds eight weeks into **Swap & Drop**. Losing weight more quickly than that means also losing muscle tissue, slowing your metabolism and making it harder to keep the pounds off.

If you've started exercising more than before, you may be losing fat while also adding muscle. Therefore, you may not see as much difference on the scale as you had hoped. But if your waist size is going down, you're doing great.

2. **Energy low? Have a snack–and get moving.** If you're feeling deep fatigue every day, talk to your doctor. But if you just have occasional slumps, try eating smaller meals and snacking more frequently during the day. Eating more frequently can steady your blood-sugar levels, so you won't crash when your energy supplies run low. Research also shows that physical activity can actually give you an energy boost, banish the blues and increase your

YOU HOLD THE POWER

Good health should always be the goal. Most of us have a pretty good idea what it takes to be healthy; we just don't always bother to take the right steps. Rely on your inner strength to change your ways. The source of that strength will be different for everyone—it could be your children, spouse or interests. Think of them everytime you're tempted to eat more than you need.

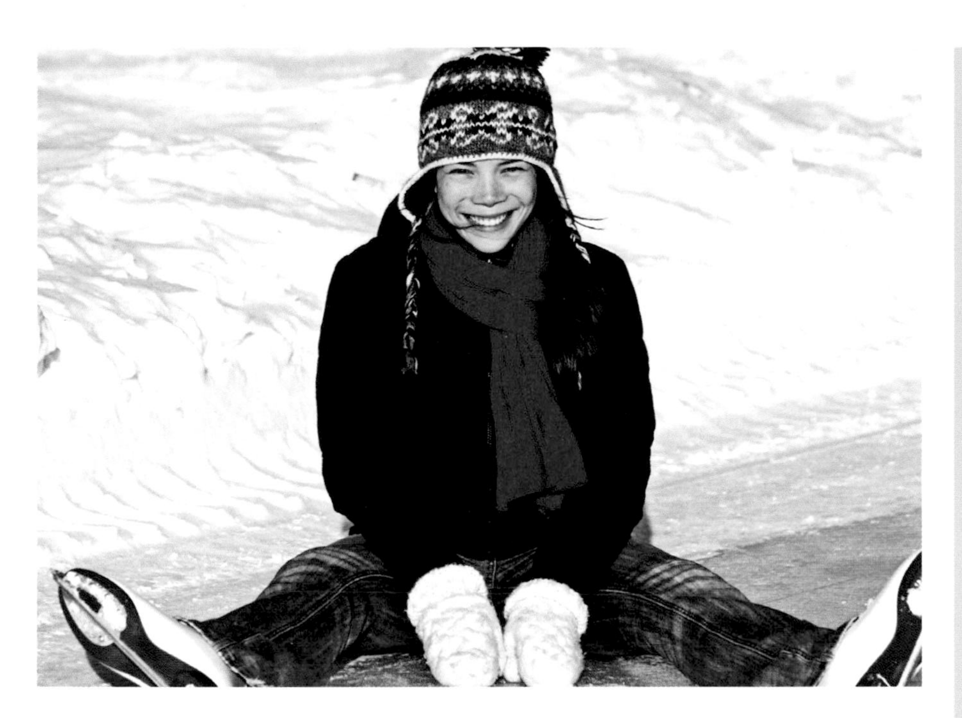

self-confidence. Plus, regular exercise increases stamina, so you'll add to your energy reserves.

3. **Need a shot of self-confidence? Celebrate small victories.** It's easy to lose confidence when you're not reaching your goals, so focus on your successes.

Let's say you've managed to lose five pounds so far, and you'd hoped to lose more by this point. Well, pounds aren't the only measure of success.

Maybe your clothes feel a little more comfortable. Maybe you're simply eating a healthier diet. You should feel a sense of accomplishment.

4. **Struggling with a particular swap? Go back for seconds.** Pounds not coming off fast enough? Go back to the swap that's giving you trouble and take another week to master it. Follow that chapter's tips to the letter and try a few suggestions you didn't try the first time around.

5. **Is dining out your downfall? Zero in on portion control.** Don't let the sizes of restaurant servings determine how much you eat. Keep in mind the portion-size visuals we've been using (page 18) and turn to the **Swap & Drop** restaurant section, which begins on page 190.

6. **Trouble planning ahead? Make a list, check it twice.** Set aside 15 minutes the night before or first thing in the morning to make a list of what you'll need to do that day to stick with **Swap & Drop**. That might include a quick shopping trip to buy what you'll need for dinner, a reminder of when and where you plan to exercise or a reminder to make a reservation at a

:) YOU CAN GET OVER THE PLATEAU!

There's nothing more frustrating than hitting a weight-loss plateau, particularly if you're doing everything right, eating well and exercising. What happened?

First, it's not your fault. Weight-loss plateaus are perfectly normal and easily explained. Your basal metabolism, or the energy your body consumes just to survive, accounts for about 70 percent of all the calories you burn—and it depends on how much you weigh.

The less you weigh, the lower your basal metabolic rate (BMR). Lose enough weight, and boom! Your metabolism slows down and you hit the weight-loss plateau.

The only way to lose more weight is to decrease the calories you take in, increase the calories you burn or both. You can also improve your BMR by building up muscle. Muscle tissue requires more energy than fat does, even at rest.

Basal Metabolic Rate

To find out how many calories your body needs just to stay alive (without all the other activity you do during the day), calculate your basal metabolic rate.

The easiest way to figure out your BMR is to use one of the free BMR calculators available online—just search "basal metabolic rate." Once you find your BMR, remember that it refers to how many calories you'd need if you were just lying in bed all day (which we're sure you rarely do!), and still maintain a healthy diet.

restaurant where you know you'll be able to order something healthy. If you're having trouble finding time to pack a lunch, choose a meal that's quicker and easier to prepare: for instance, a salad you can make in advance.

7. **Famished? Eat more often.** It's fine to be hungry before a meal, but if you're getting so famished that you're tempted to give up the whole idea of dieting, it's time for a reassessment. Begin by helping yourself to low-calorie, high-fibre snacks during those ravenous moments. You're more likely to stick to a diet that doesn't force you to go hungry.

8. **Caving in to cravings? Forge new associations.** Sometimes food cravings are part of emotional eating or reactions to environmental triggers—craving popcorn at the movie theatre, for example.

It's time to create some healthier associations. Instead of eating popcorn at the movies, bring along a **Swap & Drop** snack. For more on food triggers, emotional eating, and environmental cues, look back to Swap 4, which begins on page 42.

9. **Need a helping hand or a friendly word? Ask for it.** When the going gets tough, the tough call on close friends and family. If you're not getting the support you need, explore ways to enlist help or encouragement.

Look back to Swap 7's advice on dealing with friends and family (page 60).

10. **Motivation in need of a tune-up? Think back to the beginning.** Now's the time to remind yourself why you wanted to lose weight in the first place. Write down your three top reasons for starting **Swap & Drop**, then make a list of the benefits you've noticed so far, such as the way your clothes fit or the fact that you get more exercise than before.

11. **Feeling frazzled? Find a way to let off steam.** Dieting can be stressful, so this week, think of one change you can make in your life that will relieve some of the pressure. Ask someone to take on one of your responsibilities at home or the office. Relax by listening to music and concentrating on your breathing.

Or go for a walk—it'll ease stress and burn calories. Turn to page 210 to get started on a stress-busting routine.

12. **Surrounded by temptations? Take control of your surroundings.** If your willpower is tested every time you turn around, take charge of your environment. Put treats out of sight and make sure that calorie-efficient choices like fruits and vegetables are the centrepiece of your

People who drum their fingers or bounce their knees burn at least 500 calories a day. That alone could add up to losing about one pound per week!

THE TRIMMEST MEATS

Eat your chicken and turkey naked—as in, remove the skin. Well-trimmed pork tenderloin is also lean.

Are you !#*@%?& kidding me?

You know that excess weight puts you at higher risk for heart disease and diabetes, but obesity is also linked to an increased risk of most types of cancer, too. Digestion creates destructive particules called free radicals that play a role in a host of health problems. More food + more digestion = more free radicals. Yikes!

If you're overweight, you probably burn more calories at rest than someone who's thin. In other words, if you can stand to lose a few pounds, you're more likely to have a faster basal metabolic rate than a slower one. As you age, however, your muscle mass decreases, which slows down the rate at which you burn calories.

kitchen. If you can't remove the temptations, remove yourself–go for a walk or run errands. Remember, the less you have to rely on sheer willpower to avoid temptation, the more likely you are to reach your goals.

13. **Eating all over the house? Practice the one-room, one-chair rule.** Set aside one room and one chair for eating at home. This week make a pact with yourself to go to the designated spot for every meal and snack you eat at home–it makes it easier to resist temptation.

14. **Sitting on the sidelines? Get in on the action.** You don't have to start running marathons–all you have to do is find time to walk.

This week, find a way to add at least 10 extra minutes of walking during the day. Do it before breakfast, during lunch, or while doing errands, or go for an evening stroll. To get started, turn to page 210 and begin our Walk it Off exercise program.

Don't mistake success for failure

It's easy to have unrealistic expectations when you begin a diet–especially when it's the first time you've tried it in earnest. Even people who have dieted in the past tend to set tough goals and give up when they don't reach them. But chances are you're doing great–without even realizing it! Give yourself some credit.

Here's an interesting study. To test the reality of the typical dieter's expectations, researchers at the weight-loss clinic of the University of Pennsylvania asked a group of women at the start of a diet program to describe four different goals:

- Their dream weight: The ideal amount they would like to weigh.
- Their happy weight: A number on the scale that, even if it wasn't perfect, would make them happy.
- Their acceptable weight: The num-

Divide big goals into milestones

When you have a lot of weight you'd like to lose, it's helpful to think in terms of gradual milestones. This approach helps you gain confidence along the way. Many experts say you should first set your sights on losing about 10 percent of your starting weight. If you first weighed 222 pounds, 10 percent is about 22 pounds.

Once you've reached that goal, set the next milestone. For many people, weight loss slows as you shed pounds, so to avoid becoming discouraged, set subsequent milestones at about 5 percent of your starting weight—11 pounds if you started out at 222, for instance.

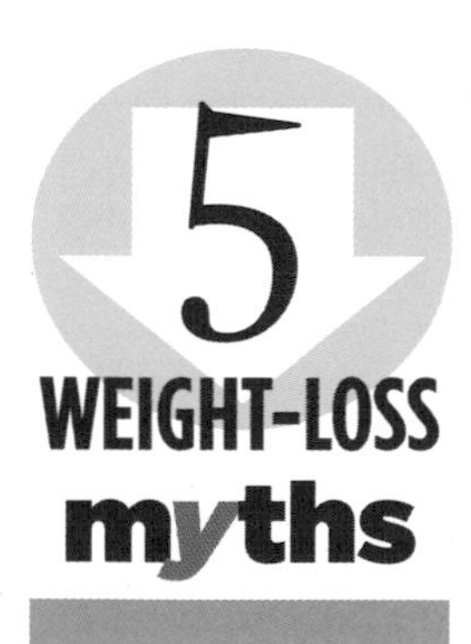

WEIGHT-LOSS MYTH 1
Your ideal weight was when you graduated from college, or before you had children.
If you're hoping to get back to what you weighed a few years ago, fine. But if we're talking 15 or 20 years ago, you might want to reconsider. Many people put on weight as they get older. Set a weight-loss goal that's appropriate for the way you live now.

WEIGHT-LOSS MYTH 2
Your ideal weight is the number listed on a standard height-and-weight chart.
Many other factors play a role in determining your weight, such as your body type, the number of fat cells you have and how much your parents weigh. The numbers listed on a standard height-and-weight chart are just approximations. Don't let them determine whether you've succeeded.

WEIGHT-LOSS MYTH 3
Your ideal weight is the lowest number you've been able to achieve on past diets.
The fact that you're dieting again means you gained at least some, if not all, of the weight back. If you set a weight-loss goal that's too low to maintain, you'll get caught in yo-yo dieting—losing weight, gaining it back and trying to lose it again. The best goal is one you can live with.

WEIGHT-LOSS MYTH 4
The less you weigh, the healthier you'll be.
Not true. In fact, many studies show that if you're overweight, losing just 5 to 10 percent of your current weight is all you have to do to get the bulk of the health benefits associated with weight loss: lower risks of heart disease, stroke, diabetes and even some forms of cancer.

WEIGHT-LOSS MYTH 5
If you don't hit your dream weight, you'll never be happy.
You don't believe that, do you? A number is just a number. And if it's a number that leaves you frustrated and stuck in an endless cycle of losing and gaining weight, it's time to replace that number with a more reasonable one.

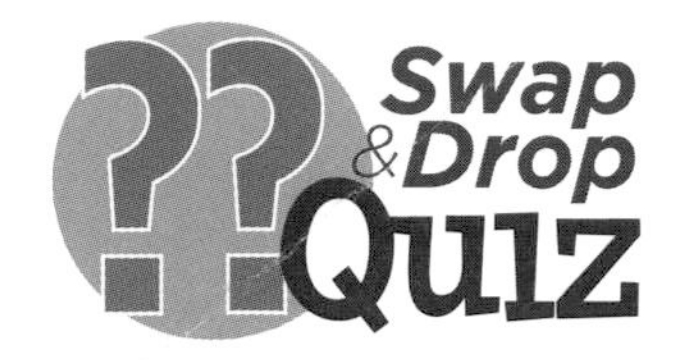

How motivated are you? Now that you're on Swap 8 of **Swap & Drop**, it's time to check your level of engagement. Circle the appropriate number in the right-hand column to track your score.

1. **How do you feel about your weight-loss progress so far?**
   Very satisfied 3
   Satisfied 2
   Disappointed 1
2. **How would you rate your energy level since you began Swap & Drop?**
   Improved 3
   About the same 2
   Slumped 1
3. **How would you rate your self-confidence while on this program?**
   Improved 3
   About the same 2
   Worse 1
4. **How many days last week did you closely follow the Swap & Drop meal plan for breakfast, lunch, dinner and snacks?**
   All or most 3
   About half 2
   Fewer than half 1
5. **How often are you able to stick to sensible portions when you eat out?**
   All or most of the time 3
   About half the time 2
   Less than half the time 1
6. **Planning is crucial to dieting success. How well are you doing when it comes to planning where and what you'll eat?**
   Very well 3
   Good 2
   So-so 1
7. **Feeling hungry can whittle away at anyone's willpower. How would you describe your experience on Swap & Drop so far?**
   Hunger isn't a problem for me 3
   Now and then I get so hungry that I eat more than I should 2
   Hunger is a problem for me a lot of the time 1
8. **How often do you experience strong cravings for specific foods (chocolate, ice cream, salty snacks or candy, for instance)?**
   Never 3
   Now and then 2
   Frequently 1
9. **What phrase best describes your family and close friends?**
   Behind me 100 percent 3
   Somewhat supportive 2
   Not very helpful 1
10. **How would you rate your overall motivation right now?**
    Excellent 3
    Good 2
    Shaky 1
11. **Stress can often get in the way when people are trying to change; how are you dealing with it?**
    Very well 3
    Well enough 2
    Not very well 1
12. **Sometimes it seems there's food everywhere. How would you rate your ability to deal with temptation?**
    I'm getting better at eating only when I'm hungry 3
    I give in to temptation now and then, but not as much as before 2
    I still have a very tough time saying no 1
13. **Where did you eat in your house during the past week?**
    Kitchen and dining room only 3
    In front of TV or in the bedroom 2
    Both in front of TV and in the bedroom 1
14. **How many days during the past week did you do at least 20 minutes of brisk walking or movement?**
    All or most 3
    About half 2
    Fewer than half 1

Score

Add up the combined score of your answers and use the guide below to start evaluating your progress.

A score of 32 to 42: A big gold star for you! Still, put a check beside any questions that you scored as 1 and read the corresponding numbered tips in this week's chapter for advice on how to move ahead.

21 to 31: You're doing well and should be proud of yourself. But the numbers also show that with a little extra help, you could be doing even better. Mark the questions you scored as 1 and read the tips in this week's chapter for advice.

14 to 20: Okay, you're having a tough time. Many people do when they first try to lose weight. Read the following advice for doing better, with a particular focus on questions which you answered with a 1. But first, remember to be kind to yourself! Don't feel bad about your score. Making changes in how you eat can be very hard emotionally, and you're not alone. But the long-term benefits of sticking with **Swap & Drop** are huge. Do all you can to stay committed, and you *will* succeed!

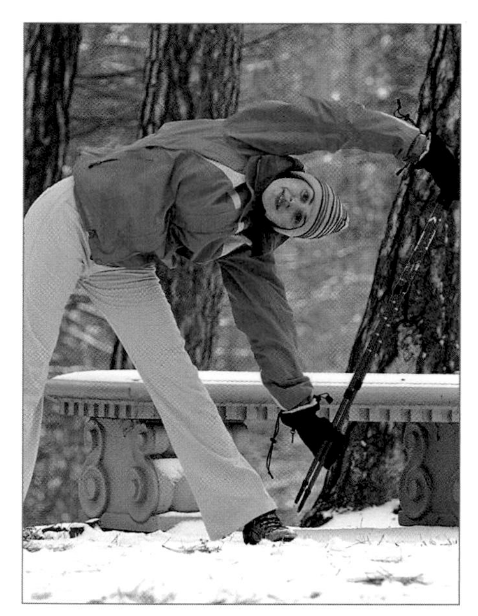

Don't hibernate during winter! Dress properly in layers of clothing that keep you warm while doing a fun outdoor activity.

ber that they would be willing to accept if they couldn't reach either their happy weight or dream weight.

- Their disappointed weight: A number that would leave them feeling as if they hadn't done well at all.

The women in the experiment had high hopes. They began the program weighing an average of 218 pounds. Their average "dream weight" was 149—a 69-pound loss. Short of that, the women said they'd be happy at an average of 155 pounds. If all else failed, they'd accept a final weight of 163 pounds. And they'd be disappointed if they ended the diet at a weight of 181 pounds—an average loss of 37 pounds.

So how did they do? The women in the six-month program lost an average of 16 percent of their starting weight, or 35 pounds. The average loss at that point in a successful diet is around 10 percent to 15 percent, so they were doing great.

The researchers were thrilled, but the women were not. On average they had fallen just short of their "disappointed weight," which would have required them to lose 17 percent. Their dream weight required a 32 percent loss—more than double what experts deem a success. Clearly, their goals were wildly unrealistic.

These women were successful and lost a lot of weight—but most of them considered it a failure. Take this to heart when setting your own weight-loss goals.

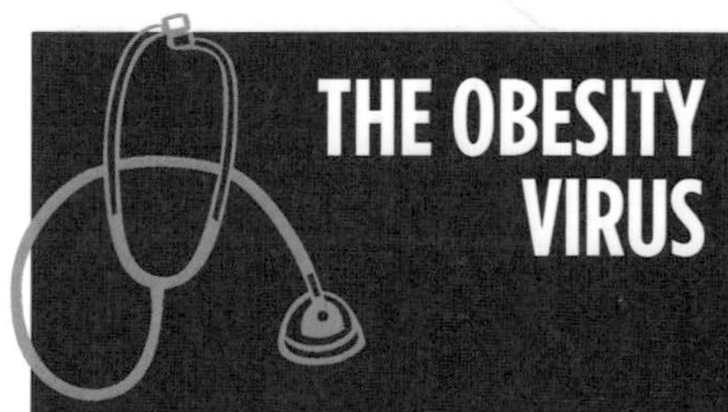

THE OBESITY VIRUS

A virus known as human adenovirus-36 may be partly responsible for obesity in some people. A study found that 30 percent of those who were obese had at one point been infected with adenovirus-36, compared with 11 percent of those who were not obese.

The researchers also looked at 28 pairs of twins and found that people who had been infected at some point tended to weigh more than their identical siblings who didn't have the antibodies.

This explanation is still controversial, so take it with a grain of salt. For the most part, you are responsible for your own weight and health.

DIETING DURING THE COLD DAYS OF WINTER CAN BE BLEAK.

Blame it on our frigid Canadian weather, which makes getting outdoors to exercise less appealing. (Plus, it's easy to camouflage an expanding waistline under layers of sweaters.) Here are several ways to cope with winter's intrusion into your diet routine:

- Go walking at an indoor location, like a mall. If you need extra motivation, join a walking group.
- Join a gym and choose from a variety of physical activities including swimming and dance.
- Go to your local library and borrow a fitness DVD for free. Do the workout at least three times per week.
- Make a healthy soup. Nothing satisfies our cravings for comfort food like a hot bowl of delicious vegetable soup, and it's a lot healthier than buttery, cheesy meals. Start by making one of the **Swap & Drop** soups in the recipe section, beginning on page 142.

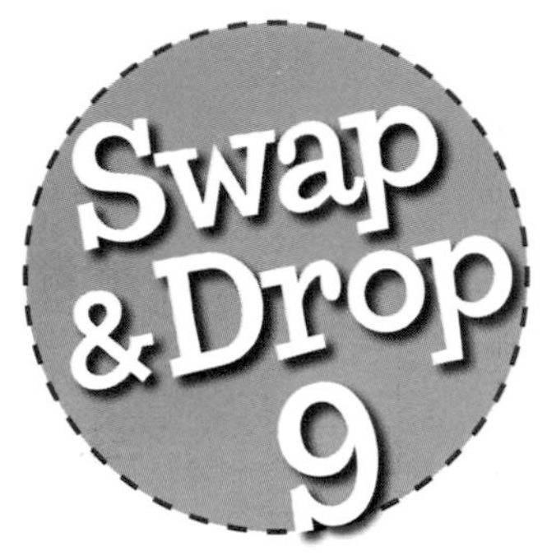

WEEK▸NINE

Fixing your kitchen

This week, take stock of your pantry and refrigerator to ensure they reflect the new, healthier you

Now that you're well-ahead on your diet, it's time to start overhauling the kitchen. If you've been following **Swap & Drop** all the way through, you'll know there's no reason to stop enjoying food when you're trying to lose weight. A kitchen makeover will get you ready for even more delicious meals.

> On days when warmth is the most important need of the human heart, the kitchen is the place you can find it.
>
> — *E. B. White*

BUY IN BULK, WITHOUT ADDING BULK

Are you addicted to the savings you get from bulk or warehouse-style food stores? Watch out—those places can be landmines of unhealthy pantry items. During your next trip, make the best of those bargains by stocking up on pricier pantry items such as unsalted nuts or extra-virgin olive oil, instead of buying snacks.

We don't ever want you to think of your kitchen as a place to be avoided. It should remain a place of warmth–one that encourages both happiness and healthy eating. This week, you'll transform your kitchen by replacing the items in your refrigerator and pantry with choices that will make it easy to whip up a **Swap & Drop**-friendly meal anytime.

Stocking up

Filling your house with food may sound like strange diet advice, but a bare cupboard is just asking for trouble. No matter how scant your provisions are, chances are there's a bag of chips from last week's party or a half-eaten box of candy lurking somewhere. And if that's all there is to eat, guess what you're going to grab if you get hungry enough?

By keeping plenty of healthy foods around and organizing your kitchen well, you can make sure the best choices are right in front of you when you open the refrigerator door. With the right selection of essentials on hand, you can put together a simple and delicious meal without having to make a run to the grocery store.

However, the first step in designing a diet-friendly kitchen isn't shopping–it's clearing your shelves. Start with the pantry, focusing especially on items that have sat around for more than six months. Move to the refrigerator and freezer next. (See "How to clear out your pantry" on page 75 for more tips.)

For every item, ask yourself, "Would I eat this?" If yes, then ask, "*Should* I eat this?" Keep your family's tastes in mind, of course–but if you shouldn't eat it, chances are your loved ones shouldn't, either.

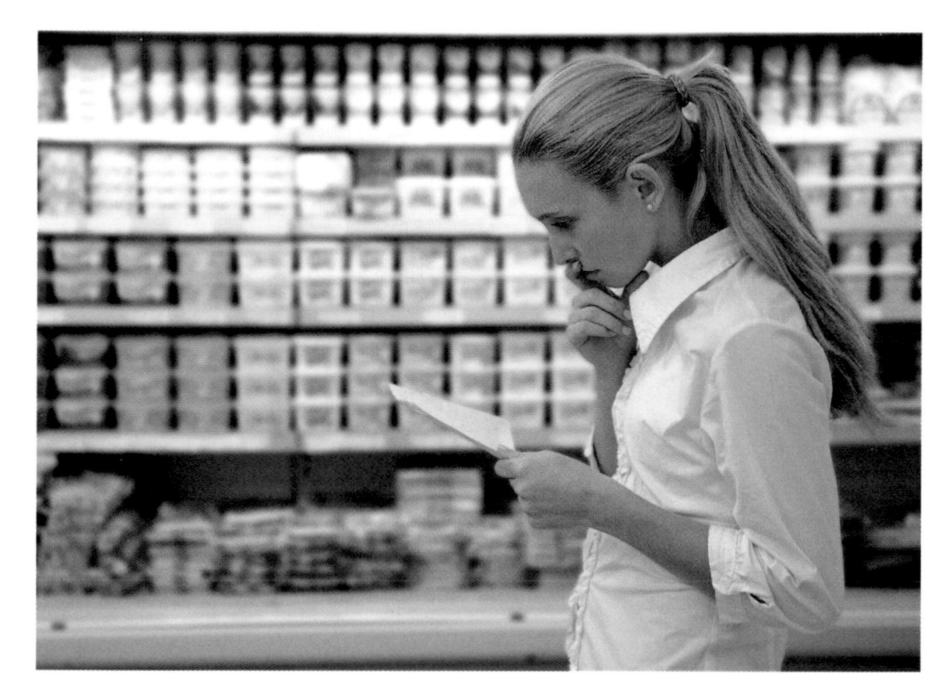

Go shopping

Next, make a run to the grocery store to buy essentials. Take into account your tastes, how often you prepare meals at home and which foods your family likes. The more choices you have on hand, the easier it will be to put together a **Swap & Drop** meal or snack at the drop of a hat. For a comprehensive guide to healthy pantry essentials, see page 77.

Before you head for the grocery store this week, keep in mind six essential strategies for smart shopping:

1. **Have a snack before you go.** Nothing weakens willpower faster than hunger, so avoid temptation by shopping only after you've eaten a meal or a healthy, energy-boosting snack.

2. **Start with a list—and stick with it.** Steer your cart down almost any supermarket aisle, and you'll be surrounded by brightly coloured packages designed to make their way into your cart. To avoid the hard sell, put together a shopping list before you leave the house, building it around recipes and meal plans.

However, you don't have to be afraid to tinker with your meal plan if there's a good bargain at the fish counter or something irresistible in the produce aisle; if, say, local peaches or tomatoes are in season, help yourself. But don't reach for that enormous bag of cheddar popcorn just because it's on sale this week.

3. **Steer your cart around the outside.** In most grocery stores, the healthiest

Breaking the chain

Researchers talk about chains of behaviour: individual decisions that connect like links on a chain. Let's say you give in to temptation one night and eat the whole pint of fudge-brownie ice cream you found in the fridge. That pint didn't get into the freezer on its own. You probably went shopping while hungry, succumbed to a sale on ice cream then ended up eating it while watching TV.

In theory, you could have brought that ice cream home and ignored it, or eaten it in small amounts when you really needed a treat. But if you're like most people, the best time to stop this chain is at the store. You don't have to resist eating something you didn't buy.

:) CLEAR YOUR PANTRY, CLEAR YOUR MIND!

Overhauling your kitchen will do more than just help you lose weight: Researchers have found that a messy home adds significant stress to people's lives, so this change will feel good for more than one reason!

FAMILY AFFAIR

If your partner or kids like to keep pop and chips around the house, ask them to keep their snack foods on upper shelves in the pantry or lower shelves in the fridge—anywhere they're more difficult to access. Insist on reserving the most accessible shelf in the refrigerator for foods that are part of the ***Swap & Drop*** *menus. Ask your kids to stash their snacks away in the designated places when they're done eating.*

Don't stop there: *Sit down with your children and explain why losing weight really matters to you. If they're still young, you'll be helping to nudge their tastes in the right direction. And since weight problems typically begin early on, you'll also be setting them up for lifelong healthy eating habits.*

choices are arranged around the perimeter of the store. That's where you'll find dairy products, produce, meat and fish. As a general rule, then, the more shopping you do around the edges, the less processed, calorie-laden food you're likely to run across.

4. **Bigger is not always better.** Giant food warehouses let you save money by buying in bulk, and that can be helpful. But you should only take advantage of those deals if they're on healthy items that fit your diet. (See "Buy in Bulk Without Adding Bulk" on page 72.)

If you really want to buy jumbo-sized bags of snacks to save money, just divide them into single-serving bags as soon as you get home.

5. **Read the fine print.** When your goal is to lose weight, the most important number on a product's nutritional label is calories per serving–but check how much one serving actually is. Some cereal boxes list ¾ cup, for example, while others use 1 cup. Some foods may look as if they're low in calories–until you discover that a serving size would probably fit in a thimble. Be realistic about how much you would eat.

6. **Keep treats at a distance.** To ensure that treats remain just that, don't buy them at the grocery store. Either bake them yourself using **Swap & Drop** recipes, or make them part of a special occasion or family outing.

When the family wants ice cream, for example, go to your local ice cream parlour. Decide in advance how much you'll have; one small bite of everyone else's ice cream will let you sample a bunch of flavours and still keep you within the recommended serving size for dessert.

Put food in its place

Once you're back from your shopping spree, it's time to take a serious look at your kitchen. The strategy is simple: Keep the healthiest choices in the most prominent spots on kitchen shelves and in the refrigerator. Put "treat" foods, or those which you know might tempt you, out of sight or even out of reach.

Keep a bowl of fruit on the counter and a few containers with carrot and celery sticks front and centre in the refrigerator. Try chopping up some carrots and celery as soon as you get home from the grocery store, so they're ready in advance for the

STOCKING UP ON WHOLE FOODS

Is your pantry full of snack foods that boast "10 percent less sodium!" and "Now with more fibre"? Ditch those products in favour of more whole foods. That means choosing packages that list only one or two ingredients—such as whole-wheat couscous or unsalted, sugar-free peanut butter.

IS YOUR KITCHEN DIET-FRIENDLY?

For a detailed analysis of your kitchen and tips on how to make it work better for you, take our "Inspection Time" quiz on page 76.

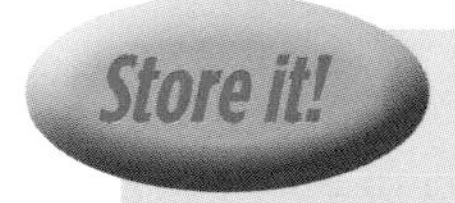

If your drawer is full of scratched-up plastic storage containers, consider investing in glass or metal versions instead—some older plastics might leach the harmful chemical bisphenol-A into your food.

moment when hunger strikes. A lot of snacking is compulsive: If you're bored or upset and unhealthy snacks are just staring you in the face, you might end up reaching for something you would have avoided otherwise.

By contrast, keep those chips, crackers and cookies safely stored away on the very top shelf of the pantry, high enough that you need to get the stepladder out when you want them. By the end of this week, your kitchen will feel relaxing, not like a place where you have to constantly fight through temptation.

Check-in

Is someone in your life making it harder for you to eat right? If you realized in Swap 7 (page 60) that you have a saboteur working against you, consider taking an extra week to resolve the situation.

Keep a record: Write down every time someone says something or does something that seems designed to sabotage your efforts.

At the end of each day, look over your entries and brainstorm ways to free yourself. We gave you tips for strategic confrontations in Swap 7. It's important to remain calm. Don't get accusatory. Remember: the other person might not realize what effect his or her actions have on you.

Sometimes the best approach is to talk it out. At other times, separating yourself from the source of trouble is a better solution. (Your family may be putting you in the line of temptation without meaning to–see the "Family Affair" sidebar.)

Just remember that it's you–and no one else– who is in charge of what you eat. Be considerate of other people's feelings, but stick to your resolution. ■

Are you !#*@%?& kidding me?

Surprisingly, some commercially processed food may actually be more nutritious than fresh versions. Produce used for freezing or canning is often harvested in peak condition and processed quickly to preserve its appearance and nutritional value. Many fresh fruits and vegetables, however, are picked before they're ripe, and they mature under refrigeration, never reaching peak flavour. Buying fresh produce in season will help you get the most out of it.

HOW TO ▸ CLEAR OUT YOUR PANTRY

1▸ TOSS

Take a look at the best-before date on every package and can (yes, canned food goes bad, too) and throw out anything expired. Move the foods that will expire soon to the front of your shelves so you'll know to use them first.

2▸ DONATE

If you have non-perishable food you know you're never going to use, donate it to a food bank. Make sure it hasn't expired, that the packages are still in good condition and that the cans aren't dented.

3▸ STOCK UP

Pick up a variety of whole grains such as amaranth, barley and quinoa—they're great in everything from salads to stews. Once opened, whole grains should be stored in an airtight container. (They'll keep even longer in the fridge.)

4▸ ACCESSORIZE

Keep a good selection of herbs, spices, low-sodium sauces and even canned tomatoes on hand to add an instant pick-me-up to any dish.

5▸ TAKE INVENTORY

Try keeping an inventory sheet on the inside of your pantry door to keep track of what you have on hand and in what amount. Every time you use up an item, cross it off the list so you know when to stock up.

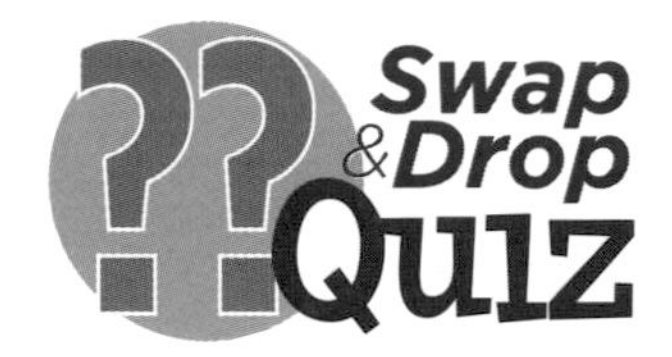

Inspection time. How diet-friendly is your kitchen? There's only one way to find out. Put on your kitchen inspector's cap, and fill out the following checklist. Be honest!

1. **What are the first three things you see when you open your refrigerator door?**
   1. ____________________
   2. ____________________
   3. ____________________
2. **What are the first three things you see when you open the freezer?**
   1. ____________________
   2. ____________________
   3. ____________________
3. **List the three handiest snacks in your kitchen:**
   1. ____________________
   2. ____________________
   3. ____________________
4. **How many kinds of fresh vegetables does your refrigerator crisper contain?**
   ❑ None ❑ One or two
   ❑ Three or more
5. **Is there a bowl of fruit on the counter?**
   ❑ Yes ❑ No ❑ Usually, but not today
6. **Do you have the makings of a Swap & Drop dinner in your cupboard and refrigerator?**
   ❑ Yes ❑ No ❑ Usually, but not today
7. **Where do you usually keep your grocery list?**
   ❑ Posted on the refrigerator door or in another prominent place
   ❑ Tucked away somewhere in the kitchen
   ❑ What list?
8. **Rate your collection of storage containers:**
   ❑ Plentiful and in a variety of different sizes
   ❑ Enough for a few leftovers
   ❑ What storage containers?
9. **How many "too-tempting-to-resist" foods are in your kitchen right now?**
   ❑ None ❑ One or two
   ❑ Three or more
10. **Which of the following do you have in your freezer?**
    ❑ Skinless, boneless chicken breasts
    ❑ Shrimp or fish fillets
    ❑ Berries or fruit slices
    ❑ Vegetables
    ❑ Frozen yogourt
    ❑ Meal-size containers of homemade chili, soup or stew
    ❑ Homemade soup stock
11. **And which of the following can be found in your kitchen?**
    ❑ Potato chips
    ❑ Premium ice cream
    ❑ Store-bought cookies
    ❑ Whole milk
    ❑ Doughnuts or cupcakes
    ❑ Salami, bologna, bacon or breakfast sausage

Score

Assessing your answers:

1, 2, 3. If the first items you see fit on the **Swap & Drop** menu, your kitchen's in great shape. If not, your kitchen is working against you. Either get rid of the stuff you'd rather not be tempted by, or tuck it away where you have to work to get it.

4. Most vegetables are super-low in calories, so stock a tempting variety. That will make it easy to throw together a low-calorie meal without running to the store.

5. Keep a bowl of fruit where everyone in the family can see it. That way it will be the first place everyone goes when a snack attack strikes.

6. If you don't have the makings of a **Swap & Drop** meal on your pantry shelf, it's time to go shopping. You'll be ready for anything, from a stormy night to a surprise visitor.

7. Invest in an erasable message board. It's a great way to keep a grocery list so that you won't be caught short whenever you want to cook a quick and simple meal.

8. Keep plenty of storage containers handy. Sure, they're great for leftovers. But you can also use them to divvy up giant food packages from the store into reasonably sized portions when you get home.

9. Why drive yourself crazy keeping foods you can't resist? Toss 'em. Or put them so far out of reach that you'll have to make a big effort to get them.

10. The freezer should be your ally in managing your diet, not your personal ice-cream parlour. Consider stocking more of these foods for fast, healthy meals and treats.

11. As we've said before, you can't eat what you don't have on hand. Fatty, sugary, low-nutrition foods stop being an issue when there aren't any around to eat. If you must have some every now and then, keep it out of the house by buying a single portion.

PANTRY ESSENTIALS

1. **SODIUM-REDUCED BROTH** It tastes just as great as the regular broth, but has 25 percent less sodium.
2. **CANNED SALMON OR TUNA** Choose sodium-reduced versions (packed in water where possible).
3. **PLAIN PASTA SAUCE** A great all-purpose staple for making spaghetti and pizza. Choose a low-sodium brand.
4. **CANOLA OIL** It should be your choice of cooking oil. It has the lowest saturated fat content of any vegetable oil, and is high in heart-healthy monounsaturated fats.
5. **GREEN TEA** It's calorie-free and filled with antioxidants. Use loose-leaf tea, as it's more flavourful than bagged. Once open, it should be stored in a dark, dry, airtight container.
6. **SPAGHETTI** Enriched whole-grain pasta has more iron, folacin and B vitamins than whole-wheat.
7. **WHOLE-WHEAT COUSCOUS** This is hands-down the fastest-cooking whole-grain food—perfect for a busy night.
8. **BARLEY** Like all whole grains, barley is packed with selenium and magnesium. It contains soluble fibre, which helps to lower cholesterol levels, and vitamin E.
9. **STEWED TOMATOES** These turn boring dishes into zestier ones. For example, add stewed tomatoes to a skillet of browned chicken. Throw in some green peas and brown rice.
10. **CANNED CHICKPEAS, BLACK BEANS OR KIDNEY BEANS** They're a speedy way to add fibre and protein to salads, soups, wraps or stews. Rinse beans first to wash off some of the sodium they're packed in.
11. **LOW-SODIUM SOY SAUCE** Punch up the flavour of a stir-fry with this low-sodium sauce.
12. **EXTRA-VIRGIN OLIVE OIL** Containing a high proportion of monounsaturated fat compared to other foods, olive oil is a staple of the healthy Mediterranean-style diet.
13. **DRIED RED AND GREEN LENTILS** These fibre-rich legumes are full of protein and don't need to be soaked before cooking. Red lentils turn soft when cooked and are great for thickening soups. Green lentils hold their shape and are perfect for rice pilafs, salads and soups.
14. **BROWN RICE** A whole grain that has about four times more fibre and magnesium than white rice.
15. **LOW-FAT GRANOLA CEREAL** Sprinkle it over yogourt and add diced apple for a nutritious breakfast. When buying, look for brands with less than 3 g of fat per serving.
16. **QUINOA** This whole grain is gluten-free and a complete protein. Make quinoa salads with veggies and nuts.
17. **HIGH-FIBRE BRAN CEREAL** Bran is one of the best sources of fibre. This makes for a filling breakfast.
18. **PEANUT BUTTER** Spread peanut butter on a whole-wheat tortilla, add some banana slices and roll it up.
19. **OATMEAL** Studies find that people who eat oatmeal on a regular basis are more likely to maintain a stable weight and healthy cholesterol level.
20. **HERBS AND SPICES** They put the kick in your vegetarian chili and the yum in your omelettes. Use them lavishly to add flavour. And cinnamon, cayenne, cloves, nutmeg, garlic, ginger and so many more boast surprising health benefits.

REFRIGERATOR ESSENTIALS

1. **SALAD FIXINGS** Always have prewashed salad greens, cucumbers and chopped onions onhand.
2. **RAW VEGETABLES FOR SNACKING** Buy celery, carrots and a variety of coloured peppers weekly. Wash thoroughly, then cut into sticks and store in resealable plastic bags.
3. **VARIETY OF FRESH FRUIT** Pears, for example, are one of the most fibre-rich fruits you can eat. One medium pear has 5 g of fibre, as long as you leave the skin on.
4. **EGGS** A nutrient powerhouse, one egg has about 85 calories, with protein, B vitamins, vitamins A and D, zinc and iron. Eggs are good sources of omega-3s and antioxidants, too.
5. **MILK** Just be sure to choose skim or 1% milk.
6. **WATER** Always keep a nice, cold pitcher of fresh water in the fridge. Try flavouring it with a slice of lemon or cucumber.
7. **SALMON** Salmon is head-and-shoulders above other fish when it comes to vitamin D and omega-3 fatty acids.
8. **GROUND FLAXSEED** One of the best sources of the plant version of omega-3s, it also contains lignans, a plant chemical similar to estrogen that is thought to protect against breast cancer. Grind it and sprinkle it on yogourt. Women don't need a lot—just 1 to 2 tbsp a day.
9. **FRESH VEGETABLES, INCLUDING BROCCOLI** This is one of the best veggies you can eat because it's so high in phytochemicals. Stock up on ultra-healthy spinach and kale, too.
10. **PEANUT BUTTER** It has protein, folate and vitamin E as well as zero trans fats. Instead, it contains the good fats: mono- and polyunsaturated.
11. **CONDIMENTS** Keep a large selection of low-fat, fat-free or low-sugar condiments on hand to add flavour to your dishes, including Dijon mustard, mayonnaise and salsa. Also keep a few low-sodium, sugar-free pickle choices in the fridge, such as garlic dill pickles, sauerkraut and pickled asparagus.
12. **WHOLE-WHEAT FLOUR** It has almost four times more fibre, two times more calcium, six times more magnesium and four times more zinc than enriched white flour. Storing it in the fridge prevents it from going rancid.
13. **TOFU** Look for tofu set with calcium sulphate: One serving (150 g) of medium-firm tofu has about 345 g of calcium, about the same as 1 cup of skim milk.
14. **CHEESE** Go for low-fat cheese or cheese sticks, as well as parmesan to add flavour. Swiss cheese offers more calcium per slice than either cheddar or Monterey Jack.
15. **HUMMUS** A healthy, vegetarian-friendly, low-fat dip or spread made from chickpeas. Serve with pita or veggies.

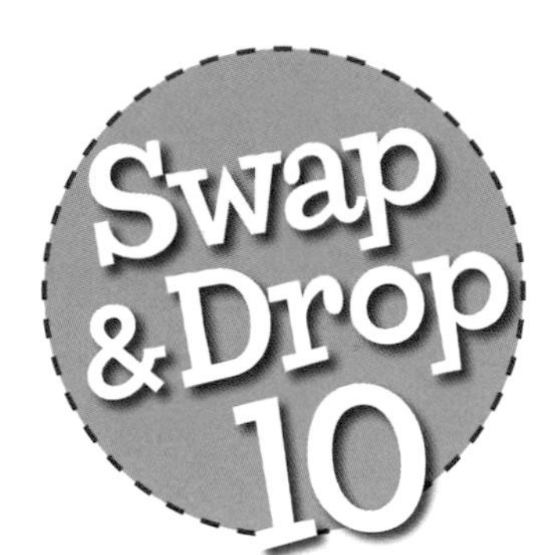

WEEK▶TEN

Stress relief

All we're asking you to do for **Swap & Drop** this week is lean back and relax—that's right, relax

Most of us know that's easier said than done. But it's extra important to de-stress while you're following **Swap & Drop**. If the pressure gets fierce enough, you may be tempted to say, "Forget it, I just can't do it," and give up your best intentions to stick to a healthier diet. Nip that stress in the bud!

"A crust eaten in peace is better than a banquet partaken in anxiety."

—*Aesop's Fables*

This week, you'll identify the different sources of stress in your life and try out techniques to manage or even eliminate them.

Take the pressure off

Like a lot of people, you may find yourself reaching for food when you're under pressure. That's hardly surprising: Recent studies have shown that eating–especially eating foods that are high in carbohydrates–can lower your levels of stress hormones and make you feel less frazzled.

Scientists are also learning that stress itself can trigger hunger. When faced with a stressful situation, the brain signals the adrenal glands to churn out a variety of hormones, including the stress hormone cortisol. One of cortisol's jobs is to trigger the release of glucose and fatty acids, in case your muscles need energy to deal with the perceived threat. This results in an increase in appetite, as a way of guaranteeing that your body will be able to replace the energy it released. A steady influx of tense situations can keep cortisol levels high all day, making you feel hungry almost all the time. As if that's not bad enough, cortisol also triggers enzymes that activate fat cells, priming them to store energy as fat–especially around your middle. Ouch!

If stress is getting the better of you, remember that everyone deals with hassles, small and large. One major difference between people who succeed and those who don't, psychologists say, is in how they deal with those tribulations. To see how well you handle stress, take a few minutes to fill out the Stress Test on page 82. Your answers will help you analyze how you cope with the challenges of daily life.

THE #1 TRUTH ABOUT STRESS

Stress isn't defined as a large workload, a difficult child or financial problems. Stress is your physical and mental reaction to external stimuli. Like in alcoholism, admitting to being a stress-aholic is half the cure. You can't change a crazy world, but you can change your reaction to it. Handle it with humour and hope.

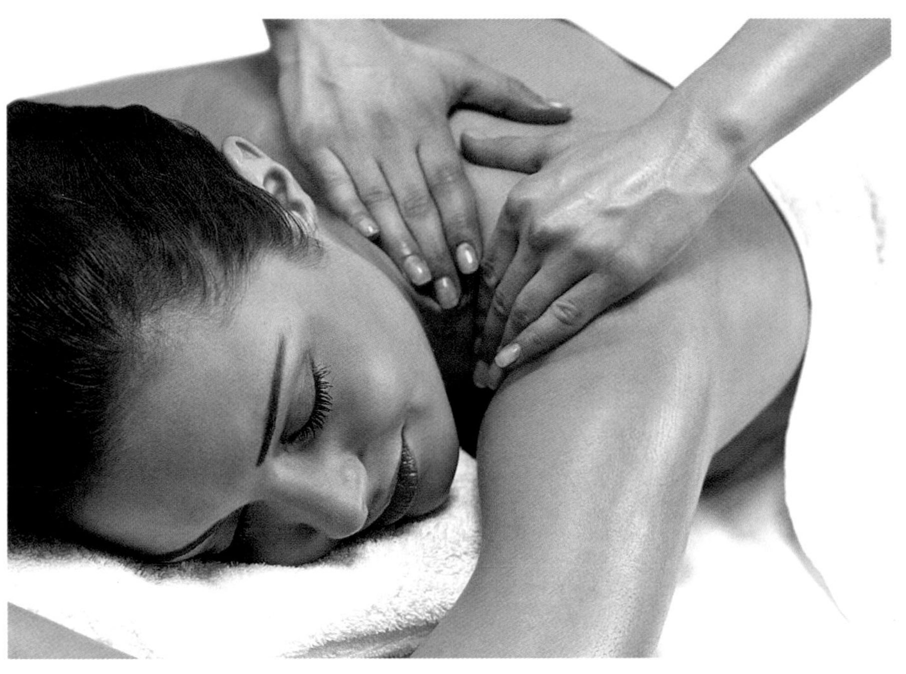

WALK IT OFF *The healthiest way to respond to a rush of stress is go for a brisk walk and burn off nervous energy. Use the time spent walking to think through issues at hand. See page 210 for more walking tips.*

For tips on dealing with the stress of the holiday season—especially the meals—turn back to Swap 7 (page 60).

Step one: solve problems that can be solved

The most direct way to deal with stress is to eliminate minor annoyances. Yes, that's easier said than done, but you may find there are plenty of petty aggravations you can fix quickly once you start paying attention to them.

For example, you could establish a designated spot to put your keys, glasses or cellphone every time you come home. Take a couple hours this Sunday to stock the pantry for the week so you'll always have dinner fixings on hand (turn back to Swap 9, on page 72, for more tips). Make double batches of storable meals to cut your cooking time.

Not all problems are that simple to eliminate, of course. Let's say your boss gives you more work than you can manage, but you haven't been given the authority you need to do the job. That's a classic high-stress dilemma. The direct solution is to talk to the boss and explain the problem. Don't frame it as a complaint, but rather as a search for solutions. ("It would help me if we could decide on priorities, and if I had your support for making key decisions," you might say.)

Or say your problems are at home–tension in your marriage, for instance, or trouble with one of your kids. You need to talk through those problems, but it might also help to explain to your family members why reducing tension is extra important to you now. If the problems are more complicated than you can handle alone, consider enlisting a counsellor.

Work out and de-stress

Think about some ways to make your workout even more relaxing. If you're a walker, be aware of the way your arms swing from front to back and the rhythm of your gait. Repeat a soothing word or phrase each time you exhale. When working out indoors, ignore the TV: Researchers have found that watching television makes people more jittery, so concentrate instead on your breathing and the repetitive movement of your arms and legs. Listening to music on a portable mp3 player can also help keep you motivated.

Are you !#*@%?& kidding me?

Stress is an accepted part of the modern work world, but it can be deadly: A sobering 2002 poll found that one in six Canadians had been under so much stress, they had considered committing suicide.

WOMEN MORE LIKELY TO SEEK COMFORT IN FOOD

Researchers at Montclair State University in New Jersey gave men and women a variety of healthy and unhealthy snacks, and asked them to complete a series of puzzles—some of which were unsolvable. When the women felt frustrated, they became much more likely to dip into the chocolate, while men were the opposite: They were more likely to only eat unhealthy treats after solving a puzzle, as a reward.

EXERCISE VS *Caffeine*

YOU'RE STRESSED and exhausted, so it's no wonder you keep reaching for the espresso every afternoon. But the coffee jitters do you no favours. Try taking a quick walk outside instead—it'll wake you up, giving you your second wind.

Step two: accept what you can't change

Researchers don't understand all the reasons why different people react so differently to stress. Having a sense of humour seems to help, as does the ability to distract oneself by socializing or enjoying a hobby. You can't completely change your personality, but you can change the way you react to hassles and frustrations.

This week, try each of our seven tips for stress reduction. If one doesn't seem to work for you, move on to the next. Your goal: to have at least two stress-busting techniques you can turn to when the pressure starts to build.

1. **Run away!** One of the most effective ways to defuse stress is to run away from it–or at least walk quickly. A 1998 study which asked men and women to keep diaries of activity, mood and stress found that respondents felt less anxious on days when they were physically active than when they didn't exercise. Even when stressful events occurred, people in the study said they felt less troubled on their physically active days.

Exercise is a simple distraction from problems, and it may even change your body chemistry, blunting the effects of thestress hormone cortisol. Exercise has also been shown to ease the symptoms of moderate depression. Virtually any kind of physical activity seems to help, although some researchers think that activities involving repetitive movements–walking, running, cycling or swimming, for instance–may offer the best defences.

Check out the **Swap & Drop** walking plan on page 210 to get started.

2. **Do one thing at a time.** Multitasking can be stressful–such as when you're trying to talk on the phone, send an email and prepare lunch, all at once. This week, make an effort to do just one thing at a time. For example, if you're constantly being interrupted by phone calls while you're trying to work on something, let those calls go to your voice mail. Call people back when the time is right for you.

3. **Put out the fire.** Anger can be harmful, especially if you have a temper. But bottling it up can be dangerous as well. If you feel your temper about to flare, stop,

An ancient cure for frayed nerves

Looking for a simple way to relax, refresh your energy, become more limber and strengthen muscles at the same time? Yoga may be just the ticket. At Oxford University, a psychologist divided 71 men and women into three groups, with three different approaches:

- **One group practiced simple relaxation techniques like deep breathing.**
- **The second visualized themselves feeling less tense.**
- **The third did a half-hour yoga routine.**

The relaxers and the visualizers felt sluggish afterward, but the people in the yoga group reported feeling more energetic and content after their class. Consider signing up for a yoga class in your area.

take a deep breath, and ask yourself three quick questions suggested by Redford Williams, a Duke University researcher who has pioneered work on anger control:

- ***Is this really important to me?*** If the answer is no, leave it behind. If the answer is yes, then ask yourself...
- ***Am I justified in being angry in this situation?*** Weigh the pros and cons, as if both sides are making their case in court. If the answer is no, you're likely to feel your anger and stress begin to melt away. Of course, the answer may be yes. If so, ask yourself just one more question...
- ***Is there anything I can really do about it?*** Say you're driving next to someone who is obviously not paying attention; they're swerving in and out of your lane, and did you just see them *texting?* Honking like crazy probably isn't going to change anything–it'll only make you angrier. So in this case, the best response is to let it go, take a deep breath, and keep out of the other driver's way.

But if your answer to the last question is another yes, then you're in luck. You have the chance to make a real change for the better. If you've done your best to remedy the situation, and you're still having trouble letting your frustration go, ask yourself, "What do I get out of staying angry?" (Usually, nothing.)

4. **Call a friend.** Talking to someone who cares does more than take your mind off your troubles: Swedish researchers have reported that people with strong social connections were almost one-third less likely to die after they'd had a heart attack than those who were socially isolated. This is most likely because enjoying close relationships reduces stress.

If you don't have a circle of friends you feel like you can turn to, work on building one by joining a fitness or art class. Go out on a limb–invite your neighbour over for a coffee. What have you got to lose?

5. **Talk to yourself.** Sometimes we're our own worst enemies. If you find yourself mumbling discouraging messages to yourself, counter your own naysaying with a steady dose of positivity–and don't be embarrassed to encourage yourself out loud when you're alone. Just remember that things go wrong for everyone some-

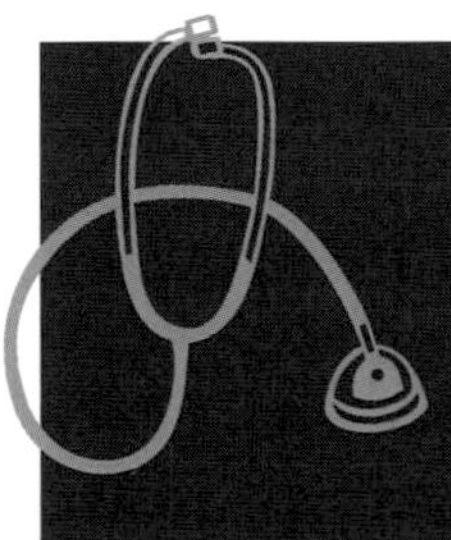

THE BEST MEDICINE

In a study published in 2001, the Center for Preventive Cardiology at the University of Maryland Medical Center tested 300 volunteers for their propensity to laugh at everyday events. Those with a ready laugh were less likely to have heart problems than those who rarely cracked a smile, the scientists found. Even among people with elevated blood pressure or cholesterol, the ability to laugh offered protection against heart attacks.

SWITCH IT UP

Stirring a big pot of delicious soup or chopping vegetables can be very relaxing—and trying new dishes is easy and fun! ***Swap & Drop****'s* *recipes start on page 104.*

8 SUPER-EASY STRATEGIES for a less-stressed workday

1. **Get ready for work the night before. Prepare and pack a healthy lunch and lay out your clothes.**
2. **Set your alarm clock a little earlier so your morning isn't always a mad dash.**
3. **Take advantage of pre-settings—set your coffeemaker to start when your alarm goes off.**
4. **When you get to work, make a point of smiling at and greeting your colleagues. It'll make both you and other people feel good.**
5. **Keep a full water bottle next to you at all times, and refill it as soon as you finish. Nothing worsens stress like dehydration.**
6. **If the weather's nice, eat your lunch outside. The fresh air will give you a natural energy boost.**
7. **Mid-afternoon, get up, go outside and take a brisk walk around the block. It'll burn calories and wake you up if you're feeling sleepy.**
8. **One hour before you're done, make a checklist of everything you need to wrap up. Even if you don't get everything done, tomorrow will be no mystery—you'll know exactly what you need to finish.**

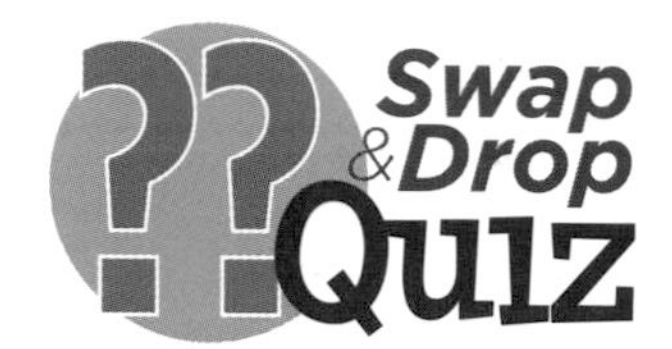

Stress test. Read each statement below and check those that apply to you right now:

- ● A lot of things in my life seem to be out of control right now.
- ▲ I have several good friends I can call if I need to talk something through.
- ● When I'm feeling frazzled, I often have the urge to eat.
- ▲ I'm feeling pretty good about my life right now.
- ● I often feel overwhelmed with the thought of everything that has to get done during the day.
- ▲ I feel better once I've made a list of what I have to do.
- ● Trying to lose weight has definitely added to the pressures I feel.
- ● It's really been frustrating for me to try to find time to be more active.
- ▲ Taking control of my diet has made me feel better about myself.
- ● Sometimes I resent all the responsibilities I have.
- ▲ I'm pretty good at taking my problems in stride.
- ● Lately I notice myself losing my temper when even little things go wrong.
- ▲ Even when things get a little crazy, I still feel as if I'm in control of what's going on in my life.
- ● If someone puts me on hold while we're talking and then doesn't come back on the line soon, it really makes me mad—mad enough to hang up sometimes.
- ● I don't have much patience for people who make mistakes.
- ▲ Even though my life can be pretty hectic, I think I'm good at keeping my priorities straight.
- ▲ I don't worry much about things I can't control.
- ● When I'm under a lot of pressure, I sometimes find myself running in three different directions at once.
- ● I frequently wake up at night feeling anxious about my life.
- ▲ No matter how hectic the day has been, it's easy for me to relax and unwind once I get home.
- ● I wish I had more control over what happens in my life.
- ▲ Exercise is a good way for me to let off steam.
- ● Social situations often make me uncomfortable and nervous.
- ▲ Frankly, I don't tend to sweat the little things—I figure they'll take care of themselves.

Score

What your score means:

How many of each colour did you check? If you tallied more blue triangles than red circles, your responses indicate that you've got the pressures of everyday life under control.

But if the **red circles** outnumber the blue, it could spell trouble. Stress could really be hurting your life. If the numbers are about equal (even if the blues slightly outnumber the reds), be aware that a bad day could set you off. Whatever your score, there are plenty of effective ways to keep cool, calm and collected.

times–nobody's life is perfect. We all have to learn to move on.

6. **Laugh it off.** The act of laughing eases muscle tension, relieves stress and has even been shown to lower the risk of stress-related illnesses such as heart disease. (See "The Best Medicine," on page 81.) It's not always easy to laugh when things go wrong. But if you need a good chuckle, try renting a favourite comedy, watching your favourite sitcom or keeping a funny book handy.

7. **Practice relaxation.** Another proven way to ease stress is what Harvard cardiologist Herbert Benson calls the "relaxation response." The method taps into an innate internal mechanism that can be used to counteract your stress-promoting fight-or-flight response.

Benson suggests setting aside 20 minutes on an especially stressful day and following these six simple steps:

- Find a quiet place where you won't be disturbed. Sit in a comfortable position, one that allows you to relax your body. Close your eyes.
- Starting with your feet and moving up, relax each of your muscle groups. End with the muscles of your face. Take a moment to experience the feeling of being relaxed.
- With your eyes still closed, breathe in and out through your nose, concentrating on each breath.
- As you exhale, begin to silently repeat a short phrase or single word, such as "peace," "calmness" or even just the meditation classic, "om." Choose a word that helps you focus your mind and banish any and all distracting thoughts.
- Continue repeating your soothing

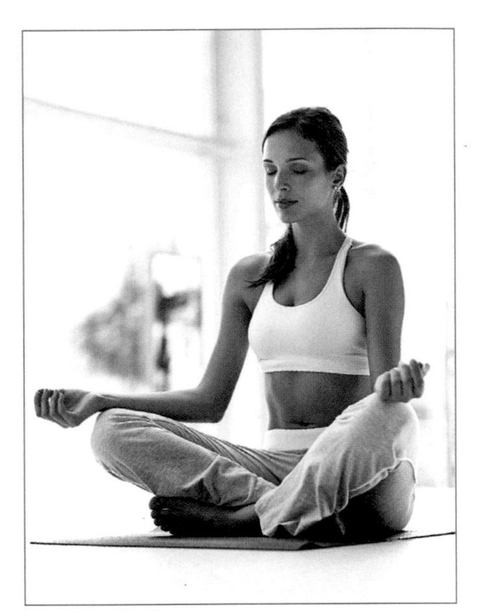

When the going gets tough, the tough...sit cross-legged and concentrate on their breathing.

word or phrase and concentrating on breathing. Try doing this exercise for 10 to 15 minutes. Don't set an alarm, though, or you'll constantly be thinking about it. Have a watch or clock handy and slowly open your eyes now and then to check the time. Don't be discouraged from doing this relaxation routine if you don't have a full 15 minutes—even a few minutes will help.

- Sit quietly for a few more minutes, first with your eyes closed and then with them open. Savour the way your body and mind feel.

Most of us have a hard time letting our minds go quiet, and you may need to practice this technique a few times before you master the art. But soon you'll find that you can slip quickly into relaxation.

Be realistic, and relax

If you're feeling frustrated at this point in your diet, focus on changes that feel more doable right now. If fitting in activity everyday just isn't in the cards, don't worry—concentrate instead on reining in portions. Build gradually to a more active lifestyle that has staying power.

If paying attention to hunger cues has made a big difference for you, channel your energy there, and don't worry that you're missing breakfast now and then. Target the changes that offer the biggest payoff and concentrate on turning them into easy habits. Most of all, go easy on yourself. ■

Stress: it's all in the family

●●● Many new parents are plagued not only by a bad case of the Terrible Twos, but also the guilty suspicion that a child's misbehaviour is all their fault. Don't blame yourself. Open up to a friend about your child-raising woes, or call up your mom if you can. Trust us—she's seen it all before.

●●● Do you find yourself blowing up at your partner for no reason? Try harder to take a deep breath and count to ten before you yell or say something snide. Is it worth it? Remember: This person loves you. But don't ignore any real problems you two may be having—force yourself to talk about them.

CRY IT OUT

Crying makes it easier to think clearly, helps heal wounds and leaves you with a sense of peace. Studies find that crying boosts the immune system and reduces levels of stress hormones. It's okay to get weepy!

:) TAKE A MULTIVITAMIN CHILL PILL

Studies have shown that chronically stressed people have lower levels of nutrients in their bodies, which can be corrected with a multivitamin and mineral supplement. There is no pill that will make stress go away, but taking a multivitamin and mineral supplement is a good idea if you're stressed.

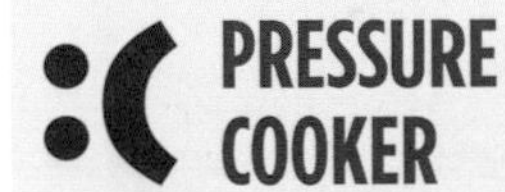

PRESSURE COOKER

For people who compulsively reach for snacks when tensions reach the boiling point, the simplest solution is the ultimate in common sense: Get away from food. If there are problems at home, don't deal with them in the kitchen. Go to another room of the house to hash them out. Under tons of pressure at work? Keep snacks out of easy reach. This week remember our rule: Don't eat to relax. Try one of our techniques first, then wait 5 or 10 minutes to see if you're still hungry.

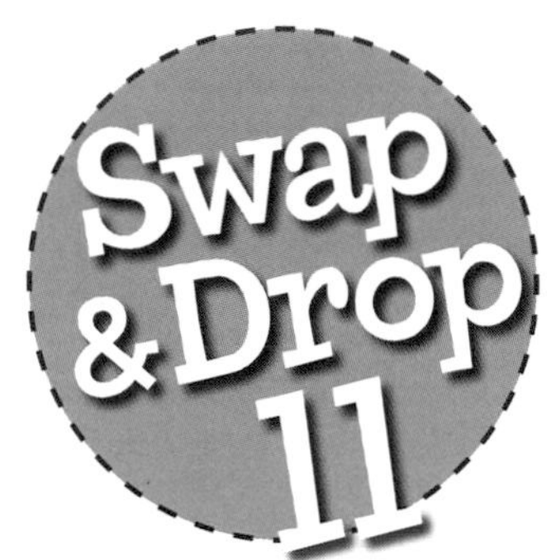

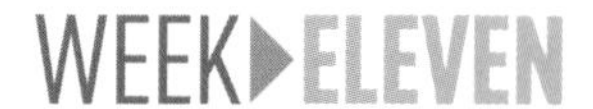

Keeping on track

This week, you should be hitting your stride. You're dropping pounds, and success should feel sweet!

Still, it's crucial that you monitor your progress. The pressure to eat, eat, eat doesn't go away. Plans to go for a walk or hit the gym can fall by the wayside. And those lost pounds sometimes have a way of sneaking back. Just keep this mantra at the back of your mind: Nothing tastes as good as being healthy feels.

"When friends tell you how awesome you look, drop the 'I still have more to go' crap. You worked hard and you deserve the compliment!"

—Jillian Michaels, fitness coach

TELL ME SOMETHING I DON'T KNOW!

Studies prove that happy people are usually more active and tend to burn more calories than their unhappy counterparts, and there's extensive research suggesting that depression contributes to obesity. Many people tend to eat more unhealthy foods when dealing with negative thoughts (as you may already be aware).

This week on **Swap & Drop**, you'll devise your own way to keep yourself on track–for life. We're not suggesting that you measure every bowl of cereal or pasta serving for the rest of your days. But by staying alert to how you're feeling, what you're doing and how much you're eating, you'll get to enjoy a huge payoff in terms of weight, health and self-confidence.

Take a reality check

With the end of the 12-week program just around the corner, you may have already reached your target weight. If so, it's time to transition from a diet that contains fewer calories than you need to one that balances your calorie intake with how many calories you burn.

If you began **Swap & Drop** hoping to lose a significant amount of weight, you may still have some pounds to take care of–and that's fine. Slow and steady is the way to go. What's important is that you prepare for the future. Almost any diet program will help you lose weight during the first few months, but the real trick is maintaining that weight loss.

Many people fall into the "on-off" trap: As soon as they finish their diet, they go right back to the way they were eating before–and the pounds pile back on. Other people, as they near their desired weight, start to lose motivation. It's nothing dramatic: They just stop paying as much attention to portion sizes, or splurge a little more often on rich desserts. Before they know it, they've gained back a chunk of the weight they lost.

If you begin to gain weight back again, it's natural to assume that the diet isn't working and to abandon it completely.

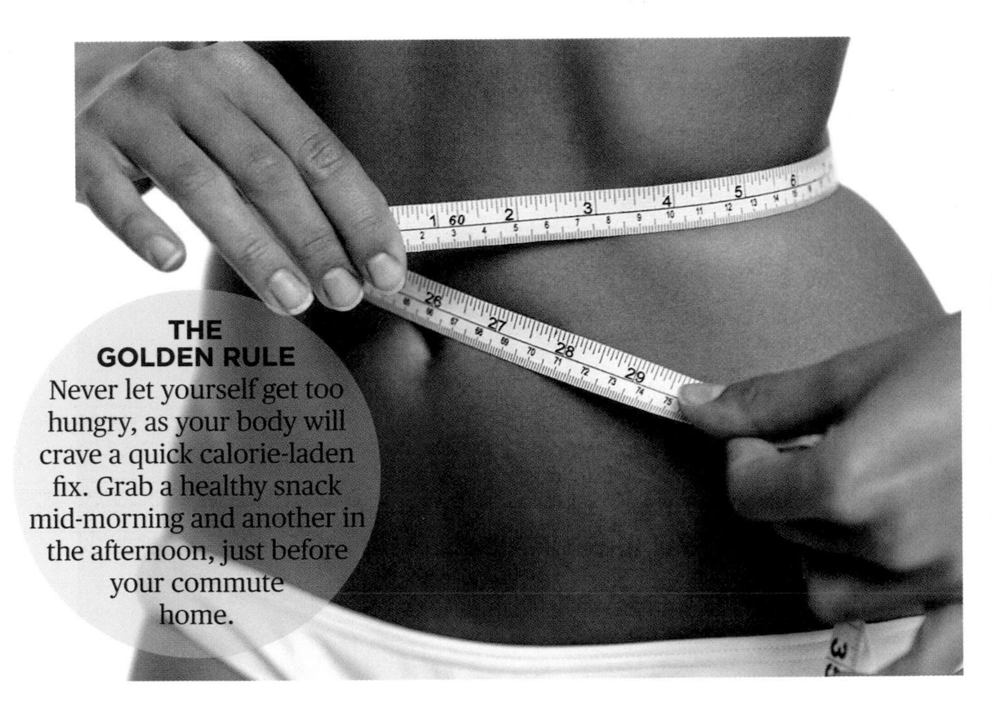

THE GOLDEN RULE
Never let yourself get too hungry, as your body will crave a quick calorie-laden fix. Grab a healthy snack mid-morning and another in the afternoon, just before your commute home.

Worse, it's easy to begin to blame yourself and feel reluctant to try again.

You've learned that eating should be pleasurable–even while trying to lose weight–and found out which changes make the biggest difference for you. Now you just need to keep a watchful eye on your daily routine.

Swap & Drop action plan

Take a few minutes once a week to do a quick self-check-up, starting now. Record your weight, estimate about how much activity you were able to do, rate your overall mood and jot down any problems you may be having.

Don't worry. You don't have to fill out weight-monitoring forms for the rest of your life. Just keep track of your progress for the next two months. If your weight is holding steady and you're comfortable with how things are going, forget the form–just pay attention to how you feel and get on with your life. If you then notice a change for the worse, start filling in progress reports again.

Remember, it's normal for your weight to go up or down a little, week by week. But if the scale creeps up more than five pounds from your desired weight, take action. Don't panic or give up. You've lost weight before, and you can do it again.

Tally your activity

Keeping track of exercise isn't as easy as watching your weight. If you follow the **Swap & Drop** walking plan (page 210), you'll be exercising each and every day

TRY A DINNER BELT

Wear one belt that gauges your level of fullness. Wear it buckled firmly around your waist when you're about to eat dinner, using the same hole every evening. As soon as you feel the least amount of strain against the belt, put your fork down.

Stepping up your efforts

Walking is an excellent way to burn calories, and pedometers are an excellent way to motivate yourself to walk more. These little gadgets clip onto your belt or waistband (some pricier models even work when you put them in your pocket) and count every step you take, motivating you to take more of them. Knowing it's there, tracking your every move, gives you the extra push you need to take the stairs instead of the elevator or walk that extra block.

On average, most people take only 2,000 to 3,000 steps a day. Studies find adding 2,000 steps a day helps maintain your current weight, while 12,000 to 15,000 steps a day (or about 10-12 km) helps drop pounds.

Have you been following the 12-week Walk it Off plan, beginning on page 210? If you haven't, now's the time to start!

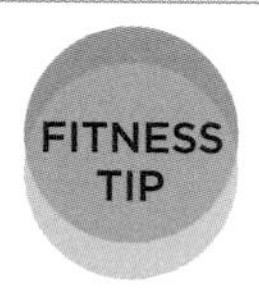

Using a pedometer, keep track of your step count on a progress log—that way you'll easily be able to see how much exercise you've been getting.

EARLY EXERCISE

Studies show that most people who wear pedometers clock more steps before lunch compared to after lunch. Morning exercise raises your heart rate and metabolism early to give you physical energy for hours. From that perspective, it also helps burn more calories throughout the day. If you live in an urban area, note that there are also generally lower pollution levels in the morning, so you can breathe easy.

CREATE A SOFT-DRINK FREE ZONE

A Harvard study of 6,000 people found that drinking just one soft drink a day (diet or regular) increased the risk of obesity by 31 percent. Another study found that rats fed artificially sweetened drinks for ten days gained more weight than those fed sugar-sweetened drinks. Researchers theorize that drinking the diet drinks makes your body prepare for a large intake of calories. When these fail to materialize, your body demands food by making you feel hungry.

in short but effective bursts. But if your exercise mostly consists of everyday activities–such as taking the stairs or walking from the far end of the parking lot–keeping track can be trickier.

One approach is to fill out an activity log, tallying up the time you spend. Your goal should be to add at least 30 minutes of moderately intense activity daily.

Another strategy is using a pedometer or step-counter. Pedometers are inexpensive devices about the size of a cellphone that can be attached to your belt or waistband. A mechanical pendulum inside moves with each step you take, automatically recording every step you take. Go for one that just counts steps, as the ones that claim to measure distance and calories burned are unreliable.

When you first start wearing the pedometer, go about your usual day and, before going to bed, jot down how many steps you took. This number will serve as your baseline. Without doing

DIAGNOSTIC CHECKLIST

Use this checklist to identify sources of trouble in your diet. Be honest, and pick the face that applies to each area of your life.

☺ A smile means you're doing just fine.

😐 A neutral expression means you're holding your own.

☹ A frown—well, you know what that means. After you're done, look over the categories that scored a frown. These are the areas to focus your troubleshooting efforts.

	☺	😐	☹	**For help:**
Breakfast				Page 30
Lunch				Page 36
Snacks				Page 42
Dinner				Page 48
Dining out				Page 54
Stress				Page 78
Resisting outside pressure to eat				Page 60
Environmental triggers				Page 43
Emotional eating				Page 44
Self-esteem				Page 87
Stopping when I'm satisfied				Page 48
Motivation to stay on a diet				Page 66

anything extra, you're likely to take about 3,000 steps. Doing roughly 15 minutes' worth of walking, stair climbing and other everyday activities will add about 2,000 steps. The optimum amount for maintaining your weight is around 10,000 to 12,000 steps a day.

Scale up your weekly goals gradually. Start by shooting for 7,000 steps per day one week, then increase your goal to 9,000 steps. You may find that using a pedometer will give you a little push when you need it. From time to time each day, check to see how many steps you've taken, and get walking to add more.

Turn to page 210 for an in-depth guide to getting the most out of walking.

Monitor your moods

Now you're keeping tabs on your weight, how your clothes fit and how much exercise you get. You should also be alert to how you feel and record it on your progress log–write down whether you feel happy, energized, sad or bored.

As you already know, feeling down can be a surefire way to eat more than you need. Keeping tabs on your mental state will help you begin to see patterns: You may see that the times your weight tends to creep back up again are times when you're bored. Once you realize that, you can make a list of alternate activities you can do when boredom strikes, such as taking a walk, calling a friend or tidying up around the house.

Staying aware of your moods can also help you remedy situations before you find yourself in a deep slump. Everyone feels down now and then, whether it's due to money problems, relationship difficulties or a bad day at work. But some people find their moods dragged down again and again because of that old antagonist low self-esteem. Our society places so much emphasis on being thin, it's no surprise that those who struggle with their weight end up having negative body image. Not only that, but it's often assumed that being overweight is due to a lack of willpower, when in fact it's a complicated mix of factors, from genes and body type to family eating patterns and psychology.

If you ever start feeling self-conscious and low, remind yourself how far you've come in just 12 weeks. You've totally revamped your eating habits and outlook, and that's a major accomplishment! Healthy bodies vary tremendously in terms of size and shape. Remember that not all of us are magazine cover models, nor should we be–it just isn't realistic to

2 PRACTICE THIS SUREFIRE 2-STEP TO HELP YOU KEEP OFF weight

1. **MOVE, MOVE, MOVE** Exercise can cut your risk of every major disease, lengthen your life and even make you happier. Best of all, there's no need to run marathons or even join a gym, since a little activity goes a long way. One large-scale study of 5,000 women found that inactivity was even more life-threatening than smoking cigarettes.
2. **SNOOZE TO LOSE** An amazing study of 68,000 women conducted at Harvard Medical School reveals that women who sleep five hours a night are 32 percent more likely to gain 30 pounds or more as they get older, than women who regularly sleep seven hours or more.

544

That's how many calories you'll burn if you cycle at a steady pace for just one hour. A daily half-hour ride could burn up nearly 10 pounds over a year.

Are you !#*@%?& kidding me?

According to a Johns Hopkins study, you can add two years to your life by climbing stairs for six minutes a day!

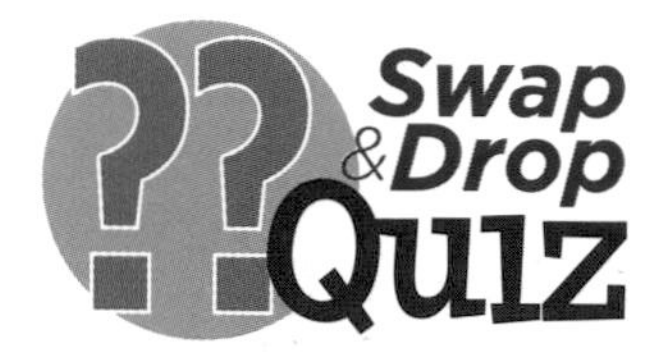

How do you spell success? Let's look back on your progress on the **Swap & Drop** diet and assess how you feel.

1. **How much did you weigh when you began the Swap & Drop diet? _____**
2. **What is your dream weight? _____**
3. **Let's say you can't reach your dream weight. What's the most you can end up weighing and still be happy with the results? _____**
4. **If you can't reach that "happy" weight, what weight would you describe as acceptable? _____**
5. **Let's say that you lose weight, but still don't reach your "acceptable" weight. What ending weight would leave you feeling disappointed? _____**
6. **Look again at your dream weight. What is the number based on?**
   - ❑ The lowest my weight has been as an adult
   - ❑ My ideal weight given my height
   - ❑ What I weighed in high school or university
   - ❑ The lowest weight I've been able to reach on a diet
   - ❑ A healthy weight for me, according to my doctor
   - ❑ Other
7. **Numbers on a scale aren't the only way to measure the success of a diet. Besides weight, what other measures are important to you? On a scale of 1 to 5—not important to very important—rate the following items:**
   - Smaller dress or pants size 1 2 3 4 5
   - How my clothes feel 1 2 3 4 5
   - How I feel (slimmer, more energetic, more attractive) 1 2 3 4 5
   - Specific health measures (lower blood pressure, for example) 1 2 3 4 5
   - Overall sense of health 1 2 3 4 5
8. **If dress or pants size is an important measure of success for you, what goal do you have in mind?**
   Dress size:
   Waist size:
9. **What else do you hope to achieve by dieting? On a scale of 1 to 5—not important to very important—rate the following motivation:**
   - Feeling more self-confident 1 2 3 4 5
   - Feeling sexier or more attractive 1 2 3 4 5
   - Being happier about myself and how I look 1 2 3 4 5
   - Feeling more in control 1 2 3 4 5
   - Not being embarrassed by my weight 1 2 3 4 5
   - Feeling fitter 1 2 3 4 5

Score

Congratulations! You got every question correct. There are no wrong answers to these questions—they're too personal for that. But your answers do say a lot about your expectations. For insights on your comments and some thoughts about whether you are being fair to yourself, read the contents of this chapter.

expect that of yourself, and deep down, you probably know that.

Of course, accepting that is easier said than done. Sometimes feelings of low self-esteem reach all the way back to childhood. Not only that, but if you find yourself struggling unsuccessfully against feelings of sadness, hopelessness or low self-esteem, you may actually be suffering from clinical depression.

Talk to your doctor if you suspect that might be the case. There is even a proven link between depression and weight gain, and studies show that treating it can actually help you lose weight.

How do your clothes fit?

If you notice that your clothes are beginning to feel a little tight again, search for the reason. You may know exactly why you're gaining weight–the notes you've made on your progress should help you out a lot.

To do more in-depth troubleshooting, fill in the diagnostic checklist on page 86. When your internal warning bell rings, use that list to identify the sources of dieting trouble.

Once you've zeroed in on the specific problem, take action–but don't try to address all your issues at once. That's what **Swap & Drop** is all about, after all: focusing on one change at a time.

Having trouble with a specific meal? Check back to the first four weeks of **Swap & Drop** for advice on how to take control of breakfast, lunch, snacks and dinner. Eating when you're not really hungry? Make a conscious effort to stop and ask

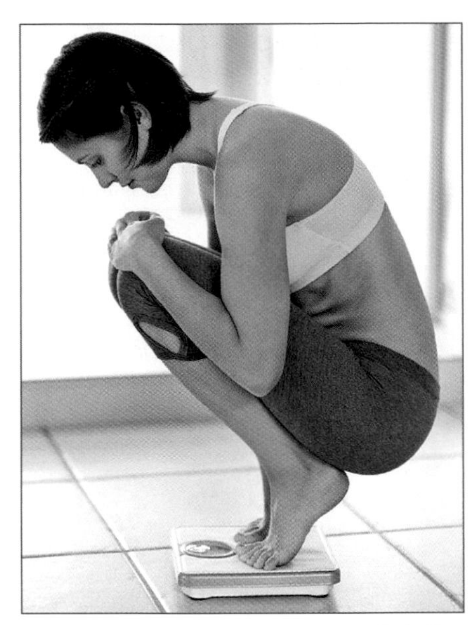

Be sure to weigh yourself daily or weekly—and be sure to keep a food and exercise diary.

yourself whether you're actually responding to an emotional or environmental cue. If you don't really need to eat, distract yourself by doing something else: Take a walk, do a chore, brush your teeth or grab a stick of sugar-free gum. Feeling overwhelmed? Tackle one problem at a time. Chances are you'll see progress on the scale.

Keeping track is so important that we urge you to set aside a particular time each week to conduct your **Swap & Drop** check-up. Many prefer to do theirs on Sunday evenings, but use whatever time works best for you. Put a reminder on your calendar. Post your weekly check-up form on the refrigerator or beside your desk–wherever it's easy to find. When all is going well, then you'll have several reminders to tell yourself, "Congratulations! Be proud!" By learning the **Swap & Drop** way to lose weight, you have changed your own life in wonderful ways. ■

:(THE INSIDIOUS SITTING DISEASE

The average Canadian spends more than 20 hours a week watching television. In a study of 3,000 people, a sports dietitian found that 41 percent of those surveyed did less than one hour a week of exercise, and more than half the group spent most of their day sitting down.

:) SNEAK IN FITNESS

Turn your TV break time into active time by fitting in chores during the commercial breaks. Getting up to load the washing machine, empty the garbage or wash dirty dishes can add 14 to 24 minutes of activity in an hour.

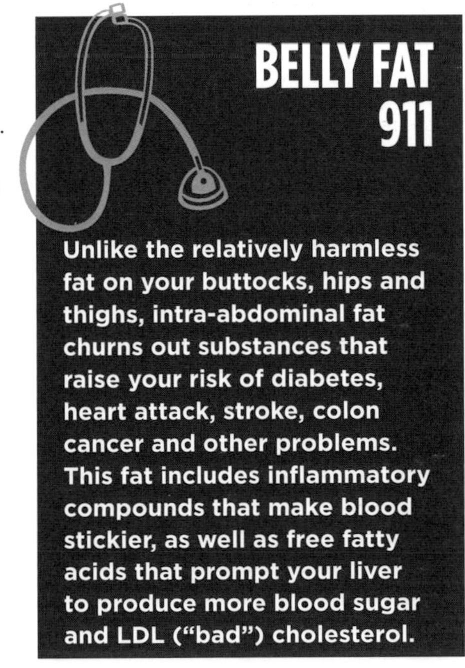

BELLY FAT 911

Unlike the relatively harmless fat on your buttocks, hips and thighs, intra-abdominal fat churns out substances that raise your risk of diabetes, heart attack, stroke, colon cancer and other problems. This fat includes inflammatory compounds that make blood stickier, as well as free fatty acids that prompt your liver to produce more blood sugar and LDL ("bad") cholesterol.

EXERCISE IN DISGUISE

People who look at exercise as one more task to add to their list almost always stop exercising (or never start at all). Those who look at it as a 24/7 attitude—full of spirit and fun—emerge as winners. You can burn calories while doing a wide range of everyday tasks. Just check out our guide:

ACTIVITY	CALORIES BURNED PER HOUR
Bicycling	544
Gardening	340
Golfing (walking with clubs)	374
Hiking	408
Ice skating/Rollerblading	408
Kayaking/Canoeing	340
Swimming	544
Tennis	476
Volleyball	204

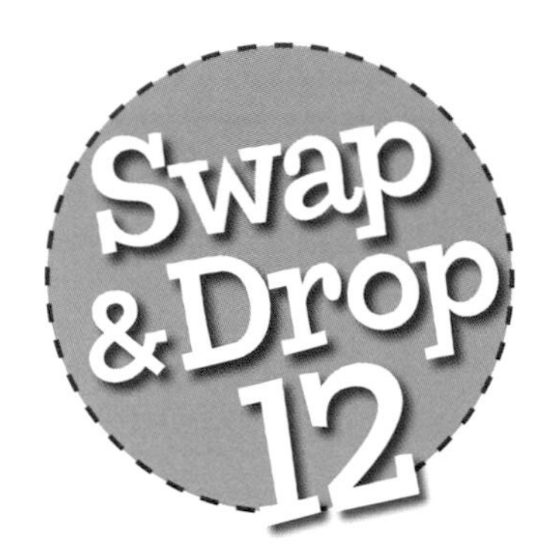

WEEK ▸ TWELVE

Swap & Drop for life!

Celebrate your success with some great new flavours, fun new activities—and a healthy promise to yourself

“Fear less, hope more; eat less, chew more; whine less, breathe more; talk less, say more; love more, and all good things will be yours.”

—*Swedish proverb*

PATTING YOURSELF ON THE BACK

You may have been taught that you should always be modest about your accomplishments. Forget that: While nobody likes a braggart, don’t be afraid to privately tell yourself, “You’re doing great. You are amazing.” Feeling a sense of accomplishment is a known happiness-booster. Take it from us: You deserve it.

It’s celebration time! You’ve reached Swap 12, the end of the formal **Swap & Drop** program. Over the past three months you’ve done something remarkable: You’ve redirected your life, changed the way you eat and, most importantly, proved to yourself that you are in control.

To celebrate, be playful with food this week–try at least two new combinations or flavours you’ve never had before. Boredom, not flavour, is the enemy of weight loss. If you always eat the same meals, under tight restrictions, you’ll want to rebel. **Swap & Drop** is all about loving and respecting food, so why not enjoy something you might never have tried otherwise?

Reward yourself

You’ve done an amazing job so far. So go ahead and reward yourself, whether it’s with something extravagant–a weekend getaway or a night on the town–or with a treat that reinforces the new you, such as running shoes, a new bike or an enticing healthy-eating cookbook.

Why make a big deal about rewarding yourself? Because too often we take our own progress for granted. Even people who have lost weight and made healthy lifestyle changes may think they’ve failed, until they take a moment to reflect on their own accomplishments. Some successes are easy to recognize–eating a healthier breakfast, for instance. Other positive changes may be more subtle, but even more important: discovering that you can make a plan and stick to it; gaining self-confidence; and learning that you can get yourself back on track after a slip-up. As helpful as other people can be, truly changing for the better is up to you and you alone–and you did it!

Trust your instincts

What’s the toughest challenge dieters face when it comes to keeping the weight off? Most people starting a diet figure the hardest part will be resisting temptation. But

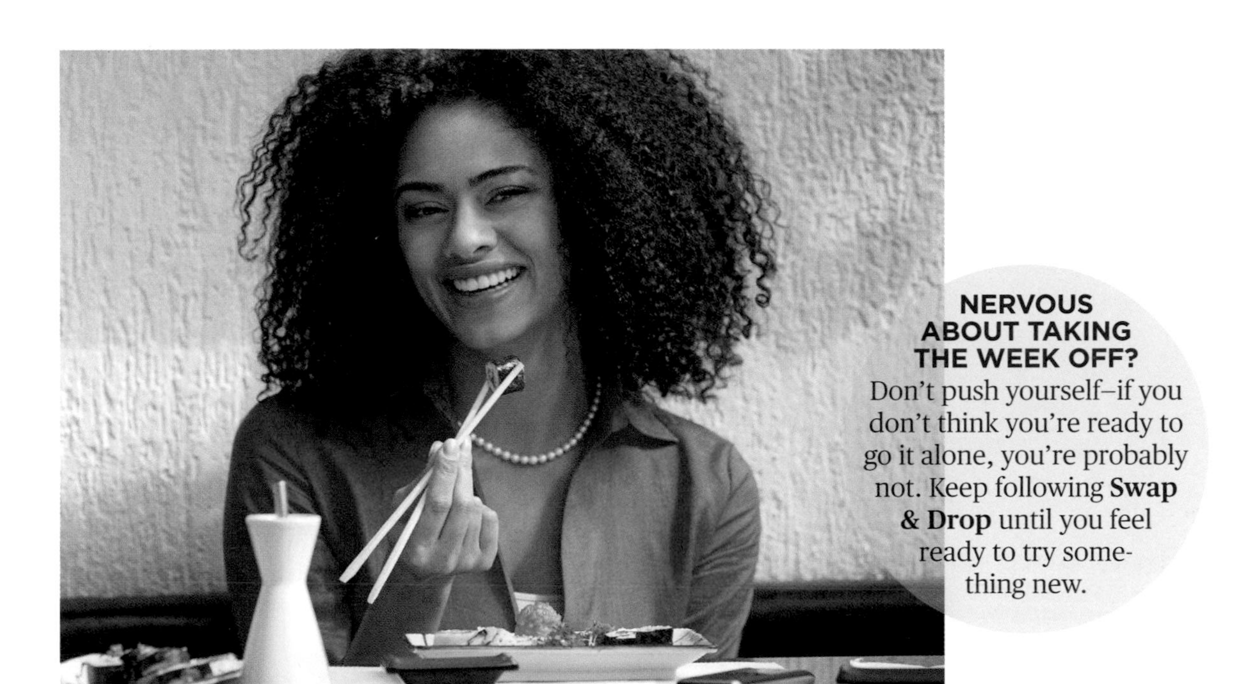

NERVOUS ABOUT TAKING THE WEEK OFF? Don't push yourself–if you don't think you're ready to go it alone, you're probably not. Keep following **Swap & Drop** until you feel ready to try something new.

as we've already mentioned, the biggest pitfall dieters face is actually something much more basic: boredom.

People often give up on diets because they're weary of tracking calories or consulting long lists of forbidden foods. But after all, a healthy diet is just about eating sensible servings of tasty and (mostly) nutritious food. More calories mean a smaller portion. Simple as that.

But even with the varied **Swap & Drop** meal plan, you could be feeling a little restless. So this week, make something you've never eaten before. Treat yourself to dinner at a restaurant you've been longing to try. Forget the **Swap & Drop** meal plan for a whole day. Heck, take the whole week off, if you want. Imagine that you're taking off the training wheels and going for a spin after 11 weeks of learning to keep your balance. This week, let healthy-eating principles guide you as you venture out on your own.

Try something new

Not sure how to add excitement to the menu this week? Check out our healthy recipes, starting page 104. Here are a few more suggestions:

Make your own salad bar. For a family dinner one night this week, put together a salad bar and invite the whole crew to create their own salads. Include at least two vegetables that aren't usually on the menu–jicama, radicchio or artichoke hearts, for instance, as well as some cooked chickpeas and lentils for protein. Warm up a loaf of whole-wheat bread. For

4 Tips for other food fun

- **At the farmer's market, ask a vendor for a cooking suggestion—and take their advice.**
- **Ever done Meatless Mondays? Try eating vegetarian just once a week—you might love it!**
- **This Saturday, pack a picnic lunch and head to the park or ski slope. You'll get fresh air, some light exercise and a delicious meal!**
- **Two words: homemade sushi. Look up a tutorial online.**

dessert, serve up a selection of colourful sorbets topped with berries.

Throw a taco party. Tacos are a terrific way to serve up vegetables such as tomatoes, lettuce and grilled peppers. Spread all the ingredients on the dining table and let everyone make their own. Use soft corn tortillas rather than hard taco shells–they contain much less fat–and mix things up by using cooked black beans instead of refried beans. Help yourself to as much salsa as you want, dab on some guacamole and skip sour cream.

Slim down an old standard. Take one of your favourite comfort meals and give it a boost by adding a few servings of vegetables. Broccoli is terrific in tuna casserole, for instance, and chickpeas make a great addition to spaghetti with tomato sauce. Green peppers can liven, and lighten, up a bowl of chili. If you'd like, use an online calorie counter to tally up the precise calories in your revamped meal.

Order a feast of appetizers. Choose a restaurant with a wide range of appetizers and vegetable sides, such as a Spanish-style tapas restaurant, and have a feast. Share the dishes with your dinner companions, and you can order practically every small dish on the menu without having to worry about portion sizes. Start with only as many dishes as there are people at the table. If you're still hungry, order more. Steer clear of fried foods, of course, and include plenty of vegetables.

Go fish. Chances are your local fish market features at least a few kinds of fish you haven't tried. Be adventurous and cook up something new–giant prawns or mahi mahi, for instance.

Once you've got the fish home, choose a recipe that involves baking or grilling, not frying. There are many low-calorie ways to give fish a burst of flavour, such as Cajun spices or a simple squeeze of lime juice. Capers and spicy salsas are also terrific on fish and other seafood.

Bake bread. This weekend, try baking your own loaf of bread. Consider investing in a breadmaker if you don't have one–then you can just pop the ingredients in, head out on a couple of errands and come back to a freshly baked loaf. Choose recipes that include whole-wheat flour and, even better, whole grains like oats.

Have a pizza extravaganza. Most markets sell do-it-yourself pizza crusts that make preparing a homemade pizza fast and easy. Get a group together for a pizza party. Include at least two vegetable toppings and use shredded cheese rather than slices, so you get more coverage with less cheese. Try grating hard goat cheese or smoked mozzarella for more flavour.

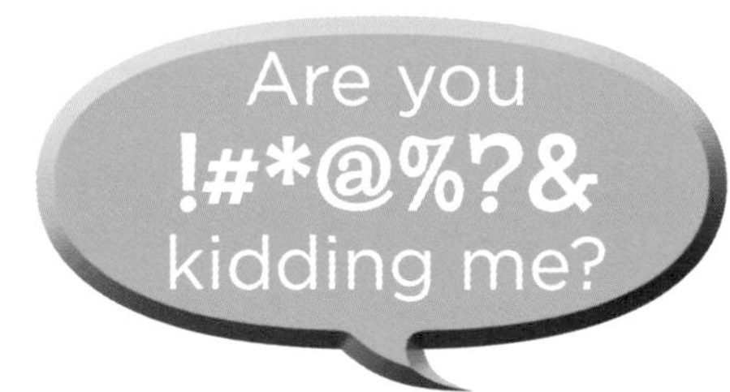

A study conducted by the University of the West of England found that 16 percent of college women polled would give up a year of their lives to be the perfect weight. Ten percent would give up five years, and 2 percent would actually forfeit a whole decade! These women aren't crazy—they're the victims of a thin-obsessed society. Don't go to extremes: If you're a healthy weight for your body type, you're doing great.

Appetizer feast

Need some ideas for a homemade appetizer dinner? Try:

- **Protein**: 1/2 cup of seafood ceviche; Thai chicken satay, 2 skewers; smoked salmon, 60 g; or 3 thin slices of prosciutto.
- **Vegetables:** Unlimited, as long as they're not prepared with added fat. Try topping with a pinch of grated cheese.
- **Other nibbles:** 10 olives, or a small handful of mixed nuts.

PIZZA-CRUST VARIATIONS

Can't find premade pizza crust at the grocery store? Any flatbread will do–just aim for whole-wheat whenever possible. Try using a pita (especially Greek-style pita–it's thicker than the thin Lebanese style) or lavash, an Armenian flatbread. Both make delicious pizza bases.

Create your own signature pasta. No other dish is as versatile, and pasta itself comes in a wide range of shapes and colours–from familiar fettuccine to fun shapes like orecchiete (shells) and cavatappi (corkscrew macaroni). And the ingredients that go with pasta are virtually limitless–from shrimp to sliced chicken, to kalamata olives, artichokes, basil, diced tomatoes, fava beans, tuna, capers, mushrooms, cauliflower, broccoli, parmesan cheese...you get the idea. Put on your chef's hat this week, and create your own pasta masterpiece.

Make new friends. This week, come home from the grocery store with a vegetable you haven't tried before. Ever eaten daikon? What about fennel? Farmer's markets are also a great source of inspiration; when you're surrounded by all that seasonal bounty, it's easy to find something delicious to try.

Travel the world. This week, sample a cuisine you haven't tried before or have never prepared at home. Check your library or local bookstore for a cookbook that specializes in a particular ethnic cuisine, or read restaurant listings for inspiration before dining out. Chances are you'll discover a world of new ingredients and tastes.

Find a new move

While you're shaking things up this week in the food department, do the same with exercise. The goal is simple: Find something fun to do this week that you haven't done before–something that involves being active. Take the plunge at a local pool. Go for a hike in a nearby park. Take the kids canoeing. Take a pilates class. If you haven't given the **Swap & Drop** strengthening routines on page 238 a try, now's the perfect time.

Don't make the excuse that you don't like sports or working out. If you think you don't like strolling in a beautiful park, walking the dog, playing catch with your kids or riding a bike around the neighborhood, changing your mind will improve your life in more ways than one.

Striking a balance

Swap & Drop is based on the simple principle that to lose weight, you have to take in fewer calories than you burn. To maintain your weight, you have to balance calories in and calories out. You can either keep track of every meal you eat, or just stay aware of what you eat throughout the day, balancing every indulgence with some restraint. If you treat yourself to

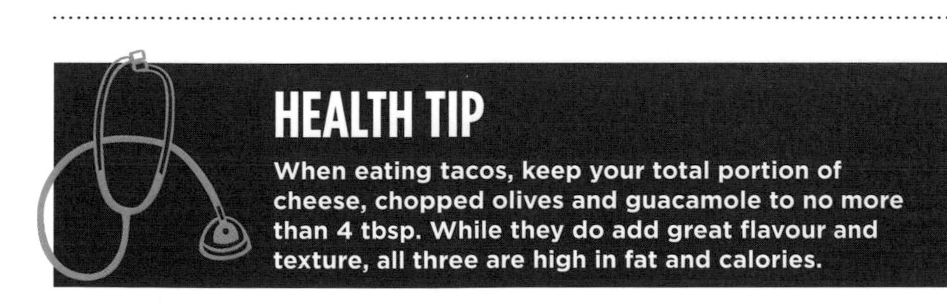

LOW-FAT REFRIED BEANS

Traditional Mexican refried beans, or frijoles refritos, are made by sautéing diced onion and sometimes garlic in lard, then adding and mashing beans. Make your own lower-fat, lower-calorie version by cooking onion in a non-stick skillet with a teaspoon or so of olive oil and a splash of chicken or vegetable broth until the onion is soft. Add a can of pinto beans plus a teaspoon of ground cumin, and mash the beans as they cook in the skillet. You might also find fat-free canned refried beans at the grocery store.

How to make a healthy taco

1. Put corn or small flour tortilla on plate.
2. Top with 1/4 cup (about the size of a golf ball) of either lean ground beef, ground turkey, shredded turkey or ground soy protein.
3. Add a total of 2 tbsp shredded reduced-fat cheddar cheese, guacamole and/or sliced olives.
4. Cover with toppings such as chopped tomatoes, shredded lettuce, diced red and green peppers, minced red onion, diced jalapeño peppers, chopped green chilies and fresh homemade salsa.
5. Fold over and eat.

(Per serving, with corn tortilla and ground beef: 430 calories, 22 g total fat, 10 g saturated fat, 80 mg cholesterol, 33 g carbohydrates, 5 g fibre, 27 g protein, 670 mg sodium.)

a sumptuous brunch with friends, for instance, go light on supper and try to fit in extra exercise.

One day of overdoing it doesn't mean the end of your diet. As long as you regain your balance shortly after, even a week off won't bring your diet crashing down—and that includes the holidays. No, we're not advising you to throw caution to the wind when holidays or special occasions roll around. Just know that you are more than capable of losing that weight again.

One (more) week at a time

Even after finishing **Swap & Drop**'s 12 essential swaps, you may still be hankering for some new goals. Most of us love making this kind of progress, so we understand if you don't want to stop now! Here are five more to try:

Conquer your cravings. It can be hard to resist the urge to snack. This week, figure out why you have cravings and try to deal with their root causes. Remember: Real hunger doesn't have food preferences, so if you are craving a particular flavour or food, it's your mind talking, not your stomach! Try to understand what those cravings might mean for you.

Eat in technicolour. This week, make sure that you eat three different colours at every meal. Every day, make sure you eat some red (peppers, tomatoes, apples) orange (carrots, oranges, cantaloupe) and plenty of green (broccoli, arugula, rapini). Different colours in natural foods means different nutrients, so brighter is better!

Get on your feet. Exercise is great, but doing some when you can doesn't mean you should sit down the rest of the time! That can be hard if you have a desk job, but there are ways to fit in some more walking and standing.

This week, stand up as much as you can—whether you're on the phone, reading the newspaper or chopping onions. Get used to being up and moving rather than sitting, and soon it will become habit.

Laugh it off. With a positive attitude, you can conquer anything! And what better in-

2 WAYS TO GET BACK ON TRACK AFTER TAKING TIME OFF FROM YOUR DIET

1. **PREPARE ALL YOUR MEALS** for one day the night before—that way, you'll already have plenty of ammo to fight hunger pangs and cravings. Make it easy for yourself.
2. **KEEP A FOOD DIARY.** We've recommended this before, and it's a great way to stay motivated about a diet. Did the holidays get you back on the overeating wagon? Writing down everything you eat will keep you accountable.

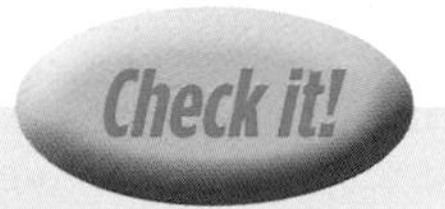

This week, take a moment to list all the reasons you want to lose or maintain your weight. (It's a good idea to return to this list every once in a while, as a reminder.) Is it because you have more energy when you eat healthy? Maybe it's because you want to stave off chronic illness. Spelling it out will strengthen your willpower even more.

HELP!

Maybe you're ready to take the plunge and try a whole bunch of new foods. Vietnamese? You're there! West African? Bring it on! But what can you do if your spouse or kids are dead-set against trying something new?

Don't let that stop you. *A lot of kids (or adults, for that matter) are uncomfortable tasting new foods. The important thing is not to bully them into trying it by saying things like, "You're so boring." Instead, start by ordering dishes that might seem more familiar—at a Thai restaurant, for example, there's a good chance everybody will love the peanut-sauce dumplings. (Split an appetizer between the whole family.) When preparing food at home, enlist the help of your family members. Once they see how something is made, they may be more willing to taste it.*

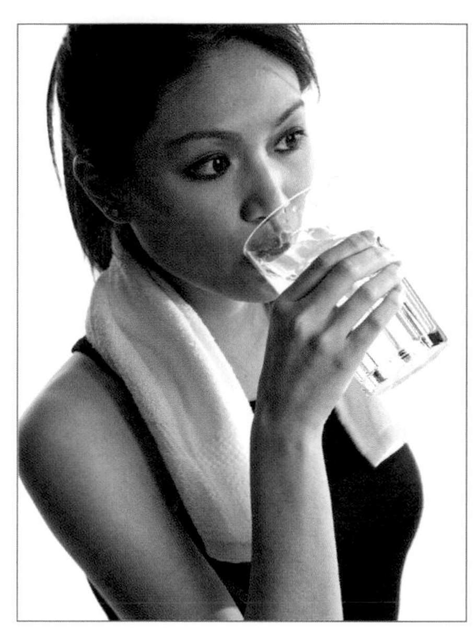

Don't forget that drinking lots of water isn't just essential for life—it's important for healthy weight loss, too.

dicator of your attitude than your laughter levels? This week, monitor how much you laugh and go in pursuit of funny. Flip to the humour section in a magazine, call up your most hilarious friend or rent the latest comedy movie. Having less than 10 or 15 good laughs in a day? You've got some *un*serious work to do!

Master your liquids. For the first few days of the week, log everything you drink in a day. Then review it for two things: Are you drinking enough, and are you drinking the right stuff? A healthy day would include at least eight glasses of water, one glass of milk, maybe a fresh-squeezed juice in the morning and one or two cups of tea or coffee. Pop should be treated like candy–a sweet treat that falls in the snack or dessert category.

Keep your perspective

Losing weight is not an all-or-nothing proposition: It's about the small choices you make every day. If you go overboard on portions one day, you have the next to restore your balance. If your weight plateaus for a while, so be it. You haven't failed, and neither has the diet. You can give yourself a little time-out and then make another change or two when you feel ready.

Keep that in mind as you relax a little this week and move into the weeks beyond, and you'll do just fine. If **Swap & Drop** has worked for you, you should already know that you've got what it takes to do almost anything you want. Just take it one step at a time. Keep your spirits up, stay positive and make time for fun. If you hit a rocky stretch, go easy on yourself–as long as your resolution is firm, you'll make it through. Set your sights on a new goal, and go for it!

Are you sure you've been eating the right portions? If you need a refresher, turn back to Swap 1 (page 18). Then flip through the whole book for a reminder of how far you've come!

30

That's how many millilitres of water you should drink per 2 pounds of your overall body weight.

:) HOLIDAY CHEER

It used to be believed that people typically gained about five pounds during the holidays. Not true: A study from the United States National Institutes of Health, which tracked 200 men and women from late September through early March using weight and other health measurements, found that the average weight gain was about one pound. And it turns out that extra pound may have had less to do with eating than with exercise; people who said they weren't physically active during the six-month-long study typically gained about 1½ pounds; those who stayed active through the cold winter months actually lost weight.

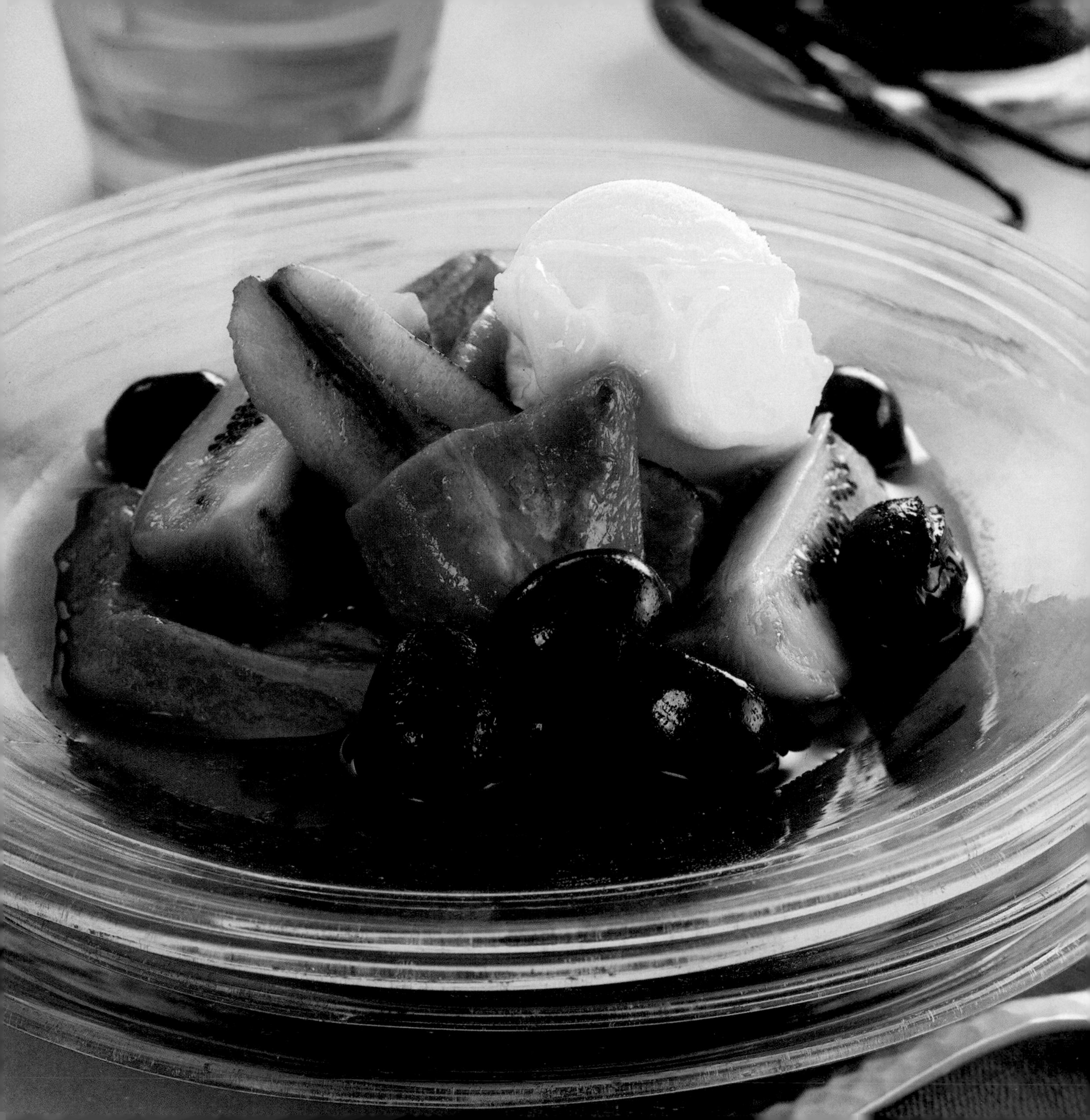

2

12-week meal planner with over 100 healthy & delicious recipes

This section of ***Swap & Drop*** *reminds me of a quote from management expert L. R. Bittel: "Good plans shape good decisions. That's why good planning helps to make elusive dreams come true."*

Our health and even our happiness are strongly influenced by how well we manage ourselves and our lives–the choices we make, the ways we spend our time and our dedication to achieving the results we dream of. Though we aren't born knowing the right foods to choose, we can learn these skills over time.

If you don't plan ahead when it comes to meals and snacks, you're likely to find yourself stuck with default options like unhealthy takeout or a high-carb, high-sugar snack from the coffee place on the corner. Though that's not the end of the world, it can't happen regularly if you want to live healthy, lose weight and look great.

Do you feel that planning sounds like more work than fun? Have a quick look at the meals and snacks laid out in the next few pages–does this look like a boring, restrictive diet plan to you?

I have to say that even I was skeptical at first–so many treats all over the place, and shouldn't there be more "serious" grains in those pancakes and muffins? Did I really see cheese ravioli on the dinner menu?

Yet these plans and recipes have been created by experts, with every calorie and gram of fat and fibre planned in for you. If you follow the meal plan, you can have those pancakes for breakfast, and still get a full 25 grams of fibre by the end of your day. Amazing!

You'll also notice the impressive variety of choices for different healthy meals and snacks. Variety is everything, for both long-term weight loss and health. It makes you less likely to get bored and give up, and will ensure you get the full spectrum of nutrients your body needs. Best of all, with a rich, diverse plan like this, you're sure to discover a passion for new foods and dishes that will persist well past the 12 weeks of this program. Bon appétit!

– Dr. Susan Biali, M.D.

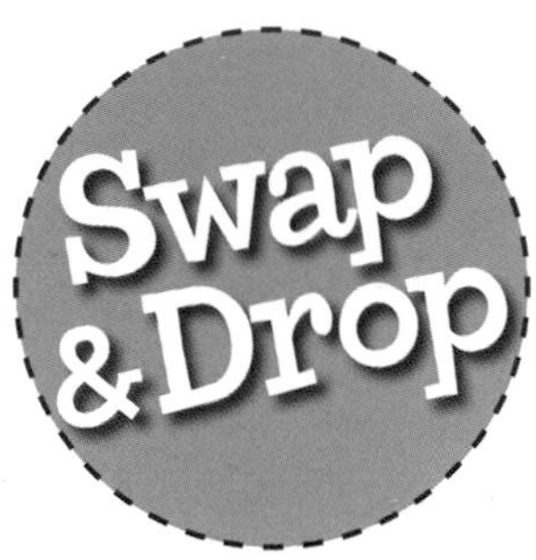

Meal Plan for WEEKS ▸ 1,4,7,10

	MONDAY	TUESDAY	WEDNESDAY
BREAKFAST	**Yogourt Parfait** *(page 104)* • Yogourt layered with granola, fruit and coconut	**Bagel Delight** • Mini whole-wheat bagel topped with jam and low-fat cream cheese • Yogourt with sliced ripe peach or other fruit	**Breakfast on the Run** • Cereal bar • Yogourt topped with blueberries or other fruit
LUNCH	**Caesar Salad Lunch** • Grilled Turkey Caesar Salad *(page 110)* • Medium whole-wheat roll • Cantaloupe cubes	**Soup and Sandwich** • Hearty Split-Pea Soup *(page 111)* • Tuna salad sandwich • Seasonal fruit	**DINING OUT:** **Harvey's** *(page 194)* • Veggie Burger • Side Garden Salad
SNACK	Handful of baked tortilla chips and salsa	Hot cocoa made with skim milk	Baked Apple *(page 124)*
DINNER	**Barbecued Halibut Steak Dinner** • Barbecued Halibut Steak *(page 118)* • Grilled onions and scallions • Penne with Zucchini *(page 120)*	**Beef Stew** *(page 115)* • Egg noodles	**Chickpea Stew Dinner** • Tomato and Chickpea Stew *(page 120)* • Garlic bread
DESSERT	Blueberry Bonanza *(page 125)*	Fudgsicle	Tropical Smoothie *(page 105)*

No need to weigh every gram or calculate every calorie—we've already done it for you. Our meal plans are designed to meet the following daily guidelines:

- Calories: from 1,300 to 1,600
- Calories from fat: 30 to 35 percent
- Saturated fats: no more than 10 percent of calories
- Fibre: at least 25 g
- Calcium: about 1,000 mg
- Fruits and vegetables: seven to eight servings a day

THURSDAY	FRIDAY	SATURDAY	SUNDAY
A Perfect Bowl of Cereal *(page 35)* • High-fibre cereal topped with raisins and chopped nuts • Skim or 1% milk	**Cottage Cheese Melba** *(page 105)* • Cottage cheese with peach slices and jam • Raisin-bread toast • Green tea	**Pancakes to Start** *(page 105)* • Silver Dollar Pancakes topped with maple syrup and sliced strawberries • Skim or 1% milk	**Cranberry Scone with Orange Glaze** *(page 107)*
Simple Sandwich Lunch • Turkey, lettuce, tomato and Swiss cheese sandwich on whole-wheat bread • Green salad • Slice of cantaloupe	**The Perfect Soup-and-Salad Lunch** • Low-sodium vegetable soup with breadsticks • Green salad topped with grilled chicken • Green or red grapes	**Pita Pizza and Salad** • Pita Pizza *(page 108)* • Green salad • Apple	**BRUNCH** • Skim or 1% milk • Crudité platter • Vegetable-Cheddar Omelette *(page 104)* • Whole-wheat toast with butter and jam • Cantaloupe wedge
Frozen yogourt	Quesadilla (corn tortilla with melted cheese)	Air-popped popcorn	
DINING OUT: **Boston Pizza** *(page 190)* • Baked Seven-Cheese Ravioli • Garden Greens	**Sweet-and-Sour Pork Dinner** • Sweet-and-Sour Pork with Pineapple *(page 115)* • Brown rice • Steamed broccoli	**DINING OUT:** **The Keg** *(page 196)* • 8 oz. Sirloin Classic • Mixed Green Salad	**Zesty Meat Loaf Dinner** • Zesty Meat Loaf *(page 114)* • Egg noodles • Steamed green beans
Brownie Bites *(page 123)*	Skim-milk, decaffeinated latte	Small container of fat-free yogourt topped with fruit	

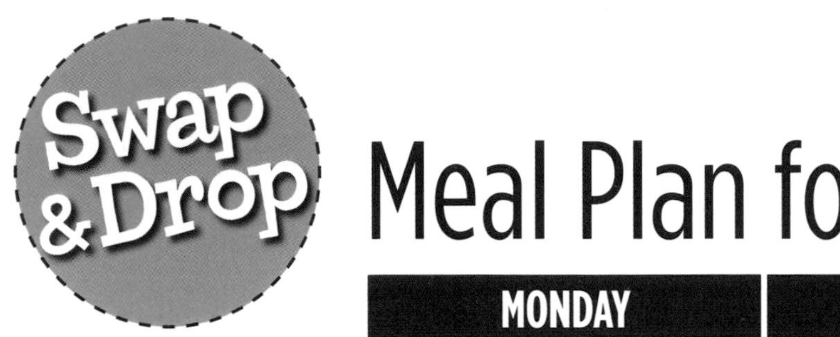

Meal Plan for WEEKS ▸ 2,5,8,11

	MONDAY	TUESDAY	WEDNESDAY
BREAKFAST	**A Smoothie Breakfast** • Tropical Smoothie *(page 105)* • Half of one toasted English muffin, with peanut butter	**A Perfect Bowl of Cereal** *(page 35)* • High-fibre cereal topped with raisins and chopped nuts • Skim or 1% milk	**Egg on a Roll Breakfast** • Scrambled egg on a whole wheat roll • Fresh fruit salad • Skim or 1% milk
LUNCH	**Tuna Salad Sandwich Lunch** • Tuna salad sandwich • Carrot and celery sticks • Banana	**Turkey Caesar Lunch** • Grilled Turkey Caesar Salad *(page 110)* • Whole-wheat flatbread crackers • Fresh fruit salad	**Baked Potato and Salad Lun** • Baked potato stuffed with broccoli and 1 tbsp cheese • Green salad • Seasonal berries
SNACK	Vegetable crudités	Chocolate Chip Oatmeal Cookie *(page 123)* with glass of skim or 1% milk	Frozen yogourt
DINNER	**Sautéed Chicken Dinner** • Sautéed Chicken with Caramelized Onions *(page 113)* • Spinach fettuccine • Green salad	**Pot Roast Dinner** • Pot Roast with Braised Vegetables *(page 114)* • Crusty sourdough bread	**Pasta Dinner** • Pasta Primavera *(page 116)* • Italian Salad *(page 120)*
DESSERT	Fruit Boats with Orange-Balsamic Glaze *(page 122)*	Apple	Fresh pineapple chunks

Review portion sizes on page 18. Here's an overview of what breakfast and lunch should include on **Swap & Drop**:

BREAKFAST

- One grain or starch: 1 cup (size of a baseball) of high-fibre cereal (check out your best cereal choices on page 35), a slice of toast or a small roll.
- One dairy or high-calcium food: 1 cup of skim or 1% milk, or 1 cup of low-fat yogourt.
- Fruit: one piece, or an equivalent amount of melon or berries.
- Variations: Pancakes, bagels and even a parfait are fine, but in small portions.

LUNCH

- One grain or starch: two slices of sandwich bread, a tennis-ball-sized potato or one serving of pasta or rice.
- One protein: thin, palm-sized slice of cheese, a small burger patty or three CD-sized pieces of lunch meat.
- Fruit: one piece, or an equivalent amount of melon or berries.
- Vegetables: as many and as much as you want.
- Variations: soups, salads, wraps and even chili, done in sensible portion sizes.

THURSDAY	FRIDAY	SATURDAY	SUNDAY
Fresh-Baked Breakfast • Blueberry Muffin with Lemon Glaze *(page 106)* • Cantaloupe wedge • Skim-milk latte	**Breakfast on the Run** • Cereal bar • Yogourt topped with blueberries	**Yogourt Parfait** *(page 104)* • Yogourt layered with granola, fruit and coconut	**Pancakes to Start** *(page 105)* • Silver Dollar Pancakes topped with maple syrup and sliced strawberries • Skim or 1% milk
Bean Salad Lunch • Black-Bean Salad *(page 109)* • Whole-wheat pita • Grapes	**Simple Sandwich Lunch** • Prosciutto, lettuce, tomato and provolone cheese sandwich on whole-wheat bread • Green salad • Slice of cantaloupe	**Pita Pizza and Salad** • Pita Pizza *(page 108)* • Green Salad • Apple	**Wrap Sandwich** • Roasted Vegetable Wraps *(page 109)* • Green salad • Honeydew melon
Peanut butter on a rice cake	Strawberry smoothie	Graham crackers with skim or 1% milk	Pretzel sticks and low-fat string cheese
DINING OUT: **Taco Bell** *(page 206)* • Two Fresco Chicken Soft Tacos	**Potpie Dinner** • One-Crust Chicken Potpie *(page 113)* • Green salad	**Dinner on the Grill** • Crudité platter • Grilled Beer-Can Chicken *(page 119)* • Grilled Summer Vegetables *(page 119)* • German Potato Salad with Dijon Vinaigrette *(page 121)* • Sesame breadsticks	**Barbecue Beef Picnic Dinner** • Barbecue Beef on a Bun *(page 118)* • Colourful Coleslaw *(page 120)*
Almond-flavoured milk	Brownie Bites *(page 123)*	Chocolate Snacking Cake *(page 125)*	Blueberry Bonanza *(page 125)*

Meal Plan for WEEKS ▸ 3,6,9,12

	MONDAY	TUESDAY	WEDNESDAY
BREAKFAST	**Quick Bread Delight** • One slice Peach Quick Bread *(page 106)* • Fresh raspberries • Skim or 1% milk	**Fresh-Baked Breakfast** • Blueberry Muffin with Lemon Glaze *(page 106)* • Cantaloupe wedge • Skim-milk latte	**Yogourt Parfait** *(page 104)* • Yogourt layered with granc fruit and coconut
LUNCH	**Soup and Sandwich** • Hearty Split-Pea Soup *(page 111)* • Tuna salad sandwich • Seasonal fruit	**Meatless Chili** • Meatless Chili Pot with Cheddar *(page 111)* • Corn tortilla • Green salad • Banana	**DINING OUT:** **McDonald's** *(page 200)* • Spicy Thai Salad with Grille Chicken and Asian Sesame dressing
SNACK	Crackers with peanut butter	Graham crackers and hot cocoa with skim milk	Edamame (steamed soybear
DINNER	**Salmon and Spanish Rice** • Salmon and Peas in a Packet *(page 117)* • Spanish Rice *(page 116)*	**DINING OUT:** **East Side Mario's** *(page 192)* • Side serving of pasta with Napolitana sauce • Side of vegetable soup	**Italian-Style Stir-Fry** • Chicken and Broccoli Stir-F Italian Style *(page 112)* • Orzo
DESSERT	Brownie Bites *(page 123)*	Two butter cookies	Frozen yogourt

Review portion sizes on page 18. Here's an overview of what snacks and dinner should include on **Swap & Drop**:

SNACKS

- Salty: a handful of chips, microwave popcorn, crackers or nuts.
- Sweet: a small palmful of M&Ms, jelly beans, chocolate almonds, raisins, hard candy or a mini candy bar.
- Baked: two small cookies, one mini cupcake or a 5 cm-square brownie.
- Frozen: two golf-ball-sized servings of frozen yogourt or sorbet. Half-a-tennis-ball-worth of regular ice cream or a Fudgsicle.

DINNER

- One protein: a tennis-ball-sized serving of shrimp, scallops or crab; one portion of chicken breast, beef, salmon or tofu; a serving of light-flesh fish the size of a chequebook; or two golf-ball-sized servings of legumes, such as chickpeas or beans.
- One grain or starch: a tennis-ball serving of pasta, rice, noodles or bread.
- Vegetables: as many and as much as you want.
- Variations: pot roasts, barbecue dinners, stir-fries.

THURSDAY	FRIDAY	SATURDAY	SUNDAY
Breakfast on the Run • Cereal bar • Yogourt topped with blueberries	**Bagel Delight** • Mini-whole-wheat bagel topped with jam and low-fat cream cheese • Yogourt with sliced ripe peach	**Hearty Frittata** • One slice Vegetable Frittata *(page 107)* • 1 slice whole-wheat toast • Fresh blueberries	**Pancakes to Start** *(page 105)* • Silver Dollar Pancakes topped with maple syrup and sliced strawberries • Skim or 1% milk
Pita Pizza and Salad • Pita Pizza *(page 108)* • Green salad • Apple	**Simple Sandwich Lunch** • Grilled chicken, lettuce, tomato and Swiss cheese sandwich on whole-wheat bread • Green salad • Slice of cantaloupe	**The Perfect Soup-and-Salad Lunch** • Vegetable soup with breadsticks • Green salad topped with grilled chicken • Green or red grapes	**BRUNCH** • Red-Pepper Crab Cakes *(page 110)* • Green salad • Crusty roll • Seasonal berries • Two Pecan Icebox Cookies *(page 124)*
Mixed dried fruit	Cranberry Trail Mix *(page 124)*	Small container of fat-free yogourt	Mixed nuts
Quick Black Beans and Rice with Chicken • Marinated grilled chicken breast *(page 119)* • Quick Black Beans and Rice *(page 117)* • Green salad	**Noodles and Greens** • Thai Noodle Salad with greens *(page 121)*	**Casserole Dinner** • Homestyle Tuna Casserole *(page 117)* • Arugula, cucumber and cherry tomato salad	**DINING OUT:** **The Keg** *(page 196)* • 8 oz. Sirloin Classic • Mixed Green Salad
Sorbet *(page 122)*	Fresh fruit	Air-popped popcorn	Fresh fruit salad

Meal Planner Recipes breakfasts

Yes, you've heard it before: Breakfast is the most important meal of the day. This is one time when you should believe the hype! Not only will a substantial, nutritious breakfast put you in a great mood, it will also help prevent you from overeating later on. For more tips on eating a healthy breakfast, see page 30.

YOGOURT PARFAIT

SERVES 1

3/4 cup fat-free plain yogourt
1/4 cup berries
1/4 cup sliced mango
1/4 cup low-fat granola
1 tbsp shredded coconut

1 In tall parfait glass, layer ingredients: Add 1/3 of yogourt, half of fruit, all of granola, another 1/3 of yogourt, remaining fruit and remaining yogourt.

2 Top with shredded coconut.

PER SERVING: 273 calories, 13 g protein, 6 g fat (5 g saturated fat), 43 g carbohydrates, 3 g fibre, 4 mg cholesterol, 199 mg sodium.

VEGETABLE-CHEDDAR OMELETTE

SERVES 1

2 medium eggs
1 tsp water
2 tsp chopped fresh herbs (such as dill, basil and parsley)
1/2 cup loosely packed, thinly sliced fresh spinach
1 plum tomato, chopped
2 tbsp shredded light cheddar cheese

1 In medium bowl, whisk eggs, water and herbs. (If desired, add pinch of salt and pepper.) In small bowl, toss together spinach, tomato and cheese; set aside.

2 Lightly coat non-stick omelette pan or small skillet with cooking spray and set over medium heat for 1 minute. Pour in egg mixture and cook until it begins to set on bottom. Lift edge with spatula, pushing cooked part toward centre of pan and letting uncooked portion run underneath. Cook until top is almost set and bottom is lightly browned.

3 Spread spinach mixture over half of omelette, leaving 1 cm border around edge and reserving 1 tbsp of filling. Lift omelette at edge and fold in half. Cook for 2 minutes. Slide onto plate and garnish with reserved filling.

PER SERVING: 166 calories, 16 g protein, 10 g fat (3 g saturated fat), 4 g carbohydrates, 1 g fibre, 375 mg cholesterol, 225 mg sodium.

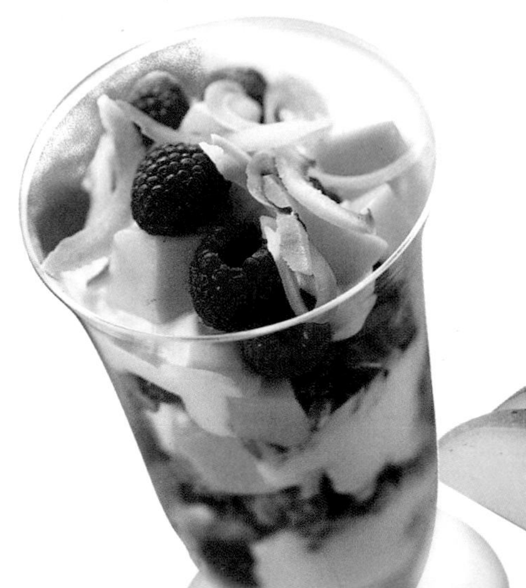

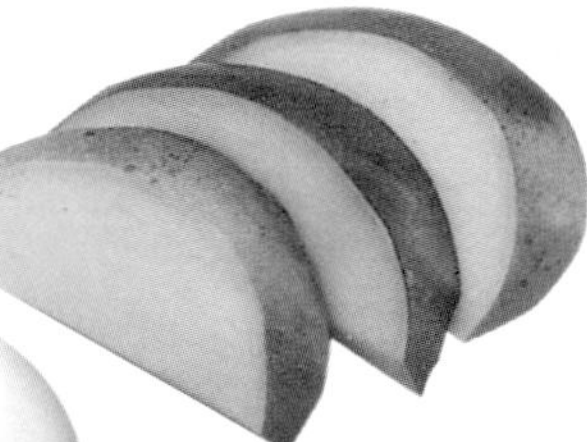

TROPICAL SMOOTHIE

SERVES 4

1 mango, cut into cubes
1 banana, cut into large chunks
1 cup pineapple chunks
1 kiwi, peeled and sliced
2 cups fat-free plain yogourt
1 cup ice cubes

1 Purée all ingredients in blender until completely smooth.

2 Freeze leftovers in sealable plastic containers. To defrost, microwave for 30 to 60 seconds and stir.

PER SERVING: 161 calories, 8 g protein, 1 g fat (0 g saturated fat), 33 g carbohydrates, 3 g fibre, 2 mg cholesterol, 97 mg sodium.

REPLACE WHITE FLOUR WITH WHOLE-WHEAT

Swap up to half of the white flour in recipes for whole-wheat flour to boost fibre.

SILVER DOLLAR PANCAKES

SERVES 4

½ cup self-rising flour
½ tbsp sugar
¼ tsp baking soda
¾ cup buttermilk
1 tbsp canola oil
1 large egg
½ tsp vanilla extract

1 In medium bowl, whisk flour, sugar and baking soda. In a small bowl, whisk buttermilk, oil, egg and vanilla until blended. Make a well in flour mixture, pour in buttermilk mixture, and whisk just until moistened. Let stand for 5 minutes.

2 Meanwhile, coat large non-stick skillet with cooking spray and set over medium heat until hot but not smoking.

3 For each pancake, pour 1 tbsp of batter into the skillet. Cook until bubbles appear all over surface and begin to burst, or about 3 minutes. Turn and cook until undersides are golden, or about 1 to 2 minutes.

PER SERVING: 144 calories, 5 g protein, 6 g fat (1 g saturated fat), 17 g carbohydrates, 0 g fibre, 57 mg cholesterol, 322 mg sodium.

COTTAGE CHEESE MELBA

SERVES 1

½ cup low-fat cottage cheese
½ cup sliced fruit of your choice
1 tsp fruit jam of your choice

1 Mix and eat on slice of raisin-bread toast with a nice cup of tea. We particularly like peach slices and raspberry jam together.

PER SERVING: 151 calories, 14 g protein, 1 g fat (1 g saturated fat), 20 g carbohydrates, 1 g fibre, 5 mg cholesterol, 474 mg sodium.

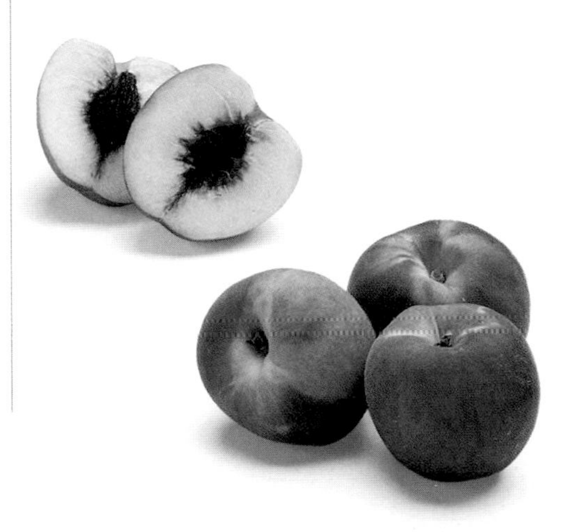

SHOPPING

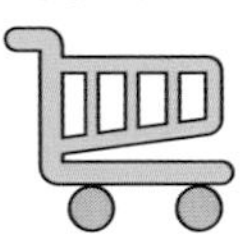

Cottage cheese is "fresh" cheese, meaning that its curds have not been aged or ripened. Its moist, loose texture and mild flavour make it ideal for all sorts of accompaniments, including fruits and jams, cereals, nuts, spices and vegetables. It comes with different amounts of fat, ranging from none to 4%. We recommend cheese that is somewhere in between: low-fat. It tastes richer than fat-free and has fewer calories than regular 4% cottage cheese.

Ricotta cheese, a fresh cousin made from whey (the liquid drained off from the semisolid curds that make up cottage cheese), is smoother and creamier than cottage cheese but higher in fat. Farmer and pot cheeses are also similar, but drier.

VARIATIONS

Instead of using blueberries in these muffins, try substituting:

- sliced strawberries
- 1 cup banana slices with ½ cup walnuts (no glaze)
- 1 cup chopped apple with ½ cup pecans (no glaze)
- 1 cup pumpkin and 1 tsp pumpkin-pie spice (no glaze).

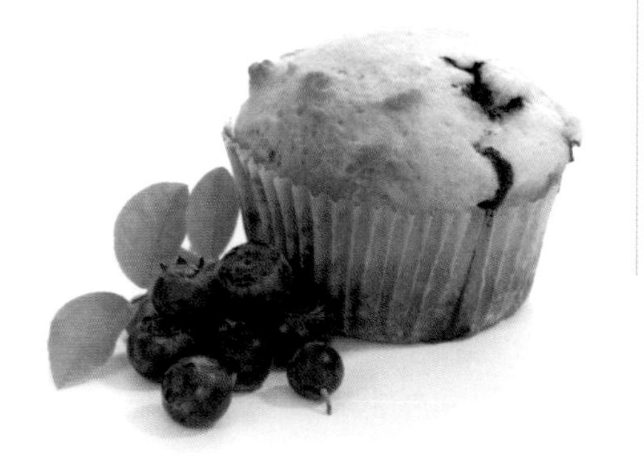

BLUEBERRY MUFFINS WITH LEMON GLAZE

MAKES 12

2 cups all-purpose flour
1 tbsp baking powder
½ tsp salt
½ cup granulated sugar
2 eggs
4 tbsp butter or margarine, melted
⅓ cup light sour cream
2 tsp vanilla extract
1 cup plus 1 tbsp skim or 1% milk
1 ½ cups fresh or frozen blueberries
½ cup sifted icing sugar
2 tsp lemon zest

1 Preheat oven to 400°F (200°C). Put paper liners in 12-cup muffin pan.

2 In large bowl, mix flour, baking powder, salt and granulated sugar. In medium bowl, combine eggs, butter, sour cream, vanilla and 1 cup of milk.

3 Make a well in centre of flour mixture. Pour in egg mixture and stir with fork until just blended; don't overmix. Fold in 1 cup of blueberries.

4 Spoon batter into muffin cups and sprinkle evenly with remaining blueberries. Bake until toothpick inserted in centre of muffin comes out clean, or about 20 minutes. Cool on wire rack for 10 minutes.

5 In small bowl, make glaze by combining icing sugar, lemon zest and milk. Only add enough milk to make glaze liquid enough to drizzle over cooled muffins.

PER SERVING: 163 calories, 4 g protein, 6 g fat (2 g saturated fat), 23 g carbohydrates, 1 g fibre, 39 mg cholesterol, 220 mg sodium.

PEACH QUICK BREAD

SERVES 16

2 medium peaches
1 ½ cups all-purpose flour
¾ cup whole-wheat flour
¼ cup toasted wheat germ
¾ cup sugar
1 tsp baking soda
½ tsp salt
½ cup fat-free plain yogourt
1 egg
2 egg whites
2 tbsp canola oil
1 tsp almond extract

1 Preheat oven to 350°F (180°C). Coat 22-by-12 cm loaf pan with cooking spray.

2 In medium saucepan, blanch peaches in boiling water for 20 seconds. Peel, pit and finely chop peaches—you should have about 1 cup.

3 In large bowl, combine all-purpose flour, whole-wheat flour, wheat germ, sugar, baking soda and salt. In small bowl, combine yogourt, egg, egg whites, oil and almond extract. Make a well in flour mixture, pour in yogourt mixture and stir just until combined—do not overmix. Fold in peaches.

4 Spoon batter into pan and smooth top. Bake until toothpick inserted in centre comes out clean, or about 1 hour. Cool in pan on wire rack for 10 minutes, then turn out onto rack to cool completely. Cut into 16 equal slices.

PER SERVING: 136 calories, 4 g protein, 2 g fat (0 g saturated fat), 26 g carbohydrates, 1 g fibre, 13 mg cholesterol, 250 mg sodium.

VEGETABLE FRITTATA

SERVES 4

125 g white mushrooms, washed, trimmed and thinly sliced
⅓ cup sliced red onion
5 eggs
4 egg whites
1 tsp chopped fresh herbs (thyme, oregano or basil)
4 small plum tomatoes, thinly sliced
8 tbsp shredded part-skim mozzarella cheese

1 Preheat broiler. Coat 25 cm non-stick ovenproof skillet with cooking spray and set over medium-high heat. Add mushrooms and onion and sauté until tender, about 5 minutes. Transfer to plate. Wipe out skillet, coat with cooking spray and return to heat.

2 In medium bowl, whisk eggs, egg whites and herbs. Season with salt and pepper. Pour into skillet and cook until eggs begin to set, or about 2 minutes. Don't stir, but lift edge of egg mixture with heatproof spatula and tilt skillet to let uncooked portion flow underneath.

3 Arrange tomatoes and sautéed vegetables in concentric circles on top. Cook until frittata is golden on the bottom and almost set on top, or 2 to 3 minutes.

4 Sprinkle cheese around the edges of frittata. Transfer skillet to oven and broil until cheese melts and begins to brown, or about 2 minutes. Cut into quarters.

PER SERVING: 154 calories, 16 g protein, 8 g fat (3 g saturated fat), 6 g carbohydrates, 1 g fibre, 242 mg cholesterol, 224 mg sodium.

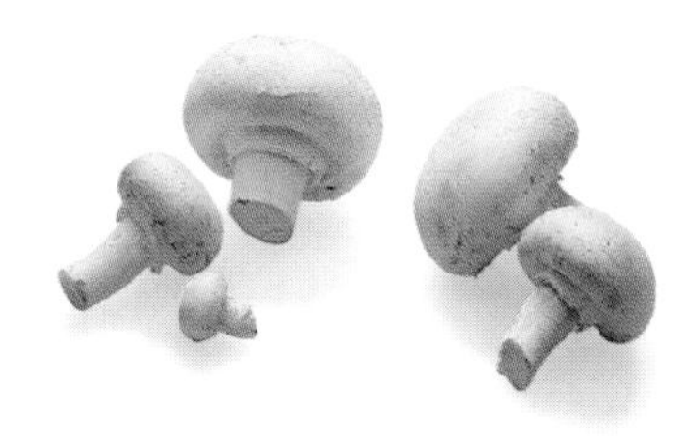

CRANBERRY SCONES WITH ORANGE GLAZE

MAKES 18

3 cups all-purpose flour
1 ½ tsp baking powder
½ tsp salt
¼ cup sugar
1 ¼ cups fat-free plain yogourt
3 tbsp butter, melted
3 tbsp margarine, melted
1 egg, lightly beaten
1 cup sweetened dried cranberries
½ cup sifted icing sugar
1 tsp orange zest
1 tbsp fresh orange juice

1 Preheat oven to 400°F (200°C). Line 2 baking sheets with parchment paper.

2 In large bowl, combine flour, baking powder, salt and sugar. In small bowl, mix the yogourt, butter, margarine and egg.

3 Make a well in centre of flour mixture, pour in yogourt mixture and blend with fork until moistened. Stir in cranberries. Flour hands and gently knead dough in bowl just until it comes together.

4 Turn dough out onto floured work surface and pat into 22 cm square about 5 cm thick. With small knife, cut into 9 squares, then cut each square into 2 triangles. Place triangles 2.5 cm apart on baking sheets and bake until golden, or about 15 minutes.

5 In small bowl, combine icing sugar, orange rind and orange juice. When scones are cool, transfer in batches to wire rack set on piece of wax paper, parchment or foil, and drizzle glaze over with small spoon.

PER SERVING: 155 calories, 4 g protein, 3 g fat (0 g saturated fat), 30 g carbohydrates, 1 g fibre, 12 mg cholesterol, 83 mg sodium.

Smooth operator

At breakfast restaurants, order the smallest smoothie available—350 mL is ideal. Any more than that just adds unnecessary calories. (Besides, smoothies can be unexpectedly filling!) And be sure to request that it be made with fat-free yogourt, skim or 1% milk or low-fat soy milk.

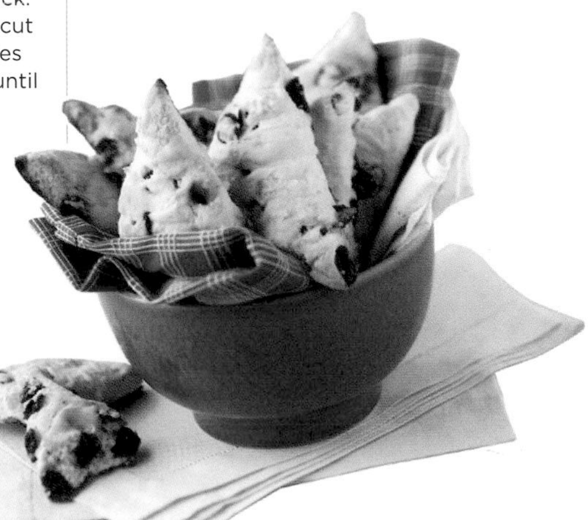

Meal Planner Recipes lunches

Lunch provides a welcome break in the middle of the day, but many of us are too stressed out or overworked to grab much more than a hamburger from the closest fast-food joint. It's time to revolutionize your lunch! Try these healthy alternatives, and you'll never want to go back to your dine-and-dash ways. For more lunch tips, see page 36.

PITA PIZZA

SERVES 1

2 tbsp tomato sauce
¼ cup grated light mozzarella cheese
Grilled or raw vegetables (such as broccoli florets, mushrooms, onions, zucchini or bell peppers)
Small whole-wheat pita

1 Preheat oven to 350°F (180°C). Spread tomato sauce on pita, and top with grated cheese and vegetables.

2 Bake in oven until cheese bubbles, or about 5 minutes.

PER SERVING: 279 calories, 20 g protein, 10 g fat (6 g saturated fat), 30 g carbohydrates, 5 g fibre, 36 mg cholesterol, 669 mg sodium.

IDEAS FOR PIZZA TOPPINGS

Stuck for inspiration about what to put on your pita pizza? Try one of these tips:

- If you have a barbecue one night, throw a few extra red peppers and zucchinis on the grill, then store them in the fridge. They make an ideal topping for a pita pizza or a delectable sandwich filling.
- When the pita pizza is about 1 minute away from being done, take it out and cover in baby spinach. You just want it to get a little cooked, but still retain its freshness.
- Go crazy with the chopped herbs! Rosemary makes a great companion for thinly sliced potato and mushrooms, while basil and tomato are a classic combo.
- Keep a can of artichoke hearts handy, and throw them on a pita alongside some crumbled feta.
- Experiment with stronger cheese. Blue cheese, feta, romano, smoked gouda or aged cheddar are delicious when grated or crumbled on a pizza. Plus, when the cheese is more flavourful, you need less of it.

MEAT LOVER?
If you want to use a little meat on your pizza—such as leftover grilled chicken or prosciutto—cut the quantity of cheese in half.

ROASTED VEGETABLE WRAPS

SERVES 4

1 tbsp olive oil
1 tbsp rice wine vinegar
1 tsp chopped fresh rosemary
1 clove garlic, minced
2 medium zucchini (total 500 g)
2 large red bell peppers
1 large red onion
4 x 17.5 cm-wide flour tortillas
3/4 cup low-fat plain yogourt
1 tbsp snipped fresh chives

1 Preheat oven to 450°F (230°C). Lightly coat jelly-roll pan or shallow-sided baking pan with cooking spray.

2 In small bowl, whisk the oil, vinegar, rosemary and garlic. (If desired, add a pinch of salt.)

3 Cut zucchinis crosswise in half, then lengthwise into 5 mm slices. Cut each red pepper into 8 strips. Cut onion into 16 wedges.

4 Pour oil mixture into pan and add vegetables. Bake, tossing frequently, until browned and tender, or about 30 minutes. Sprinkle tortillas with water, wrap in foil and place in oven during the last 5 minutes of cooking.

5 In small bowl, combine yogourt and chives. Spread evenly on each tortilla and top with vegetables. Fold in sides of tortillas and roll up.

PER SERVING: 285 calories, 12 g protein, 8 g fat (2 g saturated fat), 43 g carbohydrates, 5 g fibre, 3 mg cholesterol, 377 mg sodium.

BLACK-BEAN SALAD

SERVES 6

1/2 cup chopped red bell pepper
1/2 cup chopped green bell pepper
1/2 cup chopped cucumber
1/2 cup chopped red onion
1 1/2 cups chopped tomatoes
1 cup fresh, canned, or frozen corn kernels
1 cup rinsed and drained canned black beans
2 tbsp red wine vinegar
1 tbsp olive oil
1 tbsp lime juice
2 tbsp minced cilantro
1 jalapeño, minced (optional)

1 In large bowl, combine the red pepper, green pepper, cucumber, onion, tomatoes, corn, beans, vinegar, oil, lime juice, cilantro and jalapeño, if using.

PER SERVING: 102 calories, 4 g protein, 3 g fat (0 g saturated fat), 17 g carbohydrates, 4 g fibre, 0 mg cholesterol, 93 mg sodium.

VARIATIONS

In the Black-Bean Salad, feel free to substitute ingredients to taste, particularly among the vegetables. Instead of black beans, consider using baby shrimp, diced ham, smoked turkey breast or chickpeas. Add grilled corn when it's in season, or substitute cherry tomatoes for regular for a sweeter taste.

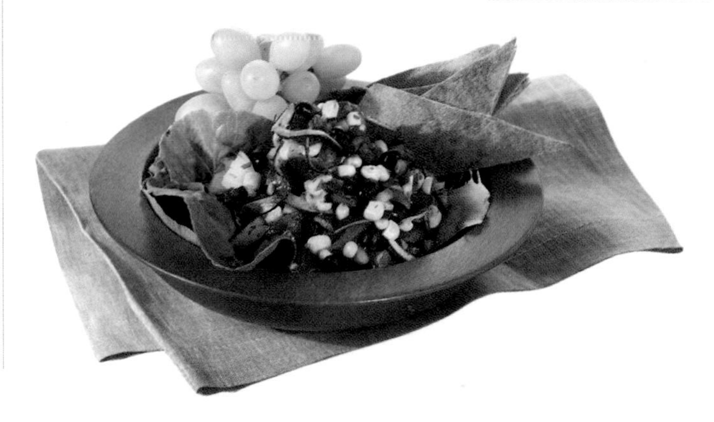

ET TU, SALAD?

● ● ● Tons of cheese, overly oily dressing, greasy croutons, insanely salty anchovies and Worcestershire sauce can make certain Caesar salads bad choices for weight loss. But if you play it light and easy with the heavier ingredients—as in our Grilled Turkey Caesar, at right—this salad is a delight.

● ● ● If you're ordering Caesar salad at a restaurant, ask that the chef halve the amount of grated cheese and dressing, and you'll probably stay right in line with your calorie plan.

● ● ● When preparing the Grilled Turkey Caesar Salad at home, consider subtituting tofu cubes, tuna, salmon or shrimp for the grilled turkey.

GRILLED TURKEY CAESAR SALAD

SERVES 4

2 cloves garlic, peeled
3 tbsp fresh lemon juice
2 tbsp fat-free plain yogourt
1 tbsp olive oil
350 g boneless, skinless turkey breast
8 cups romaine lettuce, torn into bite-size pieces
½ cup garlic croutons
30 g grated parmesan cheese

1 Preheat grill. In a small food processor, using a garlic press or with the side of a large knife, mash garlic until paste-like. Place garlic paste, lemon juice, yogourt and oil in a jar with a tight-fitting lid and shake until blended.

2 Sprinkle turkey with some salt and pepper, and lightly coat with cooking spray. Grill until cooked through, 4 to 5 minutes per side. Cut across grain into 1.25 cm-thick slices.

3 In large bowl, toss together lettuce, croutons and turkey until well-mixed. Shake dressing, drizzle onto salad and toss lightly.

4 Divide salad equally among 4 plates. With vegetable peeler, shave strips of cheese evenly over each portion.

PER SERVING: 224 calories, 31 g protein, 7 g fat (2 g saturated fat), 9 g carbohydrates, 2 g fibre, 76 mg cholesterol, 243 mg sodium.

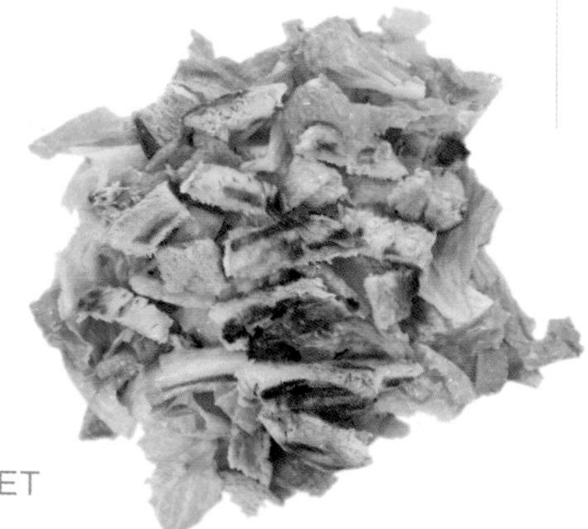

RED-PEPPER CRAB CAKES

SERVES 4

½ cup fresh breadcrumbs
1 celery stalk with leaves, finely chopped
⅓ cup finely chopped red bell pepper
2 tbsp minced shallot
1 tbsp finely chopped parsley
2 tbsp coarse-grained mustard
2 tbsp light mayonnaise
1 egg
1 tsp paprika
500 g lump crabmeat
⅓ cup all-purpose flour
2 tsp canola oil

1 In large bowl, combine bread crumbs, celery, pepper, shallot, parsley, mustard, mayonnaise, egg and paprika. Gently fold in crabmeat.

2 Preheat oven to 350°F (180°C). Spread flour on piece of wax paper. Divide crab mixture into 8 equal portions, then form into patties with floured hands. Dredge in flour.

3 Lightly coat large non-stick, ovenproof skillet with cooking spray and set over medium-high heat until hot but not smoking. Cook 4 crab cakes until browned, about 2 minutes per side. Drizzle 1 tsp of oil around crab cakes, turn crab cakes and gently shake pan to spread oil. Transfer to plate lined with paper towels. Repeat with remaining crab cakes and oil.

4 Lightly coat baking sheet with cooking spray, transfer crab cakes to baking sheet and bake until very hot in centre, or about 8 to 10 minutes.

PER SERVING: 252 calories, 29 g protein, 8 g fat (2 g saturated fat), 15 g carbohydrates, 1 g fibre, 132 mg cholesterol, 615 mg sodium.

HEARTY SPLIT-PEA SOUP

SERVES 6

1 tsp olive oil
1 cube of low-sodium stock
1 large onion, finely chopped
3 cloves garlic, minced
2 carrots, halved lengthwise and thinly sliced crosswise
3/4 cup split peas
2 tbsp tomato paste (no salt added)
250 g smoked turkey breast, chopped
1/2 tsp rubbed or ground sage
4 1/2 cups water
1/3 cup whole-wheat macaroni
1/4 cup grated parmesan cheese

1 Heat oil in a non-stick Dutch oven over medium heat. Add onion and garlic and cook, stirring frequently, until onion is golden, about 7 minutes. Add carrots and cook, stirring frequently, until crisp-tender, or about 5 minutes.

2 Stir in split peas, tomato paste, turkey, sage, stock cube and water and bring to boil. If desired, season with some salt and pepper. Reduce to simmer, cover and cook for 30 minutes.

3 Add pasta and cook until pasta and split peas are tender, or about 15 minutes. Divide equally among 6 soup bowls. (Unused portions will keep for 3 or 4 days in refrigerator and 2 to 3 months in freezer.) Sprinkle with parmesan and serve.

PER SERVING: 189 calories, 17 g protein, 3 g fat (1 g saturated fat), 25 g carbohydrates, 8 g fibre, 22 mg cholesterol, 531 mg sodium.

MEATLESS CHILI POTS WITH CHEDDAR

SERVES 4

1 medium green bell pepper, finely chopped
1 medium onion, finely chopped
2 large cloves garlic, minced
2 cans (450 mL each) low-sodium red kidney beans, rinsed and drained
1 can (796 mL) no-salt-added crushed tomatoes in purée
1/2 tsp chili powder
1/2 tsp fresh-ground black pepper
1/2 tsp ground cumin
1/4 tsp ground cinnamon
1/2 cup shredded light cheddar cheese
1/4 cup plain low-fat yogourt
1/2 cup chopped avocado

1 Lightly coat large non-stick skillet with cooking spray and set over medium-high heat. Add green pepper, onion and garlic, and sauté until onion is browned, or about 5 minutes.

2 Stir in beans, tomatoes and purée, chili powder, black pepper, cumin and cinnamon. Simmer for 5 minutes.

3 Ladle into four bowls and sprinkle each portion with 2 tbsp of cheese. Garnish with yogourt and avocado.

PER SERVING: 417 calories, 26 g protein, 5 g fat (1 g saturated fat), 72 g carbohydrates, 21 g fibre, 3 mg cholesterol, 167 mg sodium.

GET THE TEXTURE, WITHOUT THE MEAT

Do you crave the texture of ground beef in your chili? No need to visit the butcher. For a low-calorie option, pick up a package of textured vegetable protein, sometimes labelled as something like "vegetarian ground beef." Usually made of soy or other vegetables, it has the texture of meat without as much fat as the real thing. We suggest Yves Meatless Ground Round, available at supermarkets across Canada.

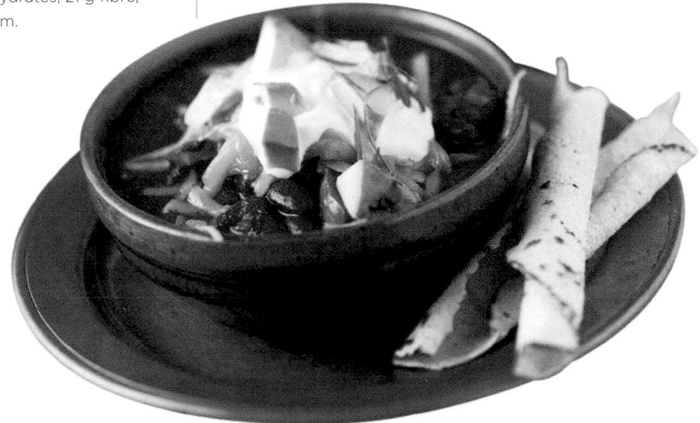

Meal Planner Recipes dinners

Dinnertime signals the end of the work day, and it should be as relaxing as possible. But that doesn't mean you should go overboard on calories. Luckily, the **Swap & Drop** meal plan includes plenty of tasty, low-calorie meals–some of which might even be lighter versions of your favourite comfort food. For even more healthy dinner tips, see page 48.

CHICKEN AND BROCCOLI STIR-FRY, ITALIAN STYLE

SERVES 4

1 tbsp peanut or canola oil
3 scallions, thinly sliced
375 g boneless, skinless chicken breasts, cut across the grain into 1 cm wide pieces
4 cups broccoli florets
1 cup chopped red bell pepper
½ cup low-sodium chicken broth
½ tsp grated lemon zest
½ cup water
1 tsp cornstarch dissolved in 1 tbsp water
1 tbsp olive oil
½ cup slivered fresh basil or ½ tsp dried
1 ⅓ cups orzo pasta

1 Heat 2 tsp of oil in a large non-stick wok or skillet over medium heat. Add scallions and sauté until wilted, about 1 minute. Add chicken and sauté until no longer pink, or about 3 minutes. Add remaining peanut oil and broccoli and sauté for 2 minutes.

2 Add pepper, broth, lemon zest and water. (You can also add salt to taste, if desired.) Bring to boil, then reduce heat and simmer until chicken and broccoli are just cooked through, about 2 minutes.

3 Stir in dissolved cornstarch, olive oil and basil. Cook, stirring, until sauce is slightly thickened, or about 1 minute.

4 Cook orzo according to package directions and drain. Divide equally among 4 plates. Divide stir-fry into 4 equal portions and serve over orzo.

PER SERVING: 420 calories, 35 g protein, 7 g fat (1 g saturated fat), 56 g carbohydrates, 3 g fibre, 54 mg cholesterol, 119 mg sodium.

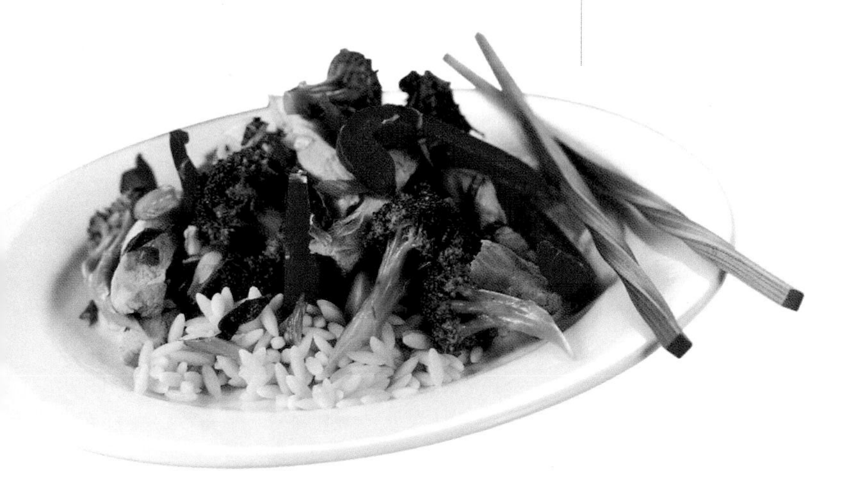

VARIATION

For an equivalent number of calories, you can substitute one of the following in this stir-fry: 275 g salmon fillet; 300 g pork tenderloin; 275 g firm tofu; 250 g beef tenderloin; 250 g boneless leg of lamb; or ½ cup cashews.

SAUTÉED CHICKEN WITH CARAMELIZED ONIONS

SERVES 4

750 g medium onions
4 boneless, skinless chicken breast halves, 125–150 g each
½ tsp salt
½ tsp fresh-ground black pepper
1 tbsp olive oil
2 tbsp sugar
⅓ cup low-sodium chicken broth
1 tsp chopped fresh rosemary
1 tsp chopped fresh thyme
1 tbsp red wine vinegar

1 Cut onions into 6 wedges each. Sprinkle chicken with ¼ tsp of salt and ¼ tsp of pepper.

2 Coat large non-stick skillet with cooking spray. Add 2 tsp of oil and heat over medium-high heat for about 30 seconds. Add chicken and sauté until browned, about 3 minutes on each side. Transfer to plate.

3 Reduce heat to medium and add remaining oil. Sauté onions, 1 tbsp of sugar, and remaining salt and pepper until onions turn golden and caramelize, about 8 minutes. Stir frequently, breaking onions apart. Add broth and boil until evaporated, about 2 minutes.

4 Stir in rosemary, thyme and remaining sugar. Return chicken to skillet and sprinkle with vinegar. Cook until chicken juices run clear, about 4 minutes. Place one chicken breast on each of four plates and top with about ½ cup onions.

PER SERVING: 271 calories, 31 g protein, 5 g fat (18 g saturated fat), 24 g carbohydrates, 3 g fibre, 72 mg cholesterol, 386 mg sodium.

ONE-CRUST CHICKEN POTPIE

SERVES 6

500 g boneless, skinless chicken breasts
¼ tsp salt
1 package (450 g) premade pie crust
1 egg white, lightly beaten with 1 tsp water
2 medium carrots, peeled and thinly sliced
1 cup frozen corn
1 cup frozen green peas
1 cup frozen small white onions
½ cup fat-free evaporated milk
3 tbsp all-purpose flour
½ tbsp butter
¼ tsp fresh-ground black pepper

1 In large saucepan, bring chicken and enough water to cover to simmer over medium-high heat. (You can also add salt if desired.) Reduce heat to low and gently poach chicken until juices run clear, about 15 minutes. Transfer to cutting board, let cool and cut into bite-size pieces. Reserve 1 cup of poaching liquid.

2 Preheat oven to 425°F (220°C). Lightly coat baking sheet and six 1-cup baking dishes with cooking spray.

3 Dust work surface lightly with flour. Unfold pie crust and cut in half. Wrap remaining half in foil or plastic wrap and store in refrigerator for future use. Roll out crust 2.5 mm thick, then cut out 6 squares to fit on top of baking dishes. Brush tops with diluted egg white. Transfer squares to baking sheet and bake until crisp and golden, or about 12 minutes. Transfer to wire rack to cool.

4 Meanwhile, cook carrots in boiling water until tender, or about 5 minutes, and drain. In colander, rinse corn, peas and onions in hot water. In small bowl, whisk milk and flour until smooth.

5 Melt butter in medium saucepan over medium heat. Whisk in milk mixture, then reserved poaching liquid. Cook until sauce thickens and boils, about 5 minutes. Stir in chicken, carrots, corn, peas, onions and pepper. Season to taste with salt if desired. Cook until heated through, or about 3 minutes. Divide among 6 baking dishes and bake until filling bubbles, or about 15 minutes. Top each with pastry square.

PER SERVING: 373 calories, 26 g protein, 12 g fat (5 g saturated fat), 40 g carbohydrates, 4 g fibre, 52 mg cholesterol, 286 mg sodium.

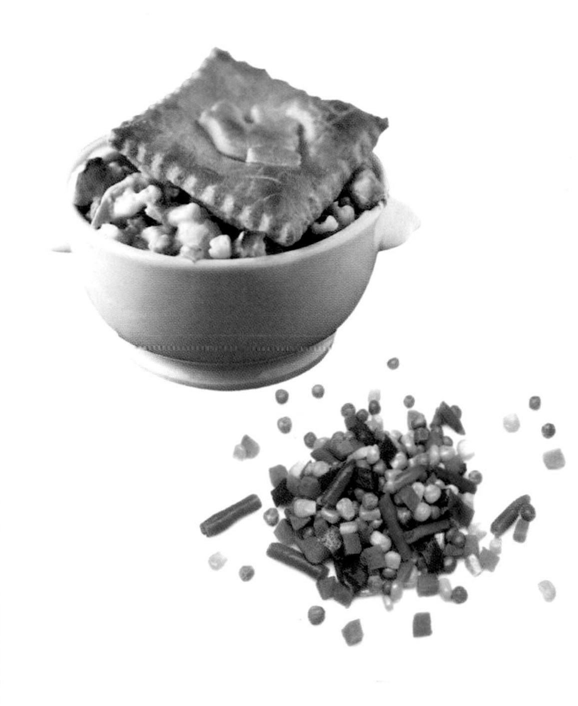

POT ROAST WITH BRAISED VEGETABLES

SERVES 12

1 boneless beef chuck roast (about 1.5 kg), trimmed of visible fat

1 ½ tsp salt

1 ½ tsp fresh-ground black pepper

8 large carrots, peeled and cut into 5 cm chunks

2 medium onions, coarsely chopped

4 cloves garlic, crushed

1 can (796 mL) whole tomatoes in purée

1 cup chopped fresh basil

2 cups dry red wine or low-sodium beef stock

1 kg small red or Yukon Gold potatoes, scrubbed

2 tsp cornstarch dissolved in 2 tbsp water

1 Preheat oven to 325°F (160°C). Tie roast and rub with 1 tsp of salt and 1 tsp of pepper. In Dutch oven, sear meat over medium-high heat until browned on all sides, about 8 minutes. Transfer to plate.

2 Add carrots, onions and garlic to pot and sauté in meat drippings until onions are browned, about 8 minutes. Stir in tomatoes and purée, ½ cup of basil and remaining salt and pepper. Cook for 5 minutes, breaking up tomatoes with a spoon.

3 Return meat to pot. Add wine and enough water to come 5 cm up side of pot. Bring to boil. Cover with foil and a lid to create tight seal. Roast for 1 hour, turning once.

4 Add potatoes and remaining basil to pot, adding more water if needed to come 5 cm up the side. Roast until meat and vegetables are tender, or about 1 hour.

5 Cut meat into small chunks and arrange on platter with vegetables. Strain braising liquid into saucepan and bring to simmer. Whisk in dissolved cornstarch, bring to boil and cook until gravy thickens, about 1 minute. Ladle over meat and vegetables.

PER SERVING: 441 calories, 34 g protein, 18 g fat (7 g saturated fat), 28 g carbohydrates, 5 g fibre, 90 mg cholesterol, 400 mg sodium.

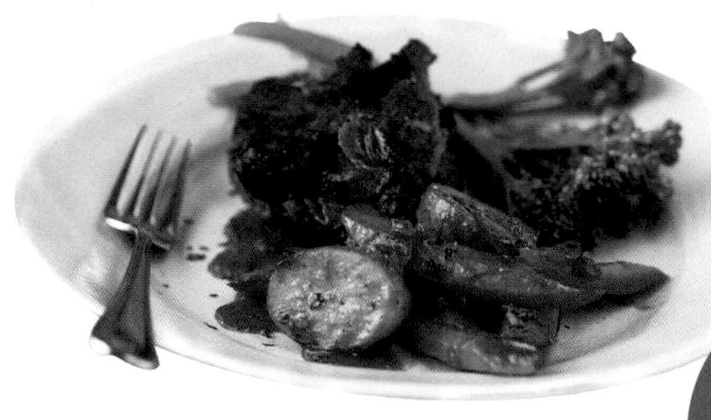

NOTE:
Cover and refrigerate leftover Pot Roast for 1 to 2 days, or divide into individual portions and freeze for up to 1 month.

ZESTY MEAT LOAF

SERVES 8

2 large onions, chopped

2 large celery stalks, chopped

1 large green bell pepper, chopped

3 cloves garlic, minced

1 kg ground lean turkey

1 cup fresh whole-wheat bread crumbs (about 2 slices)

1 egg

½ tsp fresh-ground black pepper

2 cups chopped canned tomatoes in purée

¼ cup ketchup

1 bag (375 g) egg noodles

¼ cup parsley, chopped

1 Preheat oven to 350°F (180°C). Lightly coat 22-by-33 cm baking dish and large nonstick skillet with cooking spray.

2 Add onions, celery, bell pepper and garlic to skillet and sauté over medium-high heat until soft, about 5 minutes. Transfer to large bowl. Add beef, bread crumbs, egg and black pepper; mix with clean hands.

3 In small bowl, combine tomatoes and ketchup. Add half to meat mixture and mix.

4 Transfer meat mixture to baking dish and shape into loaf about 25 by 18 cm, mounding slightly in centre. Make lengthwise groove down centre and pour remaining tomato mixture into groove. Bake until thermometer inserted in centre registers 165°F (75°C), or about 1 hour 15 minutes. Let stand for 10 minutes before slicing into 8 equal portions. Cover and refrigerate any extra for tomorrow's dinner, or wrap in foil and freeze for up to 1 month.

5 Cook noodles according to package directions. Drain, reserving ⅓ cup of cooking water. Place noodles in a bowl, add water and parsley, and toss to mix. Divide equally among four plates and top with meat loaf.

PER SERVING: 429 calories, 30 g protein, 13 g fat (3 g saturated fat), 49 g carbohydrates, 5 g fibre, 152 mg cholesterol, 274 mg sodium.

BEEF STEW

SERVES 4

1 tbsp olive oil
375 g lean stewing beef, cubed
2 cups sliced carrots (2.5 cm pieces)
2 medium onions, cut into quarters
1 cup sliced parsnips (2.5 cm pieces)
1 cup sliced celery (2.5 cm pieces)
1 cup sliced potatoes (2.5 cm pieces)
½ tsp dried thyme
Salt and pepper to taste
2 cups beef broth
4 cups egg noodles

1 Heat oil over medium heat in soup pot or baking dish large enough to hold all ingredients. Brown the beef and drain off excess fat.

2 Add carrots, onions, parsnips, celery, potatoes, thyme, salt, pepper and broth. Cover and simmer until beef and vegetables are cooked through, about 45 minutes.

3 Cook noodles according to package directions; drain. Divide into four equal portions.

4 Before serving, divide stew into 4 equal portions. Serve over the noodles.

PER SERVING: 415 calories, 24 g protein, 13 g fat (4 g saturated fat), 52 g carbohydrates, 7 g fibre, 86 mg cholesterol, 453 mg sodium.

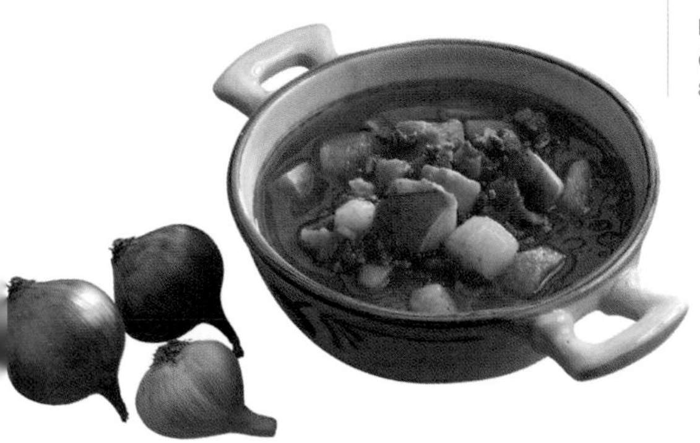

SWEET-AND-SOUR PORK WITH PINEAPPLE

SERVES 4

1 can (480 mL) juice-packed pineapple chunks
⅓ cup red currant jelly
2 tbsp plus 2 tsp Dijon mustard
500 g pork tenderloin, trimmed of all visible fat
1 tbsp lemon juice

1 Preheat the oven to 400°F (200°C). Drain pineapple, reserving juice.

2 In small saucepan, combine pineapple juice, jelly and 2 tbsp of mustard. (If desired, add salt as well.) Cook over medium heat, stirring frequently, until jelly has melted and mixture is slightly syrupy and reduced to ⅔ cup, or about 5 minutes. Remove from heat and cool to room temperature. Measure out 1 cup and set aside to be used as a sauce. Reserve the remaining mixture for basting.

3 Place pork in 17-by-28 cm baking dish. Sprinkle with lemon juice and remaining salt; brush with basting mixture. Roast, basting every 10 minutes with pan juices, until cooked through, about 30 minutes.

4 Meanwhile, in small bowl, combine pineapple chunks with remaining mustard. Let pork stand for 10 minutes before slicing into 4 equal portions. Serve with reserved sauce and pineapple-mustard mixture on the side.

PER SERVING: 282 calories, 27 g protein, 3 g fat (1 g saturated fat), 35 g carbohydrates, 1 g fibre, 81 mg cholesterol, 307 mg sodium.

Healthy pork

Have you been staying away from pork because you're worried it's fattening?

Fatty bacon and sausages have given pork a bad rep. In fact, recent analyses have found that some pork is even lower in fat than chicken. This is due to careful breeding by North American pork farmers.

So what pork should you buy? As we suggest in this recipe, go for pork tenderloin that's been trimmed of all visible fat.

HOORAY FOR PASTA!

Contrary to what many low-carb diets might dictate, pasta is actually not an unhealthy food. When eaten in moderation, it can certainly be healthy. This pasta primavera is a prime example: Packed full of vitamin-rich veggies like broccoli and mushrooms, it's an easy way to get more produce into your diet, without giving up many people's favourite comfort food.

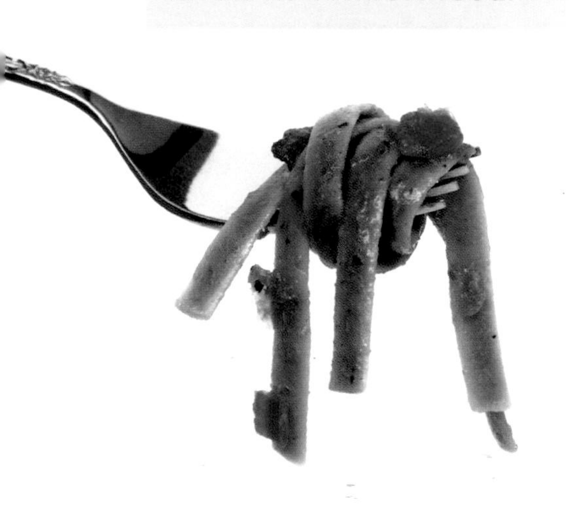

PASTA PRIMAVERA

SERVES 4

1 ⅓ cups small cauliflower florets
1 ⅓ cups small broccoli florets
200 g plain or spinach fettuccine
2 tsp olive oil
1 small red onion, diced
2 cloves garlic, minced
250 g mushrooms, thinly sliced
½ tsp salt
½ tsp dried rosemary, crumbled
1 medium tomato, cut into 1 cm cubes
2 tsp all-purpose flour
1 cup skim or 1% milk
¼ cup grated parmesan cheese
¼ cup parsley

1 In large pot of boiling water, blanch cauliflower and broccoli for 2 minutes. Transfer to plate with slotted spoon.

2 Add fettuccine to boiling water and cook according to package directions. Drain and transfer to large serving bowl.

3 Meanwhile, heat 1 tsp of oil in large non-stick skillet over medium heat. Add onion and garlic and sauté until tender, or about 5 minutes. Add mushrooms and sauté until softened, about 3 minutes.

4 Add remaining oil to skillet. Add cauliflower and broccoli, sprinkle with salt and rosemary, and sauté until heated through, for about 1 minute. Add tomato and cook until softened, or about 3 minutes.

5 Sprinkle flour over vegetables and stir to coat. Add milk and bring to boil, then reduce heat and simmer, stirring, until slightly thickened, or about 3 minutes. Stir in cheese and parsley. Add to pasta and toss to combine. Divide into 4 equal portions and refrigerate any extras.

PER SERVING: 193 calories, 12 g protein, 5 g fat (1 g saturated fat), 28 g carbohydrates, 3 g fibre, 25 mg cholesterol, 483 mg sodium.

SPANISH RICE

SERVES 4

1 medium onion, finely chopped
1 medium green bell pepper, finely chopped
1 celery stalk, finely chopped
2 cloves garlic, minced
115 g mushrooms, sliced
⅔ cup long-grain white rice
1 cup low-sodium tomato juice
1 cup low-sodium chicken broth
½ tsp salt
¼ tsp fresh-ground black pepper
1 bay leaf
4 plum tomatoes, halved, seeded, and finely chopped

1 Lightly coat deep non-stick skillet with cooking spray. Add onion, bell pepper, celery and garlic. Sauté until onion is almost soft, about 3 minutes. Stir in mushrooms and rice, and sauté until rice is golden, or about 2 minutes.

2 Stir in tomato juice, broth, salt, black pepper and bay leaf and bring to boil over medium-high heat. Reduce heat, cover and simmer, stirring occasionally, for 15 minutes. Stir in tomatoes.

3 Cover and cook until rice is tender and liquid is absorbed, or about 10 minutes. Fluff with fork to keep rice from sticking. Remove from heat and discard bay leaf.

4 Divide into 4 equal portions of 1 cup each.

PER SERVING: 165 calories, 6 g protein, 1 g fat (0 g saturated fat), 35 g carbohydrates, 3 g fibre, 0 mg cholesterol, 452 mg sodium.

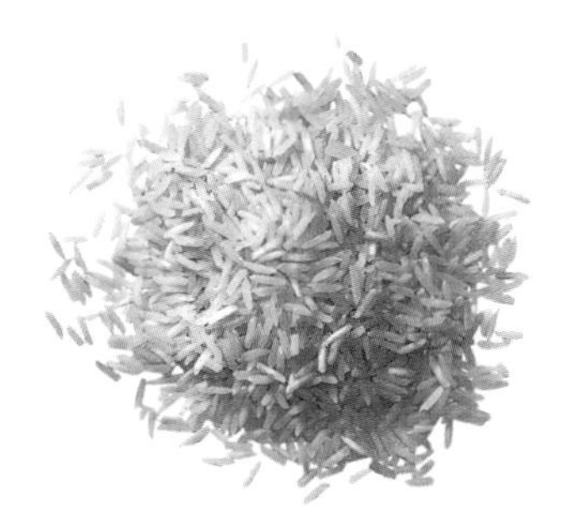

SALMON AND PEAS IN A PACKET

SERVES 4

3 cups sugar snap peas or snow peas
2 tbsp lemon juice
2 tsp olive oil
Salt and fresh-ground black pepper to taste
4 salmon fillets (about 175 g each)

1 Preheat oven to 400°F or prepare the grill.

2 In medium bowl, toss together peas, lemon juice, oil, salt and pepper.

3 Coat four 40 cm pieces of parchment or foil with cooking spray. Place fillet on bottom half of each piece and top with about ¾ cup of pea mixture. Fold parchment over fish and peas and seal by folding over edges.

4 Place packets on baking sheet in oven or directly onto grill and cook for about 10 to 12 minutes.

PER SERVING: 455 calories, 43 g protein, 28 g fat (6 g saturated fat), 6 g carbohydrates, 2 g fibre, 109 mg cholesterol, 120 mg sodium.

HOMESTYLE TUNA CASSEROLE

SERVES 4

2 cans (175 g each) water-packed tuna, no salt added
1 can (400 mL) low-sodium cream of mushroom soup
½ cup fat-free evaporated milk
¼ cup sliced black or green olives
1 can (125 mL) chopped green chilies
2 cups cooked noodles

1 Preheat the oven to 375°F (190°C). Coat a medium baking dish with cooking spray.

2 Combine the tuna, soup, milk, olives, chilies and noodles in the baking dish. Bake until bubbly, about 30 minutes.

PER SERVING: 339 calories, 31 g protein, 6 g fat (1 g saturated fat), 39 g carbohydrates, 2 g fibre, 54 mg cholesterol, 699 mg sodium.

QUICK BLACK BEANS AND RICE

SERVES 4

2 tsp olive oil
1 red bell pepper, finely chopped
½ medium onion, finely chopped
1 celery stalk, chopped
1 clove garlic, minced
1 can (398 mL) black beans, rinsed and drained
1 tsp hot sauce (optional)
2 cups cooked brown rice

1 Heat oil in large non-stick skillet. Add pepper, onion, celery and garlic and sauté until softened, about 5 minutes. Add beans and hot sauce (if using) and heat until warmed. Combine with the rice.

2 Divide into four equal portions of 1 cup each.

PER SERVING: 278 calories, 12 g protein, 4 g fat (1 g saturated fat), 50 g carbohydrates, 11 g fibre, 0 mg cholesterol, 16 mg sodium.

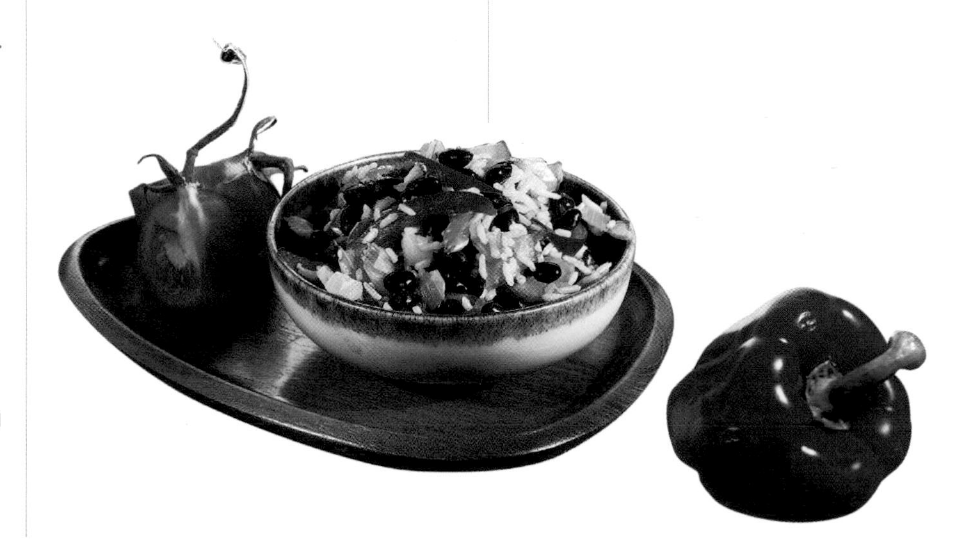

VARIATIONS

When making the Homestyle Tuna Casserole, feel free to substitute ingredients to suit your tastes (and what you have in the fridge). Instead of tuna, try tofu or leftover turkey or chicken. Instead of low-sodium cream of mushroom soup, try using the lightest variety available, or your very own homemade broth.

Also consider adding vegetables such as broccoli, onions, zucchini, carrots or celery for extra vitamins and flavour.

SHOPPING

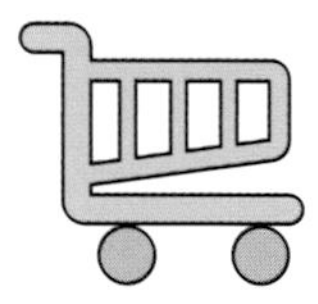

How to buy soy sauce

If you don't cook Asian-style food very often, you may not realize how versatile an ingredient soy sauce can be. Visit a Chinatown supermarket, and you'll see that there's also a wide variety of soy sauce you can buy. Should you buy dark or light, mushroom-flavoured or plain? For Swap & Drop purposes, it's best to opt for low-sodium formulas. This will probably also mean choosing a lighter-coloured variety—check the nutritional label.

BARBECUED HALIBUT STEAKS

SERVES 4

3 small scallions
1 tbsp low-sodium soy sauce
⅓ cup reduced-sugar apricot jam
3 tbsp ketchup
1 tbsp red wine vinegar
4 halibut steaks (150 g each)

1 Preheat broiler or prepare grill. Thinly slice scallions diagonally, transfer to small bowl and set aside.

2 In small bowl, combine soy sauce, jam, ketchup and vinegar. Measure out ⅓ cup and set aside to be used as sauce.

3 Place fish on broiler pan or grill rack and brush with remaining soy sauce mixture. Broil 10 cm from heat until browned and cooked through, about 5 minutes, or grill on one side just until cooked through, or about 10 minutes. Spoon reserved sauce over fish. Place bowl of sliced scallions on the table to sprinkle over the fish.

PER SERVING: 205 calories, 32 g protein, 3 g fat (0 g saturated fat), 10 g carbohydrates, 0 g fibre, 48 mg cholesterol, 347 mg sodium.

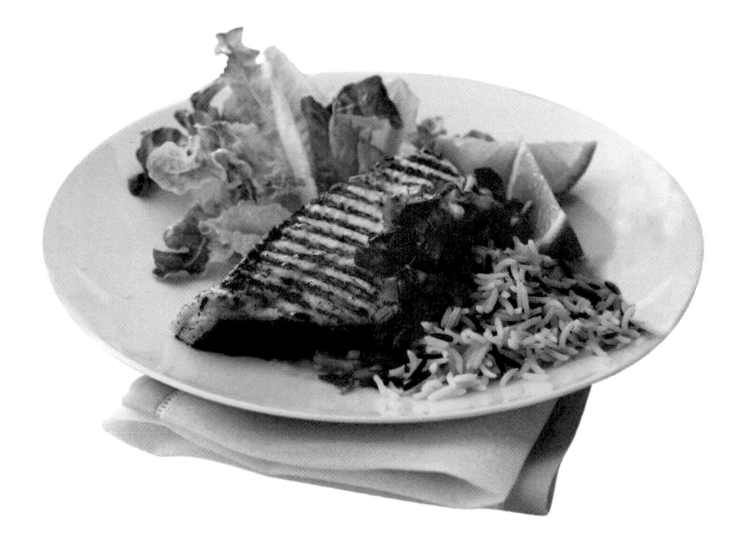

BARBECUE BEEF ON A BUN

SERVES 4

⅓ cup ketchup
1 tbsp red wine vinegar
2 tsp brown sugar
½ tsp ground ginger
½ tsp mustard
375 g sirloin steak
4 medium kaiser buns

1 Preheat broiler. In small bowl, combine ketchup, vinegar, brown sugar, ginger and mustard. Brush on one side of steak.

2 Broil steak 15 cm from heat for 4 minutes. Turn, brush with sauce and broil for 3 to 4 minutes.

3 Slice steak thinly and divide equally among buns. Refrigerate any extra portions.

PER SERVING: 336 calories, 33 g protein, 8 g fat (3 g saturated fat), 30 g carbohydrates, 1 g fibre, 62 mg cholesterol, 558 mg sodium.

VARIATIONS

● ● ● To make the Barbecue Beef on a Bun with chicken instead, use about 500 g of boneless, skinless breast or thigh meat. Cut into strips and combine with the sauce. Heat in a 350°F (180°C) oven or simmer on the stove until the sauce bubbles and the chicken is cooked through, about 15 minutes.

● ● ● To make this recipe with pork, use about 500 g of a lean cut, such as tenderloin, with fat trimmed. Prepare as with beef.

GRILLED BEER-CAN CHICKEN

SERVES 4

1 roasting chicken (1.25 kg)

3/4 tbsp dry spice rub (or make your own with equal parts paprika, onion powder and garlic powder. You can also add a pinch of salt and black pepper to taste if desired)

1 can beer

1 Prepare grill. If using charcoal grill, place coals around outside edge. If using gas grill, leave one burner off.

2 Rub chicken inside and out with dry rub.

3 Place half-full can of beer in centre of grill if using charcoal or over unlit burner if using gas. Place chicken on top of can—can should fit inside chicken cavity so it and chicken's legs form a "tripod" on grill.

4 Close grill lid and cook on medium heat until done, 45 minutes to 1 hour. Carefully remove chicken and from the grill.

5 Remove skin and cut chicken into 6 pieces—2 thighs, 2 drumsticks and 2 breast halves.

PER SERVING: 214 calories, 30 g protein, 8 g fat (2 g saturated fat), 4 g carbohydrates, 1 g fibre, 88 mg cholesterol, 90 mg sodium.

GRILLED SUMMER VEGETABLES

SERVES 4

2 small bulbs fennel (about 250 g each), cleaned

1 eggplant (about 500 g), cut lengthwise into 1 cm-thick slices

4 plum tomatoes, halved

3 large bell peppers (preferably 1 each green, red and yellow), cut into 1 cm-wide strips

1 medium red onion, cut into 8 wedges

½ tsp salt

½ tsp fresh-ground black pepper

1 tbsp orange juice

8 basil leaves, very thinly sliced

1 small clove garlic, minced

1 tsp grated orange zest

1 Preheat gas grill to high or light charcoal grill. Cut fronds from fennel and set aside. Peel bulbs and cut vertically into 1 cm slices. Coat fennel, eggplant, tomatoes, bell peppers and onion with cooking spray or very light coating of olive oil, then sprinkle with the salt and pepper.

2 Grill vegetables, turning once, until tender and evenly browned, about 4 minutes on each side. Transfer to serving platter and sprinkle with orange juice.

3 Finely chop 1 tbsp of reserved fennel fronds. In small bowl, combine with basil, garlic, and orange zest. Sprinkle over vegetables.

4 Divide into 4 equal portions and refrigerate any extra portions. One serving is 1 ½ cups (about a coffee mug).

PER SERVING: 124 calories, 5 g protein, 1 g fat (0 g saturated fat), 28 g carbohydrates, 11 g fibre, 0 mg cholesterol, 362 mg sodium.

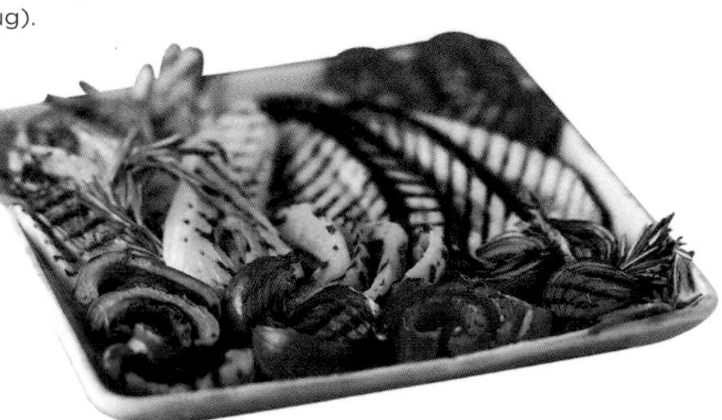

HOW TO MARINATE

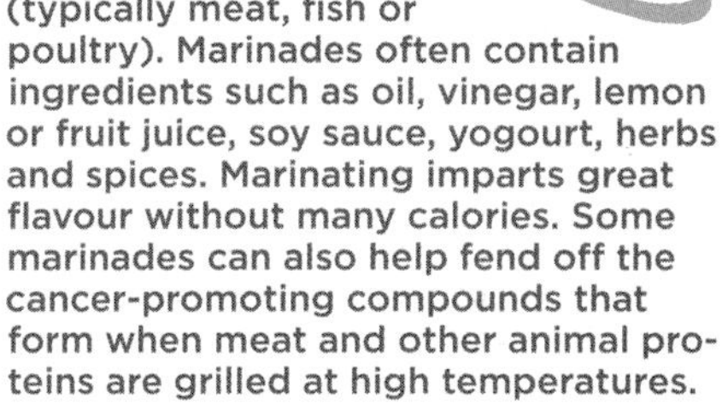

A marinade is a seasoned liquid used to flavour, tenderize and moisten food (typically meat, fish or poultry). Marinades often contain ingredients such as oil, vinegar, lemon or fruit juice, soy sauce, yogourt, herbs and spices. Marinating imparts great flavour without many calories. Some marinades can also help fend off the cancer-promoting compounds that form when meat and other animal proteins are grilled at high temperatures.

Most supermarkets stock a wide selection of marinades, but as always, check the label to make sure the calorie and fat counts aren't exorbitant. Or make your own, incorporating your favourite flavours. Marinades are perfect for improvisation, so don't get hung up on following recipes to the letter.

To marinate, place the food in a bowl or resealable plastic bag. Pour in about ¼ cup of your favourite marinade—such as teriyaki, lemon-pepper or lime-ginger—and mix well. Refrigerate for at least 1 hour.

To ensure food safety, discard remaining marinade after removing the food from the container.

Cooking with cabbage

- One head of cabbage goes a long way. To use it up, slice cabbage thinly and throw it in a soup, such as a beet borscht.
- For a super-easy Asian-flavoured side dish, stir-fry some chopped cabbage with garlic, ginger and a dash of hot sauce. Simple and delicious.

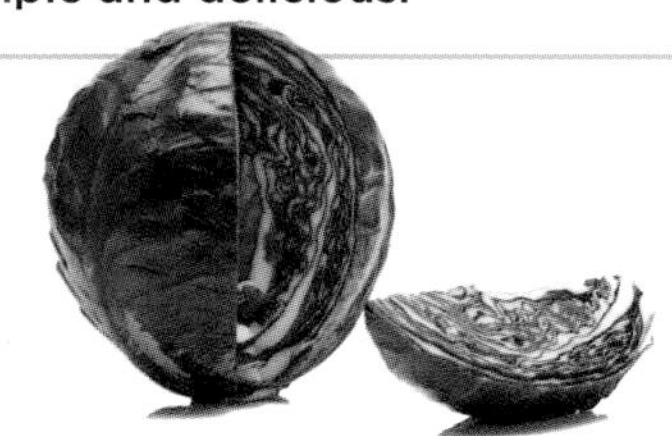

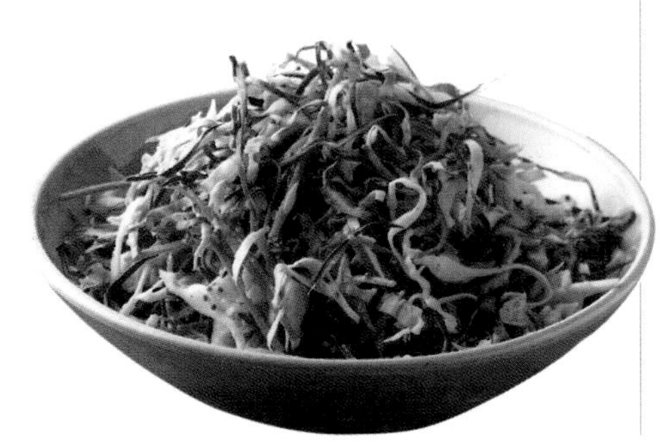

ITALIAN SALAD

SERVES 4

1 head romaine lettuce, torn into bite-size pieces
2/3 cup finely chopped red bell peppers
2/3 cup finely chopped green bell peppers
1/4 cup pine nuts
1/2 cup canned or cooked chickpeas
2 tbsp fat-free Italian dressing

1 In large salad bowl, toss together lettuce, peppers, pine nuts and chickpeas. Dress with fat-free Italian dressing (you can use low-fat dressing instead, but this will add about 30 calories per serving).

2 Divide into four equal portions of 3 cups each (about the size of three baseballs).

PER SERVING: 135 calories, 5 g protein, 7 g fat (1 g saturated fat), 16 g carbohydrates, 6 g fibre, 0 mg cholesterol, 183 mg sodium.

COLOURFUL COLESLAW

SERVES 4

1 1/4 cup shredded green cabbage
1 1/4 cup shredded red cabbage
1/2 cup shredded carrots
1/4 cup light mayonnaise
1/2 tbsp Dijon mustard
1 tbsp red wine vinegar
1/2 tbsp sugar
Salt and fresh-ground black pepper to taste

1 In a large bowl, combine green and red cabbage with carrots, mayonnaise, mustard, vinegar, sugar, salt and pepper. Mix well. Refrigerate for at least 1 hour. (Cabbage will wilt and shrink when marinated.)

2 Divide into four equal portions of 1 cup each.

PER SERVING: 91 calories, 1 g protein, 6 g fat (1 g saturated fat), 10 g carbohydrates, 1 g fibre, 7 mg cholesterol, 77 mg sodium sodium.

TOMATO AND CHICKPEA STEW

SERVES 4

1 can (796 mL) tomatoes, no salt added
1 can (796 mL) chickpeas or other beans
2 cups frozen mixed vegetables, no salt added
1 cup whole-wheat pasta (preferably elbow macaroni or small shells)
1 tsp dried herbs of your choice (such as half oregano and half basil)
2 cups water

1 Bring entire mixture to a boil over medium-high heat.

2 Reduce heat to low and simmer until pasta is cooked, about 20 to 30 minutes, depending on pasta size. Serve with slice of garlic bread, if desired.

PER SERVING: 425 calories, 16 g protein, 3 g fat (0 g saturated fat), 86 g carbohydrates, 18 g fibre, 0 mg cholesterol, 651 mg sodium.

PENNE WITH ZUCCHINI

SERVES 4

175 g penne
2 medium zucchini
2 tsp olive oil
2 tbsp slivered basil
2 tbsp grated parmesan cheese

1 Cook penne according to package directions, then drain.

2 Meanwhile, slice each zucchini in half crosswise, then slice each half into eighths lengthwise. Place in medium bowl and microwave just until softened, or about 3 minutes.

3 Add penne, oil, basil and cheese and toss to combine.

4 Divide into 4 equal portions of 1 1/2 cups each (about the size of two tennis balls).

PER SERVING: 116 calories, 6 g protein, 4 g fat (1 g saturated fat), 16 g carbohydrates, 1 g fibre, 19 mg cholesterol, 125 mg sodium.

THAI NOODLE SALAD

SERVES 4

250 g Asian rice noodles
1 tsp peanut oil
2 cloves garlic, minced
1 medium onion, thinly sliced
¼ cup vegetable stock
¼ cup sliced scallions
1 ½ cups bean sprouts, rinsed and drained
¼ cup natural peanut butter
¼ cup light coconut milk
8 cups mixed greens
¼ cup fresh cilantro, chopped
Juice of 2 limes
1 tbsp unsalted peanuts, chopped

1 Cook noodles according to package directions.

2 Meanwhile, heat oil in large non-stick skillet. Add garlic and sauté for about 30 seconds. Add onion and stock and cook until tender, about 5 minutes.

3 Drain noodles and add to skillet. Add scallions and bean sprouts and toss gently until well-mixed.

4 In small bowl, combine peanut butter and coconut milk. Add to skillet and toss to coat.

5 Divide noodles into four equal portions. Place 2 cups of greens on each plate, top with noodles and garnish with cilantro, lime juice and chopped peanuts.

PER SERVING: 425 calories, 11 g protein, 13 g fat (4 g saturated fat), 68 g carbohydrates, 5 g fibre, 0 mg cholesterol, 191 mg sodium.

GERMAN POTATO SALAD WITH DIJON VINAIGRETTE

SERVES 4

500 g small red potatoes, scrubbed and quartered
3 slices turkey bacon
1 small onion, chopped
3 tbsp cider vinegar
1 ½ tbsp sugar
1 tbsp Dijon or grainy mustard
½ tsp olive oil
½ tsp fresh-ground black pepper
¼ cup finely chopped low-sodium sweet pickles
¼ cup finely chopped red bell pepper
¼ cup minced parsley

1 Place potatoes, and enough water to cover, in large saucepan and bring to boil over high heat. Reduce heat to medium and cook until tender, about 10 minutes. Drain and keep warm.

2 Cut bacon in half crosswise. Cook in large, deep non-stick skillet until crisp, transfer to paper towels to drain, then crumble. Add onion to skillet and sauté in pan drippings until golden, about 7 minutes.

3 Place vinegar, sugar, mustard, oil, black pepper and remaining salt in jar and shake. Whisk into skillet, bring to simmer and cook until fragrant, about 2 minutes. Add potatoes, pickles, bell pepper and half of the bacon. Cook, stirring, until potatoes are coated and heated through, or about 2 minutes. Sprinkle with parsley and remaining bacon.

4 Divide into 4 equal portions (refrigerate any extra portions). One serving is ½ cup (about the size of 2 golf balls).

PER SERVING: 178 calories, 6 g protein, 4 g fat (1 g saturated fat), 30 g carbohydrates, 3 g fibre, 10 mg cholesterol, 343 mg sodium.

SHOPPING

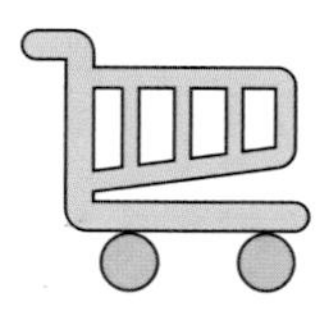

Choosing the right potato

Most of us don't give much thought to which potatoes we buy at the supermarket—a potato is a potato is a potato, right?

In fact, different varieties of potatoes are suited to different dishes. Tiny new potatoes or small red potatoes are great for potato salads, because they can keep their shape and won't fall apart. Russet potatoes, on the other hand, are great for mashing or making into baked potatoes (skip the butter that usually goes with them).

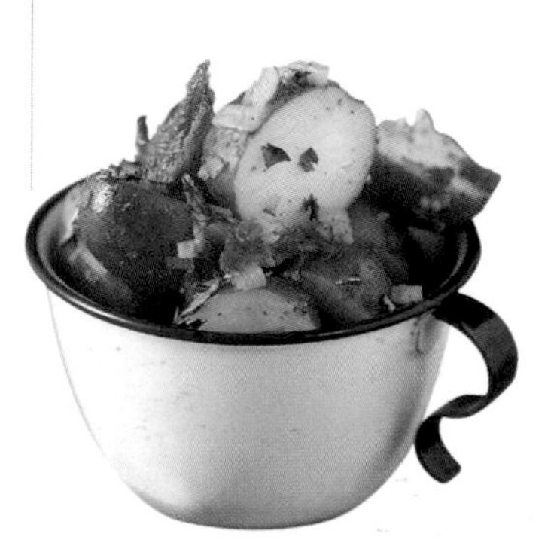

Meal Planner Recipes snacks & desserts

You may be on a diet, but that doesn't mean you can't enjoy tempting desserts and snacks! On **Swap & Drop**, you just need to remember to keep your portions reasonably sized (for more help on this, see page 18). Indulging your sweet tooth with luscious brownies and refreshing sorbet, and *still* losing weight–is there anything better?

SORBET

SERVES 2

1 can (240 g) of fruit packed in heavy syrup (blueberries, peaches or strawberries are good choices)
½ cup apple juice

1 Freeze an entire can of fruit packed in heavy syrup.

2 Take out of freezer 30 minutes ahead of time and place on counter. After 30 minutes open can on both ends and push out contents into food processor. Add apple juice and process until smooth.

3 Serve soft, or refreeze. One portion is about ½ cup.

PER SERVING: 117 calories, 1 g protein, 0 g fat (0 g saturated fat), 31 g carbohydrates, 2 g fibre, 0 mg cholesterol, 10 mg sodium.

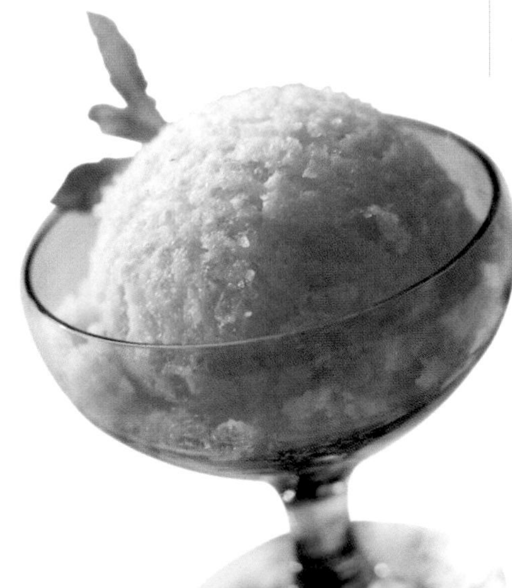

FRUIT BOATS WITH ORANGE-BALSAMIC GLAZE

SERVES 4

¼ cup balsamic vinegar
¼ tsp grated orange zest
2 tbsp fresh orange juice
2 tsp brown sugar
1 large cantaloupe
2 cups strawberries, rinsed, hulled and quartered
1 cup blueberries, rinsed
1 cup raspberries, rinsed
2 kiwis, peeled, halved and cut into thin wedges

1 In small bowl, combine vinegar, orange zest, juice and brown sugar. Microwave on high until syrupy, about 2 to 3 minutes, or cook in small saucepan over medium-high heat for 4 to 5 minutes. Set aside.

2 Cut cantaloupe into quarters and scoop out balls, leaving thin layer of flesh on rinds.

3 In large bowl, combine cantaloupe balls, strawberries, blueberries, raspberries and kiwis. Drizzle with glaze and toss to coat. Spoon into 4 cantaloupe boats and serve immediately. One serving is 1 boat.

PER SERVING: 181 calories, 4 g protein, 1 g fat (0 g saturated fat), 44 g carbohydrates, 8 g fibre, 0 mg cholesterol, 39 mg sodium.

BROWNIE BITES

MAKES 16

2/3 cup all-purpose flour
1/3 cup unsweetened cocoa powder
2 tbsp cornstarch
1 tsp baking powder
1/4 tsp baking soda
1/4 tsp salt
1 cup packed light brown sugar
1/4 cup prune butter
2 tbsp fat-free plain yogourt
2 tbsp canola oil
1 egg
3 tbsp semisweet mini chocolate chips
1/2 cup coarsely chopped walnuts

1 Preheat oven to 350°F (180°C). Coat 20 cm square baking pan with cooking spray.

2 In medium bowl, stir together the flour, cocoa, cornstarch, baking powder, baking soda and salt. Set aside.

3 In large bowl, using electric mixer, beat together brown sugar, prune butter, yogourt, oil and egg. Stir in the flour mixture just until combined.

4 Pour batter into baking pan and scatter chocolate chips and walnuts on top. Bake until toothpick inserted in centre comes out with some crumbs and sides of brownie begin to pull away from pan, or 18 to 20 minutes. Transfer pan to wire rack to cool. Cut into 16 pieces about 5 cm square. One serving is 1 brownie. You can wrap leftovers in heavy foil and freeze for up to 1 month. Well-sealed, these can last at room temperature for about 5 days.

PER SERVING: 160 calories, 3 g protein, 6 g fat (1 g saturated fat), 13 g carbohydrates, 3 g fibre, 13 mg cholesterol, 69 mg sodium.

CHOCOLATE CHIP OATMEAL COOKIES

MAKES 36

1 cup all-purpose flour
1/2 tsp baking soda
1/2 tsp salt
1 cup old-fashioned oats
4 tbsp butter
2/3 cup packed light brown sugar
1/2 cup granulated sugar
1 egg
1 1/2 tsp vanilla extract
1/3 cup light sour cream
3/4 cup semisweet chocolate chips

1 Preheat oven to 375°F (190°C). Line 2 large baking sheets with parchment paper.

2 In a medium bowl, whisk flour, baking soda, and salt. Stir in oats.

3 In a large bowl, using electric mixer on high speed, cream butter, brown sugar and granulated sugar until well blended. Add egg and vanilla and beat until light and creamy, or about 3 minutes. With wooden spoon, blend in sour cream, then add flour mixture all at once and stir until combined (don't overmix, or cookies may be tough). Stir in chocolate chips.

4 Drop heaping teaspoonfuls of dough 5 cm apart on baking sheets. Bake until golden, about 10 minutes. Cool on baking sheets for 2 minutes, then transfer to wire racks to cool completely. One serving is 1 cookie. You can store cookies in an airtight container for up to 2 weeks or freeze for up to 3 months.

PER SERVING:
62 calories, 1 g protein, 2 g fat (1 g saturated fat), 9 g carbohydrates, 1 g fibre, 8 mg cholesterol, 88 mg sodium.

CHOCOLATE: IT'S GOOD FOR THE SOUL

Researchers have known about the heart-healthy benefits of dark chocolate for years. Not only that, but its luxurious flavour activates transmitters in your brain that release serotonin, making you feel good. (No surprise there!) That's no excuse to go wild, though: You only need a small square (or one Chocolate Chip Oatmeal Cookie) to feel the love.

CRANBERRIES These little jewels are more than just tasty—they're also packed with vitamin C and can help reduce the risk of urinary tract infections.

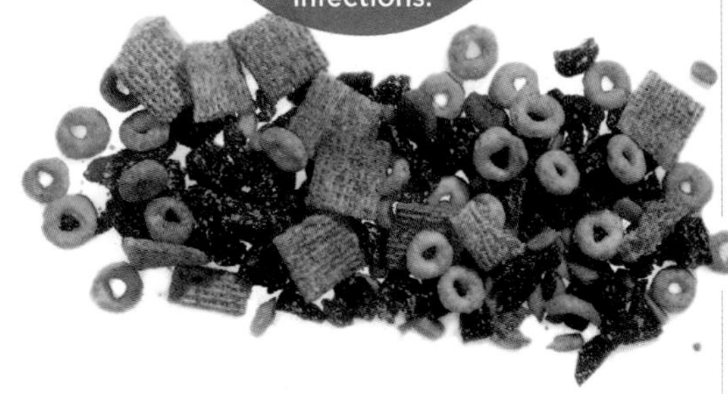

CRANBERRY TRAIL MIX

MAKES 3 CUPS

1 ½ cups square-shaped cereal (such as Shreddies)
¾ cup oat O-shaped cereal (such as Cheerios)
2 tbsp hulled sunflower seeds
¼ cup grated parmesan cheese
¾ cup dried cranberries, coarsely chopped

1 Preheat oven to 350°F (180°C). In large bowl, combine cereals and sunflower seeds. Coat lightly with cooking spray. Add parmesan and toss to combine.

2 Transfer to jelly-roll pan and bake, stirring occasionally, until crisp and slightly crusty, or about 15 minutes.

3 Let cool to room temperature, then transfer to large bowl. Add cranberries and toss to combine. One serving is ½ cup (about the size of 2 golf balls). You can store leftovers in the refrigerator in an airtight container.

PER SERVING: 140 calories, 4 g protein, 4 g fat (1 g saturated fat), 24 g carbohydrates, 3 g fibre, 4 mg cholesterol, 162 mg sodium.

For a different take on baked apples, see the recipe for Maple-Walnut Roasted Apples on page 178.

BAKED APPLE

SERVES 1

1 medium apple (any but Red Delicious—they get too watery)
1 pinch of cinnamon
1 tsp sugar

1 Core apple and sprinkle inside with cinnamon and sugar.

2 Cover and microwave 3 minutes, or until soft.

PER SERVING: 105 calories, 1 g protein, 0 g fat (0 g saturated fat), 28 g carbohydrates, 5 g fibre, 0 mg cholesterol, 2 mg sodium.

PECAN ICEBOX COOKIES

MAKES 72

1 ¾ cups all-purpose flour
½ tsp ground cinnamon
¼ tsp salt
¼ tsp baking soda
¼ cup (½ stick) butter, softened
⅔ cup granulated sugar
⅓ cup packed light brown sugar
1 egg
1 tbsp vanilla extract
⅓ cup light sour cream
⅓ cup chopped pecans, toasted

1 In medium bowl, whisk flour, cinnamon, salt and baking soda.

2 In large bowl, using electric mixer on high speed, cream butter, granulated sugar and brown sugar until light and fluffy, about 4 minutes. Add egg and vanilla and beat until well-blended. Using wooden spoon, stir in flour mixture, then sour cream and pecans.

3 Tear off 50 cm sheet of plastic wrap and sprinkle lightly with flour. Transfer dough to plastic and shape into 40 cm log. Roll tightly in plastic and refrigerate until firm, for about 2 hours.

4 Preheat oven to 375°F (190°C). Unwrap dough and cut into rounds 5 mm thick, making about 72 cookies. Working in batches, place rounds 1 cm apart on ungreased baking sheets. Bake just until crisp and golden around the edges, or about 8 minutes. Transfer to wire racks to cool. One serving is 2 cookies. You can store the cookies in airtight container for up to 2 weeks or freeze for up to 3 months.

PER SERVING: 73 calories, 1 g protein, 3 g fat (1 g saturated fat), 11 g carbohydrates, 0 g fibre, 8 mg cholesterol, 29 mg sodium.

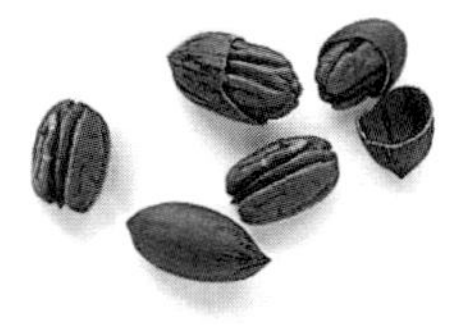

CHOCOLATE SNACKING CAKE

MAKES 36 SQUARES

1 1/3 cups all-purpose flour
1 cup plus 2 tsp unsweetened cocoa powder
1 1/2 tsp baking powder
1/2 tsp salt
1/4 cup fat-free buttermilk
1 tbsp instant espresso powder
1 cup granulated sugar
1/2 cup packed light brown sugar
1/2 cup unsweetened applesauce
2 tsp vanilla extract
2 egg whites
1/2 cup semisweet mini chocolate chips
1 tbsp icing sugar

1 Preheat oven to 325°F (160°C). Line 20 cm square baking pan with foil, leaving some overhang.

2 Sift flour and 1 cup of cocoa together into small bowl, then add baking powder and salt. In small saucepan, heat buttermilk and espresso over low heat until espresso is dissolved.

3 In medium bowl, mix granulated sugar, brown sugar, applesauce, buttermilk mixture and vanilla. Stir in flour mixture just until blended.

4 In large bowl, using electric mixer on high speed, beat egg whites just until soft peaks form. Fold into batter and stir in chocolate chips.

5 Pour batter into baking pan and bake just until set, or about 35 minutes; do not over-bake. Transfer pan to wire rack to cool for 15 minutes, then remove cake from pan and place on rack to cool completely.

6 Sift icing sugar and remaining cocoa over cake. Cut into 36 pieces. One serving is 1 square.

PER SERVING: 72 calories, 1 g protein, 1 g fat (1 g saturated fat), 16 g carbohydrates, 1 g fibre, 0 mg cholesterol, 39 mg sodium.

BLUEBERRY BONANZA

SERVES 4

1/2 cup 1% milk
2 tbsp dry skim milk
1 package (375 g) frozen blueberries, thawed
1/8 tsp salt
1/4 cup plus 1 tsp sugar
1/2 cup fat-free plain yogourt
1/2 package unflavoured gelatin
2 tbsp cold water
1/2 cup fresh blueberries

1 In small bowl, combine milk and dry milk and whisk until well blended. Place in freezer for up to 30 minutes.

2 In medium saucepan over low heat, combine frozen blueberries, salt and 1/4 cup of sugar. Bring to simmer and cook until sugar has dissolved, berries have broken up and mixture has been reduced to 1 cup, or about 10 minutes. Let cool to room temperature, then stir in 1/3 cup of yogourt.

3 Sprinkle gelatin over cold water in heat proof measuring cup. Let stand for 5 minutes to soften. Set measuring cup in a saucepan of simmering water until gelatin has melted, for about 2 minutes. Let cool.

4 With hand mixer, beat chilled milk until thick, soft peaks form. Beat in remaining sugar, then gelatin mixture. With rubber spatula, fold milk mixture into blueberry mixture.

5 Spoon into 4 dessert bowls or glasses and refrigerate until set, or about 2 hours. To serve, top each portion with a dollop of remaining yogourt and fresh blueberries. One serving is 1 bowl or glass.

PER SERVING: 151 calories, 7 g protein, 1 g fat (0 g saturated fat), 31 g carbohydrates, 3 g fibre, 2 mg cholesterol, 123 mg sodium.

BLUEBERRIES AND WEIGHT LOSS

Some animal studies have suggested that blueberries might aid in speeding weight loss, for reasons yet to be understood. We say the reasons are obvious! Blueberries are low in calories, sweet, delicious and lots of fun to eat—so of course dieters (and animals) would be inclined to snack on them!

But blueberries are also healthy for more complex reasons: They're packed full of antioxidants which can help prevent cancer. Keep a carton around for whenever you feel like a super-powerful, disease-fighting snack.

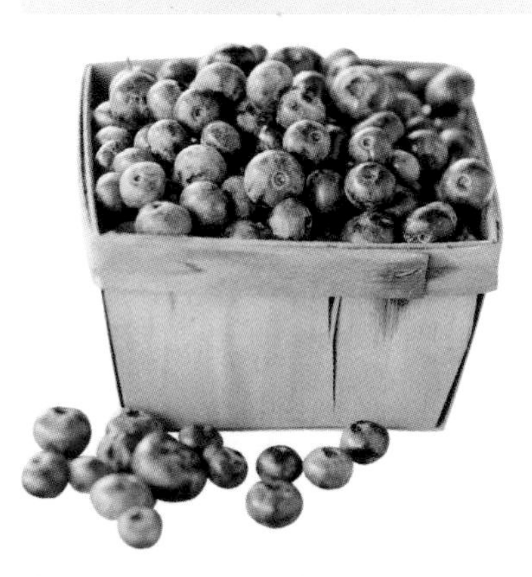

Additional Recipes breakfasts

Mix it up! Eating healthy is all about taking advantage of the whole spectrum of colourful fruits and veggies, lean proteins and healthy grains. Here are many more recipes to keep you fit and happy, **Swap & Drop**-style.

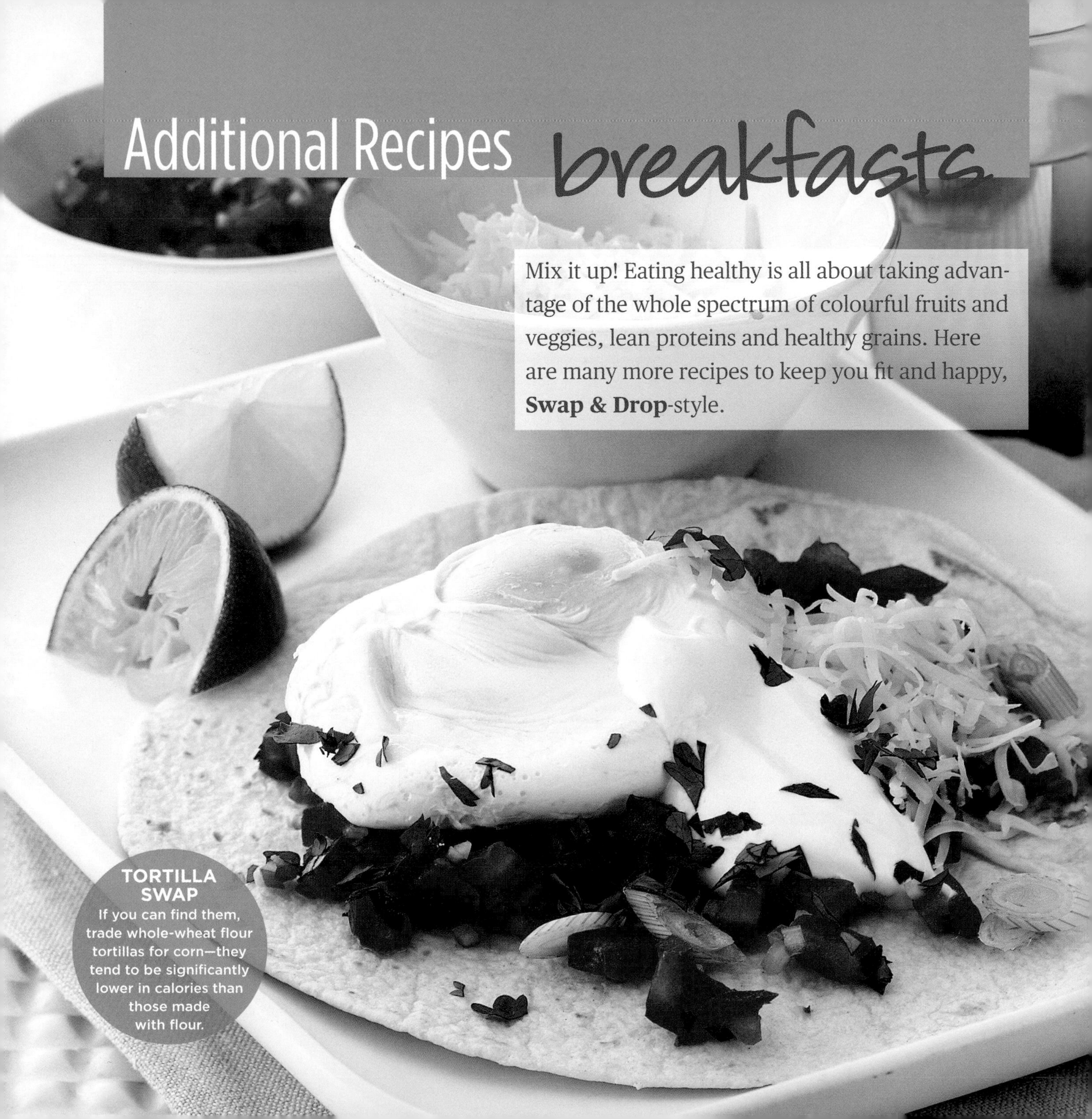

TORTILLA SWAP
If you can find them, trade whole-wheat flour tortillas for corn—they tend to be significantly lower in calories than those made with flour.

HUEVOS RANCHEROS

SERVES 4

In order to refuel and stabilize blood sugars in the morning, it is important to have a balanced breakfast consisting of a small amount of protein along with carbohydrates, dairy and fruit or vegetables. For a fun weekend brunch, serve this perfectly balanced Mexican-style dish of poached eggs, warm tortillas and a fresh tomato-and-chili salsa, topped with light, grated cheese and sour cream, scallions and fresh cilantro.

SALSA

5 medium tomatoes, finely chopped
1 mild fresh red chili pepper, seeded and finely chopped
1 small red onion, finely chopped
1 small garlic clove, finely chopped
2 tbsp finely chopped fresh cilantro
1 tbsp olive oil
2–3 tbsp lime juice
Pepper

EGGS

4 x 25-cm whole-wheat flour tortillas
1 tsp vinegar
4 eggs
60 g coarsely grated light cheddar cheese
6 tbsp light sour cream
4 scallions, chopped
Chopped fresh cilantro
Lime wedges

1 To make salsa: Place chopped tomatoes in bowl and stir in chili, pepper, red onion, garlic and cilantro. Add oil and lime juice to taste. Set aside to marinate for about 30 minutes, then season lightly with pepper to taste.

2 Preheat oven to 350°F (180°C). Wrap stacked-up tortillas in foil and put in oven to warm for 10 minutes.

3 Meanwhile, half-fill large skillet with water. Heat until just starting to simmer, then reduce heat so water does not boil. Add vinegar. Break eggs into water, one at a time, and poach for 3 minutes. Toward end of cooking, spoon water over yolks. When cooked, remove eggs with slotted spoon and drain on paper-towel-lined plate.

4 Place warmed tortillas on plates. Spoon over some salsa, then put eggs on top and season with pepper to taste. Let everyone help themselves to remaining salsa, grated cheese, sour cream and scallions, plus chopped cilantro for sprinkling over the top and lime wedges for squeezing.

PER SERVING (WITH ½ CUP SALSA): 422 calories, 16 g total fat, 5 g saturated fat, 200 mg cholesterol, 51 g carbohydrates, 3 g fibre, 11 g sugars, 19 g protein.

Healthy Swaps

You can add healthy, homemade refried beans for a full Mexican breakfast—instructions are on page 93.

Low-fat dairy products, such as the light cheddar and sour cream in Huevos Rancheros, are an excellent source of calcium. Health Canada's Food Guide recommends that most adults consume 2 to 3 servings of milk or alternatives (such as soy milk) every day.

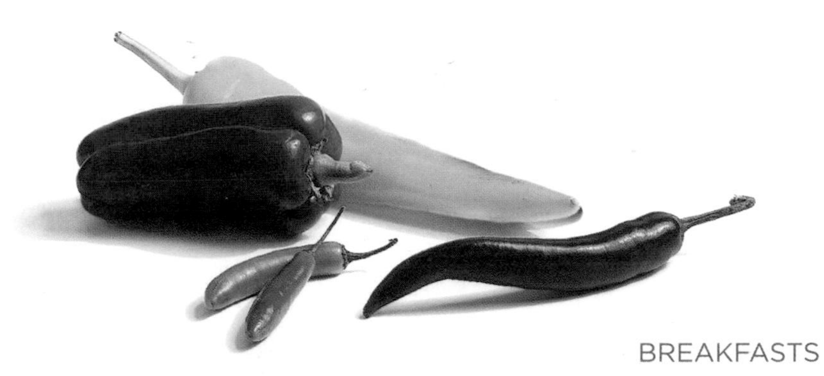

SAVOURY TREAT

This hearty breakfast dish contains fewer calories than the traditional sweet French toast, which is often served with butter and maple syrup.

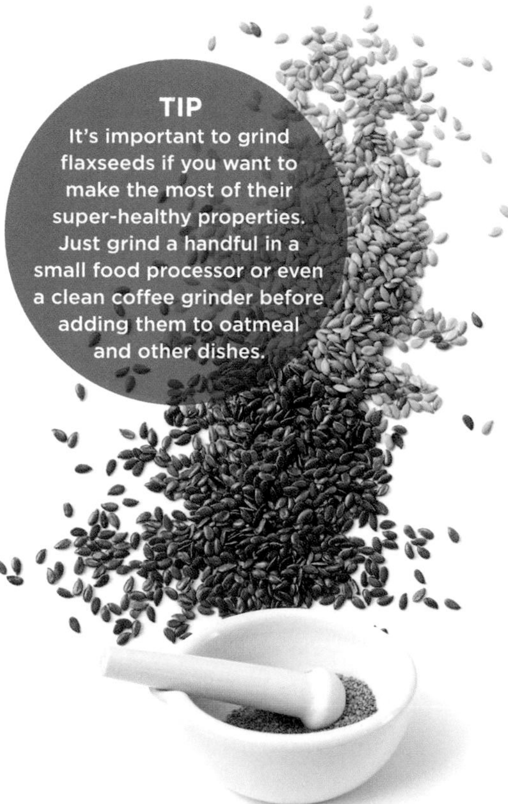

TIP

It's important to grind flaxseeds if you want to make the most of their super-healthy properties. Just grind a handful in a small food processor or even a clean coffee grinder before adding them to oatmeal and other dishes.

HERBED FRENCH TOAST WITH MUSHROOMS

SERVES 4

In this savoury French toast, bread is dipped in a fresh herb and egg mixture.

4 large eggs
5 tbsp 1% milk
1 tbsp finely chopped parsley
1 tbsp finely chopped
Fresh chives
1/2 tbsp chopped fresh thyme or 1/8 tsp dried
1/8 tsp paprika
Pepper to taste
4 large flat mushrooms (such as portobello), about 250 g in total, stalks removed
4 tbsp canola oil
4 strips bacon, trimmed of visible fat
5 thick slices whole-wheat bread

1 Preheat broiler. Combine eggs, milk, most of parsley, chives, thyme and paprika in shallow dish. Season with pepper and set aside.

2 Using 1 tbsp oil, lightly brush mushroom caps. Place them gill-side up on the broiler rack. Add bacon. Broil bacon and mushrooms until cooked, remove from oven and keep warm.

3 Meanwhile, cut each slice of bread into 4 triangles. Heat large skillet over medium heat and add 1 tbsp of remaining oil. Dip about one-third of each bread triangle into egg mixture to moisten on both sides, then place in hot pan. Cook for 1 to 2 minutes or until golden-brown. Remove from pan and keep warm while you cook the rest, adding oil as needed.

4 To serve, arrange 5 triangles of French toast on each plate. Cut mushrooms into thick slices and add to plates, together with bacon. Sprinkle with remaining parsley.

PER SERVING: 393 calories, 23 g protein, 26 g total fat, 5 g saturated fat, 275 mg cholesterol, 17 g carbohydrates, 3 g sugars, 4 g fibre, 862 mg sodium

OATMEAL WITH APPLE AND FLAXSEEDS

SERVES 4

What better way to start your day than with a comforting bowl of steaming oatmeal?

2 cups 1% milk or vanilla soy milk
3/4 cup old-fashioned rolled oats
1 medium apple, peeled, cored and chopped
1/3 cup dried cranberries or raisins
1/2 tsp cinnamon
1/4 cup whole flaxseeds, ground or 1/3 cup flaxseed meal
1/4 cup fat-free plain or vanilla yogourt
1/4 cup maple syrup, warmed, or 2 tbsp brown sugar

1 Combine milk, rolled oats, apple, dried cranberries (or raisins) and cinnamon in heavy medium saucepan. Bring to simmer over medium-high heat, stirring almost constantly.

2 Reduce heat to medium-low and cook, stirring, until creamy and thickened, 3 to 5 minutes.

3 Stir in flaxseeds. Spoon cereal into individual bowls and top each serving with dollop of yogourt and drizzle of maple syrup.

PER SERVING (2/3 CUP): 282 calories, 10 g protein, 47 g carbohydrates, 6 g fibre, 7 g total fat, 1 g saturated fat, 8 mg cholesterol, 84 mg sodium.

MINT- AND BERRY-SCENTED MELON CUP

SERVES 6

This is a perfect light summertime treat: a combination of colourful ripe fruit and pieces of crisp cucumber, drizzled with orange-flavoured liqueur and garnished with fresh mint. The salad is served in hollowed-out melon shells for an elegant presentation, and slices of starfruit add another intriguing touch. Serve the salad at an afternoon picnic or for Sunday brunch.

MELON CUP
1 small cantaloupe (about 500 g)
1 small honeydew melon (about 500 g)
1 ½ cups ripe strawberries, hulled and sliced
1 large pear, cut into 1 cm pieces
½ small cucumber, diced (½ cup)
2 starfruits, sliced 5 mm thick
6 tbsp orange brandy
2 tbsp shredded fresh mint

GARNISH
Fresh mint sprigs

1 Cut melons in half crosswise and scoop out seeds from centres. Using melon baller or a small spoon, scoop balls of melon into large bowl. With tablespoon, scoop out any remaining melon into bowl, leaving smooth shells.

2 Add strawberries, pear chunks and diced cucumber to melon in bowl. Set aside 4 starfruit slices for decoration. Dice remaining slices and add to bowl.

3 Drizzle brandy over fruit, sprinkle with mint, and toss gently to mix well. Cover with plastic wrap and let marinate in refrigerator for 20 minutes.

4 Pile fruit mixture into melon shells and decorate with reserved slices of starfruit.

PER SERVING: 109 calories, 1 g total fat, 0 mg cholesterol, 19 g carbohydrates, 3 g fibre, 9 g sugar, 1 g protein.

VARIATIONS

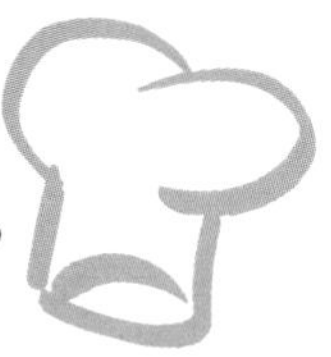

- **Non-alcoholic Melon Cup:** Substitute a mixture of 3 tbsp fresh orange juice and 3 tbsp honey for the orange brandy.

- **Luncheon Salad:** You can also change this dish into a great noon meal—just adjust the flavour balance.

For the fruits and vegetables, use 1 small honeydew melon, 1 ½ cups sliced, hulled strawberries, 1 large crisp red apple, 1 cup seedless green grapes, 2 peeled sliced kiwis and ½ cup diced cucumber. Omit the cantaloupe, pear, starfruits and brandy.

In a large bowl, toss 6 cups mesclun salad leaves, 2 cups watercress, and ½ cup chopped scallions. Arrange on 6 salad plates and spoon the fruit on top. Add a scoop of low-fat cottage cheese, if you want, and sprinkle with the shredded mint.

CINNAMON-RAISIN BREAD

MAKES 1 LARGE LOAF

This whole-wheat bread loaf studded with raisins tastes good plain or with a little light butter or margarine spread on it. It's also wonderful toasted for breakfast, when the gentle aroma of warm cinnamon makes a soothing start to the day.

5 cups whole-wheat flour
1 ½ tsp salt
2 tsp ground cinnamon
1 package instant dry yeast
⅔ cup raisins
3 tbsp sugar
3 tbsp unsalted butter
1 cup skim milk, plus 1 tbsp to glaze
1 egg, lightly beaten

1 Lightly coat 22 cm-by-13 cm loaf pan with cooking spray and flour. Sift flour, salt and cinnamon into large mixing bowl. Stir in yeast, raisins and sugar, and make a well in centre.

2 Gently heat butter and milk in small saucepan until butter has melted and mixture is just warm. Pour into well in dry ingredients and add beaten egg. Mix together to make a soft dough.

3 Turn dough out onto lightly floured surface and knead until smooth and elastic, about 10 minutes. Shape dough into loaf and place in prepared pan. Cover with clean towel or plastic wrap that has been coated with cooking spray and leave to rise in warm place until doubled in size, about 1 hour.

4 Toward end of rising time, preheat oven to 425°F (220°C). Uncover loaf and brush with milk to glaze. Bake until loaf sounds hollow when removed from pan and tapped on bottom, about 30 minutes. Cover loaf with foil toward end of cooking time if top is browning too much.

5 Turn out onto wire rack and leave to cool. Bread can be kept, wrapped in foil, for 2 to 3 days.

PER SERVING (ONE SLICE): 198 calories, 3 g total fat, 1 g saturated fat, 19 mg cholesterol, 38 g carbohydrates, 6 g fibre, 8 g sugars, 7 g protein.

Dried fruit: yea or nay?

Dried fruits, like the raisins in this bread, are a great source of fibre—but don't eat too many. Their sugars are more concentrated than those in fresh fruit, so be careful not to overdo it. A small handful of raisins combined with nuts makes a healthy homemade trail mix, and a great **Swap & Drop** snack for when you're on the go.

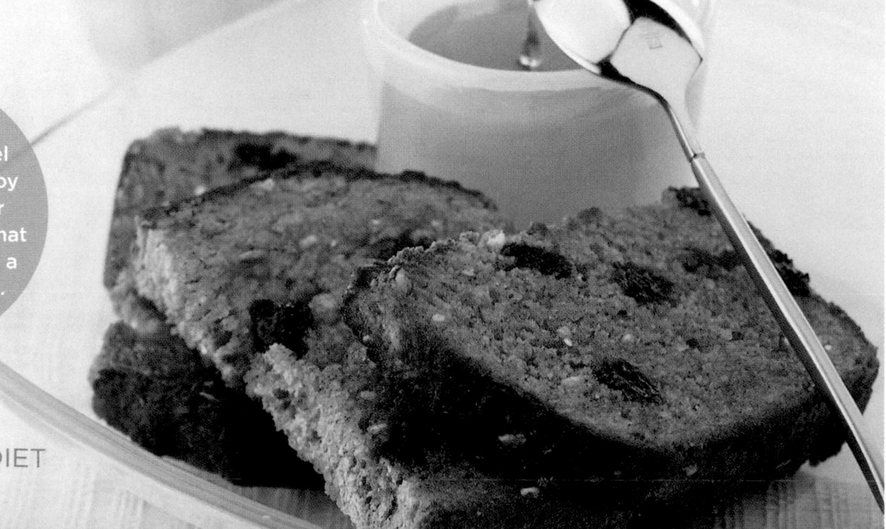

MILK SWAP
For this recipe, feel free to substitute soy or almond milk for skim milk if that's what you prefer—choose a sugar-free version.

APRICOT-PECAN MUFFINS

MAKES 12 LARGE MUFFINS

Any time can be muffin time, especially when you bake up these fresh apricot-pecan muffins. They come out of the oven light, moist and smelling of cinnamon. Wheat bran is added to the recipe for flavour and extra nutrition. If fresh apricots are not in season, any type of fresh fruit, such as blueberries, strawberries or bananas, can be used instead.

- 2 ¼ cups all-purpose flour
- 1 cup packed brown sugar
- 3 tbsp wheat bran
- 1 tbsp baking powder
- 1 tsp ground cinnamon
- ½ tsp grated lemon zest
- ¼ tsp salt
- 2 large eggs
- 6 tbsp light unsalted butter, melted and cooled
- 1 cup skim milk
- 5 apricots, peeled, pitted and coarsely chopped (about 1 cup)
- ¼ cup chopped pecans

1 Preheat oven to 375°F (190°C). Lightly coat a 12-cup muffin pan with cooking spray or line with paper baking cups.

2 In large bowl, mix flour, sugar, wheat bran, baking powder, cinnamon, lemon zest and salt. Make a well in centre of dry ingredients and set aside.

3 In large measuring cup, whisk eggs until frothy and light yellow. Beat in butter, then milk, until well blended. Pour mixture into well in centre of flour mixture. Stir just until dry ingredients are moistened—do not overmix or muffins will be tough. With rubber spatula, gently fold in apricots and pecans.

4 Spoon batter into prepared muffin pan, filling cups ¾ full. Bake until muffins are peaked and golden brown, about 20 minutes. Muffins are done when wooden toothpick inserted in centre comes out almost clean, with moist crumbs clinging to it. Let muffins cool in pan for 3 minutes before removing. Muffins are best when served piping hot or within a few hours of baking.

PER SERVING (ONE MUFFIN): 236 calories, 7 g total fat, 3 g saturated fat, 43 mg cholesterol, 40 g carbohydrates, 2 g fibre, 21 g sugars, 5 g protein.

VARIATIONS

Banana-Nut Muffins: Use 1 cup mashed ripe banana instead of the apricots.

Blueberry-Nut Muffins: Substitute 1 tsp grated orange zest for the lemon zest. Substitute 2 cups fresh blueberries for the apricots and ¼ cup chopped walnuts for the pecans.

Strawberry Muffins: Substitute 2 cups coarsely chopped, ripe strawberries for the apricots.

Peach Muffins: Use 2 cups coarsely chopped, peeled peaches instead of the apricots.

High-Fibre Muffins: Use 2 cups all-purpose flour and ¼ cup whole-wheat flour.

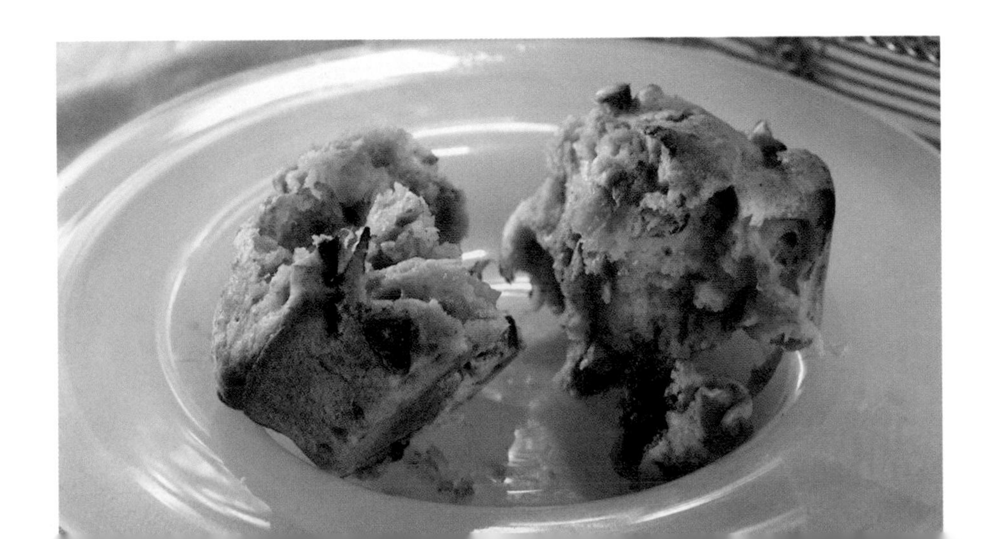

Early-morning veggies

- It might sound a bit strange, but grated beets can be a sweet garnish on your morning cereal (carrots work, too!). Just a ½ cup of grated beets puts one serving of vegetables under your belt before you even leave the house.
- Here are some other quick ways to add veggies to breakfast: Toss ½ cup of chopped peppers with your scrambled eggs, add ½ cup of chopped tomatoes to cottage cheese or throw some greens into your breakfast smoothie.

FRESH FRUIT MUESLI

SERVES 6

Fresh muesli, moist from soaking and rich with juicy fruit, is a revelation to those who have only eaten dried muesli. It has the consistency of oatmeal with the freshness of raw ingredients. It makes for a satisfying way to start the day.

½ cup bulgur
¾ cup rolled oats
1 cup apple juice
½ cup slivered unblanched almonds
4 tbsp pine nuts
2 tbsp sunflower kernels
10 dried apricots, diced
10 dried figs, stalks removed and diced
4 tbsp brown sugar
2 green apples, cored and coarsely grated
1 large or 2 small peaches or nectarines, peeled and diced
1 passionfruit
A few drops of pure almond extract
Pomegranate seeds or blueberries to garnish
Extra diced peach or nectarine to garnish

1 In a large bowl, combine bulgur with about 1 cup water and stir to combine. Cover and let soak for 30 minutes to soften bulgur. Drain well in sieve and return to bowl.

2 Add rolled oats, apple juice, almonds, pine nuts, sunflower kernels, apricots, figs, brown sugar, grated apple and diced peaches. Fold into bulgur.

3 Cut passionfruit in half. Place sieve over bowl of muesli and spoon passionfruit pulp and seeds into it. Press until juice has passed through sieve and only seeds are left behind. Discard seeds.

4 Add almond extract and more apple juice, if needed, for moist but not sloppy consistency. Keep covered in fridge until ready to eat, then serve topped with pomegranate seeds or blueberries, plus additional peach pieces. Muesli can be kept in refrigerator, tightly covered, for up to two days. Stir well before serving, and then add fresh fruit garnish.

PER SERVING: 394 calories, 8 g protein, 14 g total fat, 1 g saturated fat, 0 mg cholesterol, 60 g carbohydrates, 43 g sugar, 12 g fibre, 29 mg sodium

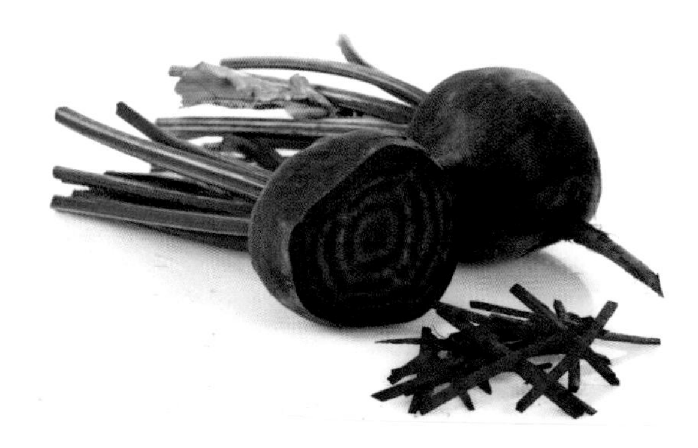

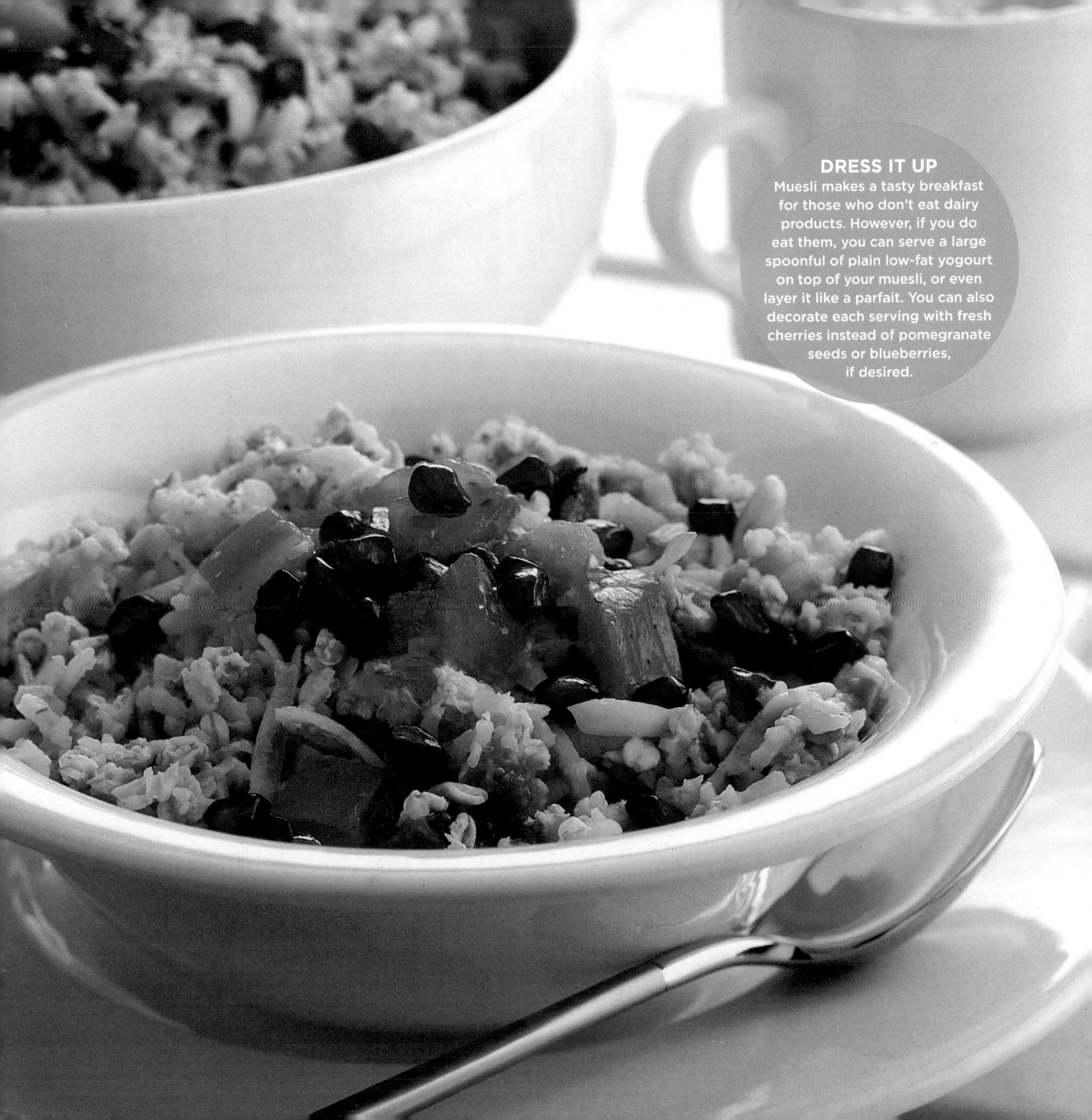

DRESS IT UP

Muesli makes a tasty breakfast for those who don't eat dairy products. However, if you do eat them, you can serve a large spoonful of plain low-fat yogourt on top of your muesli, or even layer it like a parfait. You can also decorate each serving with fresh cherries instead of pomegranate seeds or blueberries, if desired.

SHOPPING

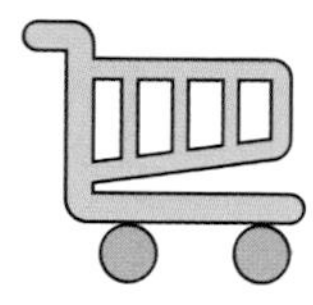

Are omega-3 eggs worth it?

Chances are you've already heard of omega-3 fatty acids. So what's all the fuss about? It's simple: Omega-3s are essential for your body—especially your brain—to function properly.

But in omega-3-fortified eggs, the benefits are all found in the yolk, something dieters tend to avoid. For your purposes, omega-3 eggs may not actually be worth the money.

If you're concerned that omelettes which contain mostly whites lack the fatty acid you want, just be sure to include fatty fish like salmon and tuna in your diet. They're great sources of omega 3s.

SPINACH AND GOAT CHEESE OMELETTE

SERVES 1

A folded omelette is one of the fastest protein-rich meals you can make. It is also an excellent strategy for healthy solo dining. Omelette filling options are limitless. (Check out the Vegetable-Cheddar Omelette on page 104 for another idea.) Improvise with whatever leftover cooked vegetables or ingredients you have on hand.

2 cups baby spinach, rinsed
2 tbsp crumbled goat cheese or feta cheese
1 tbsp chopped scallion
1 large egg
2 large egg whites
¼ tsp Tabasco sauce
Pinch of salt
Pinch of freshly ground black pepper
1 tsp olive oil

1 Bring about 25 cm of water to boil in large saucepan. Drop in spinach and cook just until wilted, or about 30 seconds. Drain, press out liquid and chop coarsely. (Alternatively, place spinach in microwave-safe bowl, cover with vented plastic wrap and microwave on high for 1 to 2 minutes.) Place spinach in small bowl. Stir in cheese and scallion.

2 Blend egg, egg whites, hot sauce, salt and pepper briskly with fork in medium bowl. Heat oil in an 18 to 25 cm non-stick skillet over medium-high heat until hot. Tilt skillet to swirl oil over surface. Pour in egg mixture. Immediately stir egg mixture with heat-resistant rubber spatula or fork for a few seconds. Then use spatula to push cooked portions at edges toward centre, tilting skillet to let uncooked egg mixture fill in areas around edges. Sprinkle spinach mixture over omelette. Continue to cook until almost set and bottom is golden. Cooking process should take about 1 minute.

3 Use spatula to fold one-third of omelette over the filling. Tip skillet and, using spatula as guide, slide omelette onto plate so that it lands, folded in thirds, seam-side down.

PER SERVING: 235 calories, 20 g protein, 4 g carbohydrates, 1 g fibre, 15 g total fat, 6 g saturated fat, 228 mg cholesterol, 471 mg sodium.

SEEING GREEN
Spinach may have been Popeye's favourite food, but other leafy greens, like kale and Swiss chard, are actually even healthier. Try them with eggs!

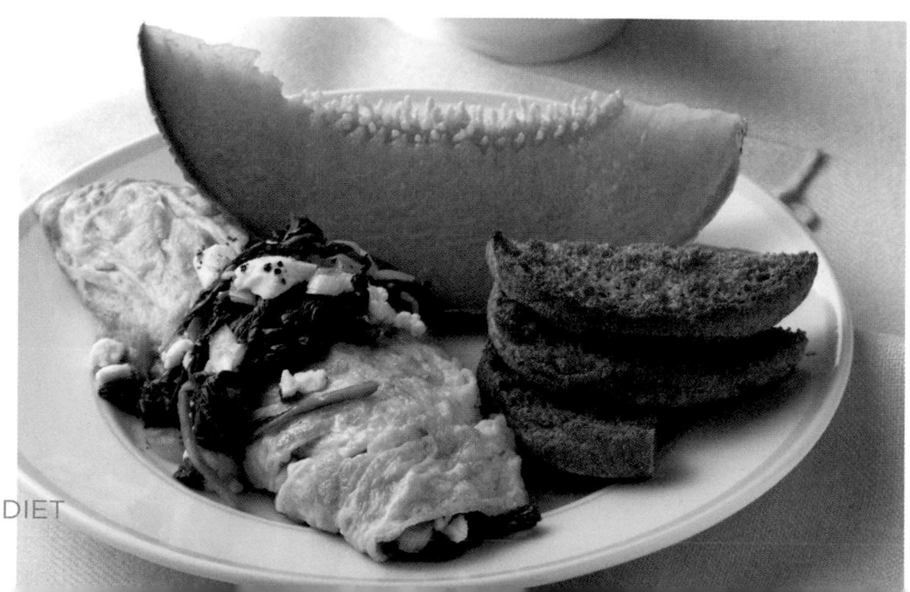

MULTI-GRAIN WAFFLES

SERVES 8

Most waffles are anything but diet-friendly, but here the weekend treats have been entirely reimagined using whole-wheat flour, oats and super-healthy wheat germ.

2 cups low-fat buttermilk
½ cup old-fashioned rolled oats
⅔ cup whole-wheat flour
⅔ cup all-purpose flour
¼ cup toasted wheat germ
1 ½ tsp baking powder
½ tsp baking soda
¼ tsp salt
1 tsp cinnamon
2 large eggs
¼ cup firmly packed brown sugar
1 tbsp canola oil
2 tsp vanilla extract
1 cup maple syrup, warmed
1 ½ cups sliced strawberries or blueberries

1 Mix buttermilk and oats in small bowl. Let stand for 15 minutes.

2 Whisk whole-wheat flour, all-purpose flour, wheat germ, baking powder, baking soda, salt and cinnamon in large bowl.

3 Whisk eggs, sugar, oil and vanilla in medium bowl. Add buttermilk mixture. Add mixture to flour mixture and mix with rubber spatula just until flour mixture is moistened.

4 Waffles: Coat waffle iron with cooking spray. Heat iron. Spoon in enough batter to cover three-quarters of surface, close iron, and cook until waffles are crisp and golden brown, or 4 to 5 minutes. Keep waffles warm in 200°F (90°C) oven while you finish cooking remaining batter.

5 Top with maple syrup and strawberries or blueberries. Wrap leftover waffles individually in plastic wrap and refrigerate for up to 2 days or freeze for up to 1 month. Reheat in toaster or toaster oven.

PER SERVING (2 WAFFLES): 292 calories, 8 g protein, 60 g carbohydrates, 3 g fibre, 3 g total fat, 1 g saturated fat, 56 mg cholesterol, 331 mg sodium.

VARIATION

Multi-Grain Pancakes
This batter produces equally great (and healthy!) pancakes.

Start by coating a large non-stick skillet with cooking spray. Heat over medium heat. Spoon about ¼ cup batter for each pancake into the skillet and cook until bottoms are golden and small bubbles start to form on top, about 3 minutes. Flip the pancakes and cook until browned and cooked through, 1 to 2 minutes. (Adjust the heat as necessary for even browning.) Keep the pancakes warm in a 200°F (90°C) oven while you finish cooking the remaining batter.

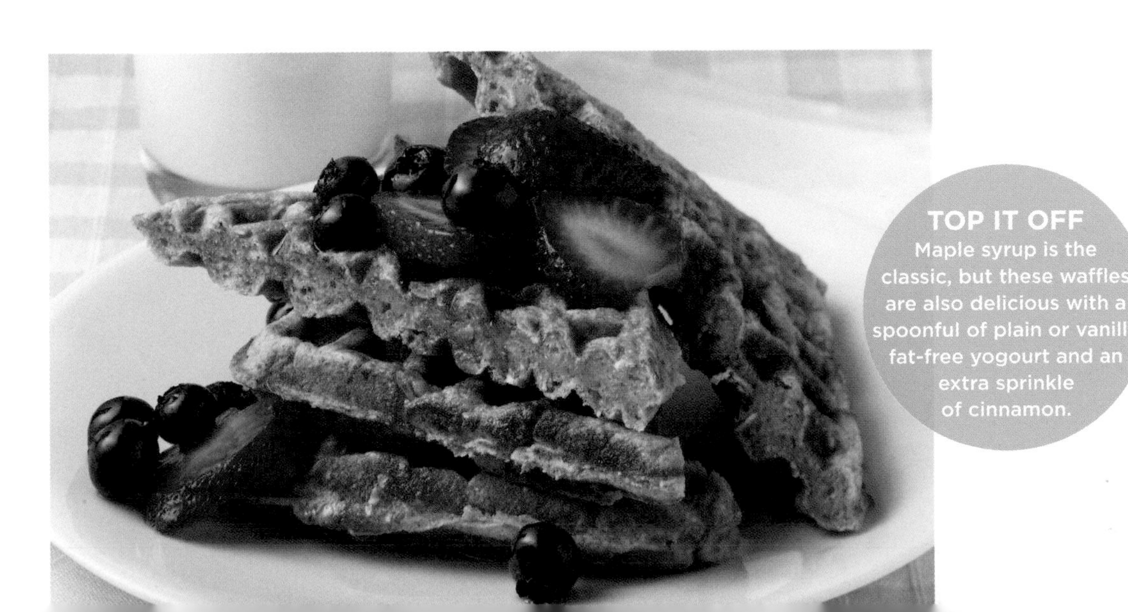

TOP IT OFF
Maple syrup is the classic, but these waffles are also delicious with a spoonful of plain or vanilla fat-free yogourt and an extra sprinkle of cinnamon.

EGGS BENEDICT

SERVES 4

This dish traditionally uses ham or bacon and a rich, butter-based hollandaise sauce. Here, a yogourt and chive hollandaise sauce contrasts with the richness of poached eggs and lean prosciutto, to make a lighter, but equally special version.

1 tsp vinegar
4 eggs
4 whole-wheat English muffins, halved
4 slices prosciutto, about 50 g in total, trimmed of all visible fat
pepper to taste
paprika to garnish
1 tbsp snipped fresh chives to garnish

HOLLANDAISE SAUCE
2 egg yolks
1 tsp Dijon mustard
150 g Greek-style yogourt
1 tbsp snipped fresh chives
pepper to taste

1 Hollandaise sauce: Whisk together egg yolks, mustard and yogourt in heatproof bowl. Set over saucepan of barely simmering water and cook for about 12 to 15 minutes, stirring constantly, until thick—sauce will actually become thinner before it starts to thicken. Stir in chives and season with pepper. Remove from heat and keep sauce warm over pan of hot water.

2 Half-fill frying pan with water. Bring to boil, then add vinegar. Reduce heat so water is just simmering gently, then carefully break eggs into water, one at a time. Poach for 3 to 4 minutes, spooning hot water over yolks toward end of cooking.

3 Meanwhile, preheat broiler. Lightly toast muffin halves for about 1 minute per side. Place one half on each of 4 warmed plates and top each with slice of prosciutto, crumpled slightly to fit. Season with pepper.

4 Using slotted spoon, remove poached eggs from pan, one at a time. Drain on paper towel. Place an egg on each prosciutto-topped muffin half.

5 Spoon the warm hollandaise sauce over the eggs, and sprinkle each serving with a pinch of paprika and chives. Serve immediately with the remaining toasted muffin halves.

PER SERVING: 291 calories, 19 g protein, 12 g total fat, 5 g saturated fat, 333 mg cholesterol, 25 g total carbohydrate, 5 g sugars, 3 g fibre, 590 mg sodium

VARIATION

Instead of chives, add 1 tbsp chopped fresh tarragon to the hollandaise, and garnish with sprigs of tarragon. You can also use thin slices of lean cooked ham instead of prosciutto.

VEGGIE SWAP
Don't eat meat? Slide some fresh, washed baby spinach or steamed asparagus onto the English muffins instead of prosciutto.

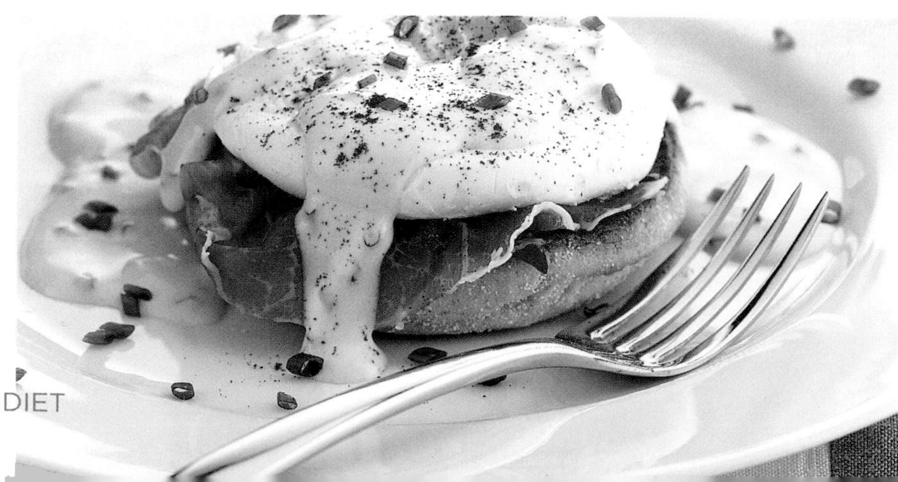

UPSIDE-DOWN NECTARINE MUFFINS

MAKES 12 MUFFINS

There is nothing ordinary about these muffins. A bit like individual upside-down cakes, they boast an irresistible caramelized fruit topping. They're tasty treats indeed, with the benefits of whole grains, stone fruit, nuts and cinnamon.

TOPPING

2 tbsp packed light brown sugar
¼ cup walnuts, chopped
340 g nectarines (about 3 medium), pitted and cut into 5 mm-thick wedges

MUFFINS

1 cup whole-wheat flour
1 cup all-purpose flour
1 ½ tsp baking powder
½ tsp baking soda
¼ tsp salt
1 ½ tsp ground cinnamon
½ tsp ground nutmeg
2 large eggs
½ cup packed light brown sugar
1 cup low-fat buttermilk
3 tbsp canola oil
1 tsp vanilla extract

1 Preheat oven to 400°F (200°C). Coat 12 standard-size (7 cm-by-3 cm) muffin cups with cooking spray.

2 To make topping: Sprinkle about ½ tsp brown sugar into each muffin cup and pat into even layer, then sprinkle about 1 tsp walnuts into each cup. Arrange 3 or 4 nectarine slices, slightly overlapping, over walnuts and brown sugar. Cover and set aside. Coarsely chop remaining nectarines (you should have about ¾ cup). Set aside.

3 To make muffins: In large bowl, whisk together whole-wheat flour, all-purpose flour, baking powder, baking soda, salt, cinnamon and nutmeg.

4 In medium bowl, whisk eggs and brown sugar until smooth. Whisk in buttermilk, oil and vanilla. Add to flour mixture and mix with rubber spatula just until dry ingredients are moistened, then fold in reserved nectarines. Spoon batter into muffin cups. They will seem quite full, but nectarine wedges will collapse during baking.

5 Bake until muffins are lightly browned and tops spring back when touched lightly, or 18 to 22 minutes. Immediately loosen edges and carefully turn the muffins out onto wire rack. Replace any stray nectarine slices and spoon on any walnut pieces remaining in muffin cups. Let cool slightly before serving.

PER SERVING (1 MUFFIN): 202 calories, 5 g protein, 32 g carbohydrates, 2 g fibre, 6 g total fat, 1 g saturated fat, 41 g cholesterol, 153 mg sodium.

HOW TO FREEZE FRUIT

There's nothing like fresh, in-season stone fruit—but sadly, Canada doesn't have an endless summer. During nectarine season, make the best of your farmers' market steals by freezing your finds. Wash and dry each fruit. Slice each fruit into small wedges or chunks. Cover a baking sheet with wax paper and line up the fruit pieces on top, being careful not to let them touch. Pop it in the freezer. The next morning, remove the fruit pieces from the tray and store in a resealable freezer bag or airtight container.

FRUIT FIX
You can also substitute 340 g plums or apricots for the nectarines.

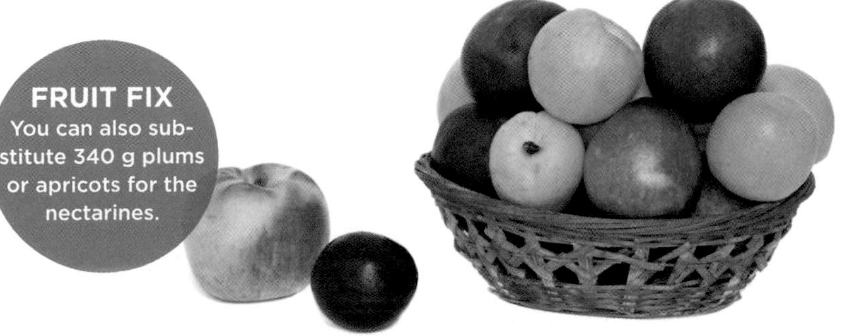

lunches

FENNEL LOVE

Fennel has a way of making other flavours seem just a little more complex, and it contains significant amounts of vitamin C and potassium.

RAINBOW SALAD

SERVES 4

This simple salad has wonderful flavours and colours. If you've never tried fennel before, this is a good place to start: It tastes similar to black licorice but has the crunch of celery. Use the stem of the broccoli in this dish—it adds a different flavour and even more crunch than the florets.

SALAD

½ head green leaf lettuce, chopped
½ medium fennel bulb, thinly julienned
1 cup red cabbage, thinly julienned
1 medium tomato, seeds removed, thinly julienned
½ yellow pepper, thinly julienned
½ cup red onion, thinly julienned
½ cup broccoli stems, peeled and thinly julienned
½ cup grated Edam cheese

VINAIGRETTE

¼ cup extra-virgin olive oil
3 tbsp fresh lemon juice
1 tsp Dijon mustard
½ tsp lemon zest
1 tsp honey

1 In medium bowl, toss together salad ingredients. In small bowl, whisk together vinaigrette ingredients.

2 Divide salad among 4 plates and drizzle with vinaigrette.

PER SERVING: 224 calories, 5 g protein, 16 g total fat, 3 g saturated fat, 16 g carbohydrates, 5 g fibre, 6 mg cholesterol, 580 mg sodium.

SHOPPING

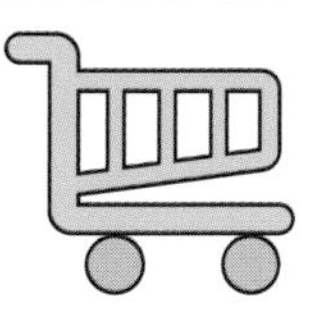

How to buy the best cabbage

Cabbage, with its many layers, can seem a little mysterious to the casual grocery shopper. How do you know if you're choosing a good one? Are all cabbages created equal?

The fastest way to tell if a cabbage is good is by its weight. Choose cabbages that seem heavy for their size, with smooth, shiny outside leaves, and you'll get a lot of bang for your buck—one head of cabbage goes a long way!

RADISH AND CUCUMBER SALAD

SERVES 4

This fresh-tasting salad is tasty and pretty, with its delicate flavours and colours. Radishes have cancer-fighting properties, while cucumbers contain vitamins C and A, as well as folic acid.

SALAD
1 large white (daikon) radish, peeled
Salt
1 medium cucumber
16 medium red radishes, thinly sliced
½ cup chopped fresh parsley
½ cup chopped chives
Mung bean sprouts, for garnish

VINAIGRETTE
1 tbsp white wine vinegar
1 tbsp lemon juice
3 tbsp canola or peanut oil
Salt and freshly ground black pepper

1 Use vegetable peeler or sharp knife to cut white radish into very thin curls. Place in colander, sprinkle with salt and leave to drain for 15 minutes. Rinse and pat dry with paper towel.

2 Peel away thin strips along the length of cucumber to create a striped effect. Slice cucumber very thinly, and arrange on serving platter or individual plates. Place red and white radishes on top of cucumber slices.

3 To make vinaigrette: Whisk vinegar, lemon juice, oil, salt and pepper to taste in a bowl. Drizzle over radishes. Top with chives and mung bean sprouts.

PER SERVING: 149 calories, 2 g protein, 14 g total fat, 1 g saturated fat, 0 mg cholesterol, 4 g carbohydrates, 3 g fibre.

4 more cucumber salads

- **Chop cucumber into matchsticks. Serve with ripe mango and red pepper, plus lime juice, olive oil and honey vinaigrette.**
- **Top round slices of cucumber with salt, dill and plain yogourt.**
- **For a refreshing summer salad, toss cucumber slices with small wedges of nectarine and plum, plus balsamic-olive oil dressing.**
- **Slice cucumbers into thin slices and arrange decoratively on a plate. Sprinkle generously with seasoned rice vinegar. Even the kids will love the flavour.**

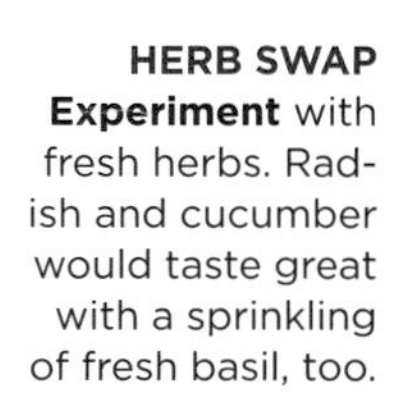
HERB SWAP
Experiment with fresh herbs. Radish and cucumber would taste great with a sprinkling of fresh basil, too.

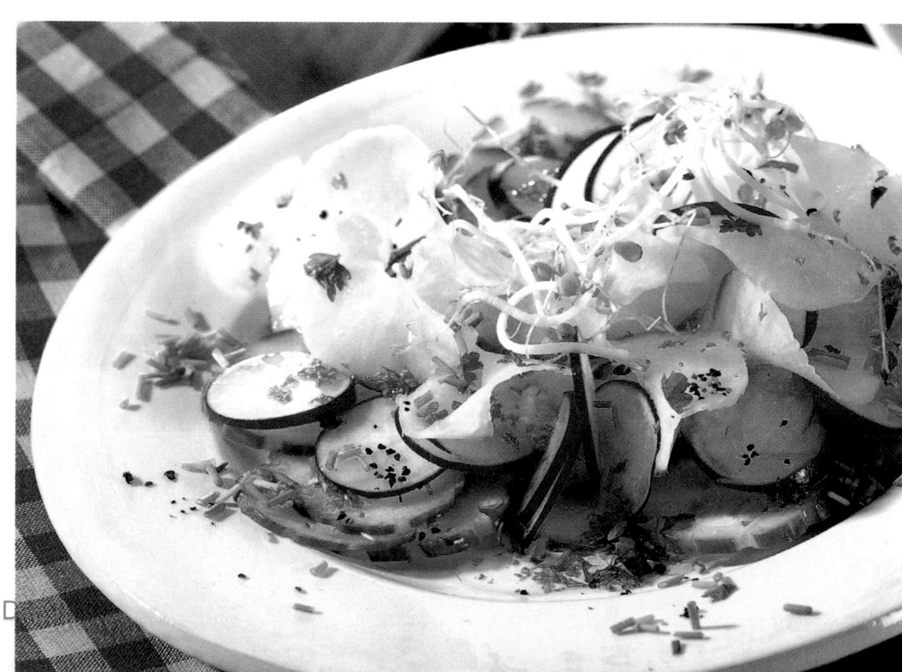

RADICCHIO AND FENNEL SALAD WITH ORANGES SERVES 4

The bitter taste of dark red radicchio complements the aniseed flavour of pale green fennel and the sweetness of oranges.

1 large head treviso radicchio
2 large oranges
1 large or 2 small fennel bulbs (about 1 kg total) with leafy fronds
2 small white onions
4 tbsp extra-virgin olive oil
1 tbsp white wine vinegar
1 tbsp lemon juice
1 sprig rosemary, leaves finely chopped
Salt and freshly ground black pepper
1 cup pitted black olives

1 Line individual plates with radicchio leaves. Peel and segment oranges.

2 Use vegetable peeler to slice fennel bulb into thin strips. Slice onions into thin rings.

3 Whisk oil, vinegar, lemon juice and rosemary in bowl until combined. Season with salt and pepper to taste.

4 Finely chop some fennel fronds. Layer fennel, oranges and onions onto radicchio. Drizzle with vinaigrette. Top with fennel fronds and olives.

PER SERVING: 272 calories, 4 g protein, 19 g total fat, 3 g saturated fat, 0 mg cholesterol, 22 g carbohydrates, 7 g fibre.

COOKING TIP:

This salad looks great if the fennel bulbs are cut into thin slices lengthwise using a vegetable peeler. First, trim the stalk so that a small amount remains. This way, the individual layers of fennel will not fall apart during slicing.

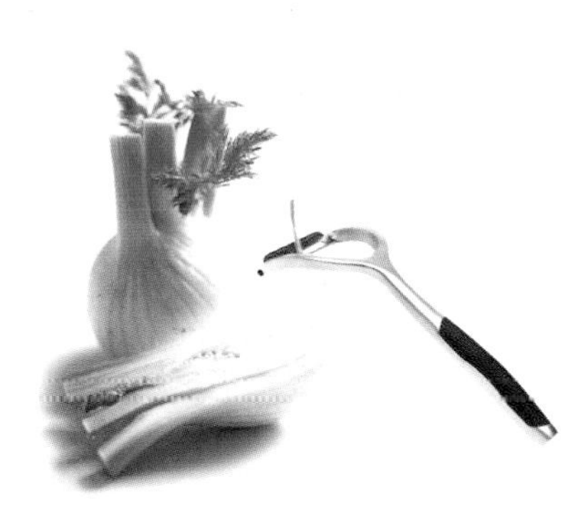

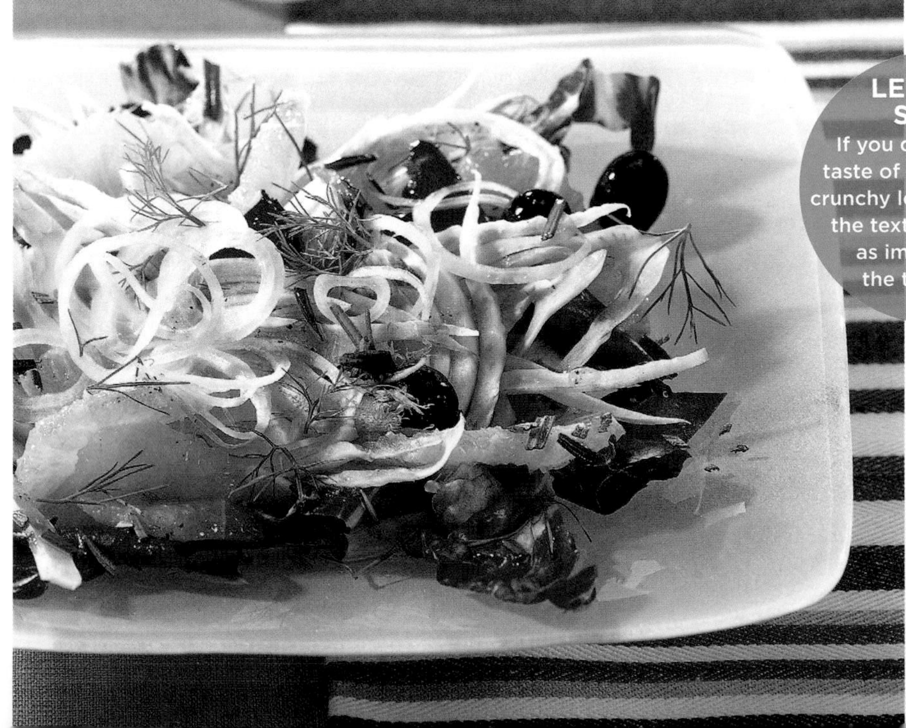

LETTUCE SWAP

If you don't like the taste of radicchio, any crunchy lettuce will do—the texture is almost as important as the taste here.

SMOKED HADDOCK AND CANNELLINI BEAN SOUP

SERVES 4

Zucchini, celery and dill combine to add depth to this swiftly prepared Italian-style dish using fresh and pantry ingredients. Serve with a slice of crusty bread.

1 tbsp extra-virgin olive oil
1 onion, chopped
1 celery stick, chopped
2 small zucchini, chopped
2 ½ cups fish or chicken stock
175 g smoked haddock fillet, skinned and diced
2 cans (398 mL each) cannellini beans, rinsed
1 tbsp chopped fresh dill

1 In saucepan, heat oil and fry onion, celery and zucchini until softened but not browned.

2 Add stock and bring to boil, then stir in haddock fillet and seasoning. Cover and simmer gently for 4 to 5 minutes, or until fish flakes easily.

3 Add beans and dill. Stir, then heat until almost boiling. Serve in wide bowls.

PER SERVING: 190 calories, 19 g protein, 2 g total fat, 0.2 g saturated fat, 24 g carbohydrates.

Try this:

● ● ● BEAN AND HALLOUMI SOUP

For a vegetarian version of the Smoked Haddock Soup, omit the fish and use 2 ½ cups vegetable stock for the base. Instead of the zucchini, dice and fry 1 small fennel bulb with the other vegetables, and simmer in the stock until tender. Mash the cannellini beans lightly with a fork before adding to the soup for a creamier, slightly thicker texture. Finally, stir in 175 g diced halloumi cheese and heat until boiling.

You can also grill the halloumi: Cut the cheese into cubes and thread on to bamboo skewers that have been soaked in water for 15 minutes. Brush with oil and grill until golden, then rest on the rim of the soup bowls to serve.

BEAN AND BARLEY SOUP

SERVES 8

A chunky soup like this one, which is big on veggies and complex carbohydrates like barley and beans, provides maximum satisfaction for relatively few calories.

7 cups low-sodium chicken or vegetable stock
6 garlic cloves, peeled and crushed
2 sprigs fresh rosemary
¼ tsp crushed red pepper
1 can (398 mL) red kidney beans, rinsed
2 tsp extra-virgin olive oil
1 cup chopped onion (1 medium)
1 cup diced peeled carrots (3–4 medium)
1 stalk celery, diced
1 can (398 mL) diced tomatoes
1 cup quick-cooking barley
10 cups baby spinach, washed
Freshly ground black pepper to taste
½ cup grated parmesan cheese

1 Bring stock to boil in large saucepan. Add garlic, rosemary and crushed red pepper. Partially cover saucepan and simmer over medium-low heat for 15 minutes to intensify flavour. Strain stock through sieve into large bowl.

2 Mash 1 cup kidney beans in small bowl with fork. Set whole and mashed beans aside. Heat oil in 4 to 6 L soup pot over medium heat. Add onion, carrots and celery. Cook, stirring often, until softened, 3 to 4 minutes. Pour in infused stock. Add tomatoes, barley and reserved mashed and whole beans. Bring to simmer, stirring occasionally. Reduce heat to medium-low, cover, and cook at a lively simmer until barley is almost tender, or about 15 minutes.

3 Stir in spinach. Cover and cook until spinach has wilted and barley is tender, or 3 to 5 minutes. Season with ground pepper. Top each serving with 1 tbsp parmesan cheese.

PER SERVING: 197 calories, 12 g protein, 30 g carbohydrates, 7 g fibre, 4 g total fat, 1 g saturated fat, 4 mg cholesterol, 757 mg sodium.

GRILLED CHICKEN SALAD WITH ORANGES

SERVES 4

Slices of grilled chicken transform a fruity Mediterranean salad into a satisfying hot-weather dinner that's packed with flavour.

⅓ cup orange juice
2 tbsp lemon juice
3 tbsp extra-virgin olive oil
1 tbsp Dijon mustard
2 garlic cloves, minced
¼ tsp salt, or to taste
Freshly ground pepper to taste
450 g boneless skinless chicken breasts, trimmed
¼ cup pistachios or slivered almonds
8 cups mesclun salad mix, rinsed and dried
½ cup thinly sliced red onion
2 medium oranges, peeled, quartered, and sliced

1 Place orange juice, lemon juice, oil, mustard, garlic, salt and pepper in small bowl or jar with a tight-fitting lid, and whisk or shake to blend. Set aside ⅓ cup of dressing for salad and 3 tbsp for basting.

2 Place remaining dressing in shallow glass dish or resealable plastic bag. Add chicken and turn to coat. Cover or seal and marinate in refrigerator for at least 20 minutes or up to 2 hours.

3 Lightly oil grill rack by rubbing with crumpled, oil-soaked paper towel (use tongs to hold paper towel). Preheat grill to medium. Remove chicken from marinade and discard marinade. Grill chicken 10 to 15 cm from heat source, basting cooked sides with 3 tbsp reserved dressing, until no longer pink in centre, and instant-read thermometer inserted in thickest part registers 170°F (75°C), or 4 to 6 minutes per side. Transfer to cutting board and let stand for 5 minutes.

4 Meanwhile, toast almonds or pistachios in small dry skillet over medium-low heat, stirring constantly until light golden, or 2 to 3 minutes. Transfer to bowl and let cool.

5 Place salad mix and onion in large bowl. Toss with dressing reserved for salad. Divide salad among 4 plates. Slice chicken and distribute over salads. Scatter orange slices over top and sprinkle with toasted nuts.

PER SERVING: 331 calories, 30 g protein, 18 g carbohydrates, 5 g fibre, 16 g total fat, 3 g saturated fat, 68 mg cholesterol, 290 mg sodium.

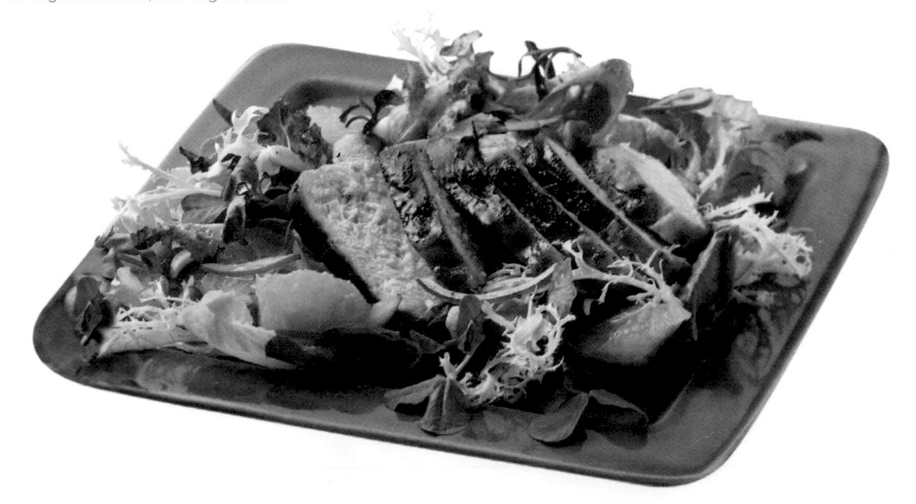

SAFE MARINADES

When marinating meat, fish or poultry, remember to set aside a few tablespoons of the marinade beforehand for basting. Do not contaminate cooked food with marinade that has been in contact with raw meat, or you could risk serious food poisoning.

SUMMER BEEF SALAD

SERVES 4

Griddling lean, tender steak gives it a smoky flavour that enhances a refreshing salad of crisp vegetables in a walnut and balsamic dressing. Enjoy with warm, crusty French bread.

½ tsp salt
1 small red onion, halved and thinly sliced
100 g radishes, sliced
1 thick-cut lean rump steak, about 375 g, trimmed of fat
1 tbsp extra-virgin olive oil
¼ tsp dried mixed herbs
2 tbsp walnut oil
1 tbsp balsamic vinegar
4 celery sticks, sliced on the diagonal
125 g bag of arugula or mixed salad greens

1 Stir salt into bowl of cold water until dissolved. Add onion and radish slices and leave to soak while cooking steak. (This will take away some of the heat and sharpness, and prevent the radishes from discolouring).

2 Heat ridged griddle or non-stick frying pan until hot. Pat steak dry with paper towel. Rub steak on both sides with 2 tsp of olive oil, then season with herbs and some ground black pepper. Cook steak for 2 ½ to 3 ½ minutes on each side, depending on whether you like it medium-rare or medium. Transfer steak to board and let rest.

3 Whisk remaining olive oil, walnut oil and vinegar together. Cut steak into slices about 5 mm thick. Pour any juices that have collected into the dressing.

4 Drain onion and radishes well, put into large bowl, then add dressing with celery and beef. Gently toss everything together. Divide arugula or salad greens among four individual plates, then spoon over beef mixture. Serve immediately.

PER SERVING: 207 calories, 20 g protein, 12 g total fat, 2 g saturated fat, 4 g carbohydrates.

Try this:

Instead of arugula or mixed greens, use chicory leaves and thinly sliced fennel. In place of the radishes, use sliced red apple.

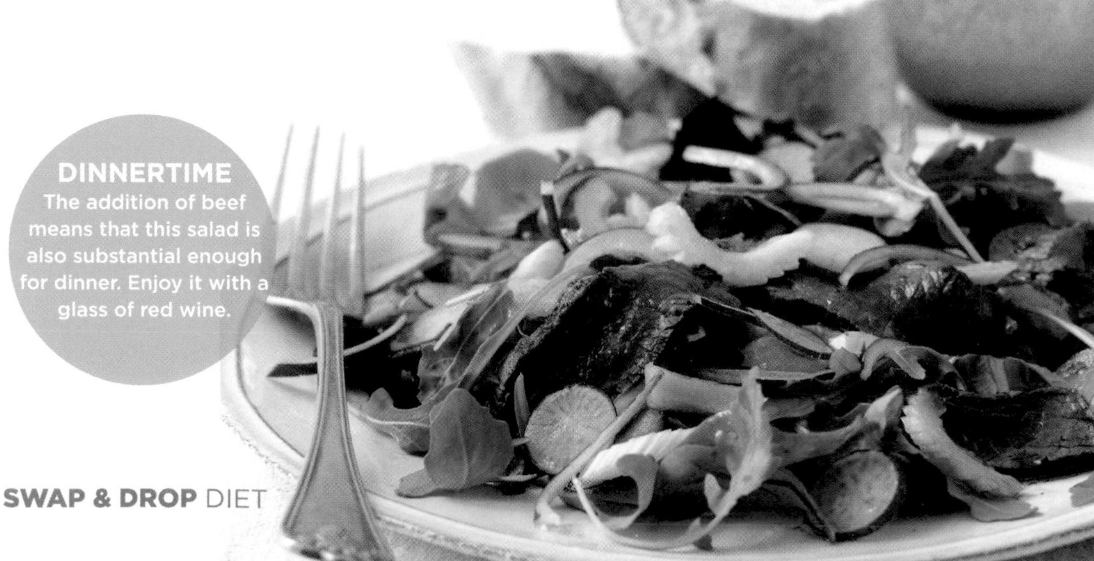

DINNERTIME
The addition of beef means that this salad is also substantial enough for dinner. Enjoy it with a glass of red wine.

CURRIED RED LENTIL SOUP

SERVES 8

You may think of lentils as something to store in the back of your pantry until a day when you have lots of time to wait for them to cook. But lentils, especially the red variety, are surprisingly convenient. They require no presoaking and cook up quickly: Red lentils cook in just 20 minutes, brown lentils in about 30 minutes.

- 2 tsp canola oil
- 2 cups chopped onions (2 medium)
- 4 garlic cloves, minced
- 4–5 tsp curry powder
- 1 ½ cups red lentils, rinsed and picked over
- 6 cups low-sodium chicken or vegetable stock
- ¾ cup water
- 2 tbsp tomato paste
- ¼ tsp cinnamon
- 2 tbsp lemon juice
- ¼ tsp salt, or to taste
- Freshly ground pepper to taste
- ½ cup nonfat plain yogourt
- ¼ cup chopped scallion greens

1 Heat oil in 4–6 L soup pot over medium heat. Add onion and cook, stirring frequently, until softened, 2 to 3 minutes. Add garlic and curry powder. Cook, stirring, for 30 seconds. Add lentils and stir to coat. Add stock, water, tomato paste, and cinnamon. Bring to simmer, reduce heat to low, cover, and simmer until lentils are very tender, about 20 minutes.

2 In batches, transfer soup to food processor or blender and purée. (Use caution when blending hot liquids.) Return purée to soup pot and heat through. Season with lemon juice, salt and pepper. Garnish each serving with dollop of yogourt and sprinkling of scallion greens.

PER SERVING (1 CUP): 187 calories, 14 g protein, 29 g carbohydrates, 12 g fiber, 2 g total fat, 1 g saturated fat, 4 mg cholesterol, 199 mg sodium.

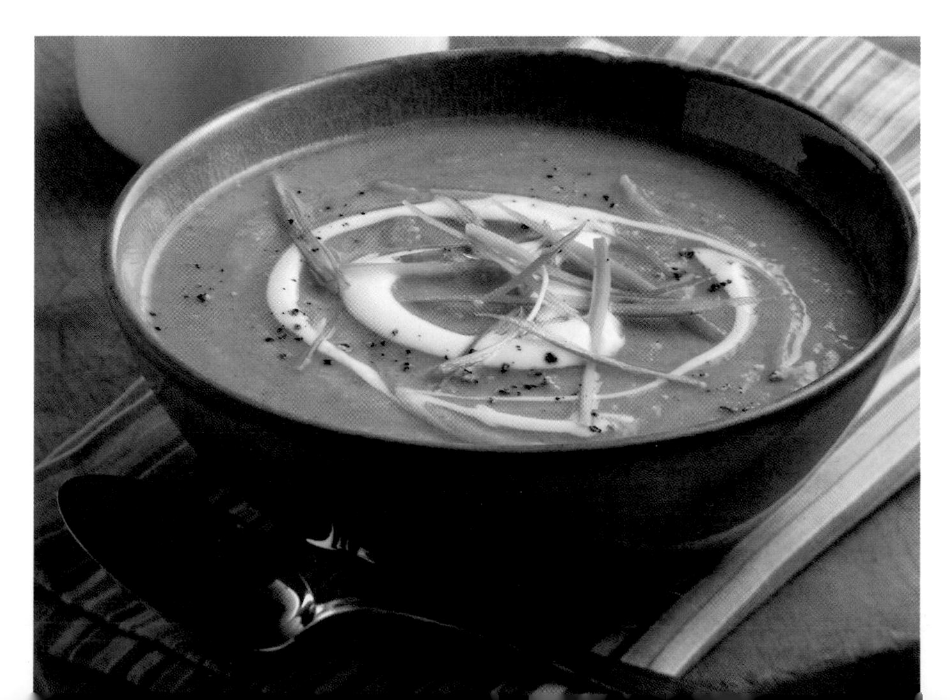

LENTIL LOVE

Lentils aren't just cheap and delicious—they're also heart-healthy. Studies have found that people who eat legumes regularly have a lower risk of heart disease than people who don't.

ANY LEFT? This lentil soup makes an especially good leftover. It should keep well in the fridge for 2–3 days.

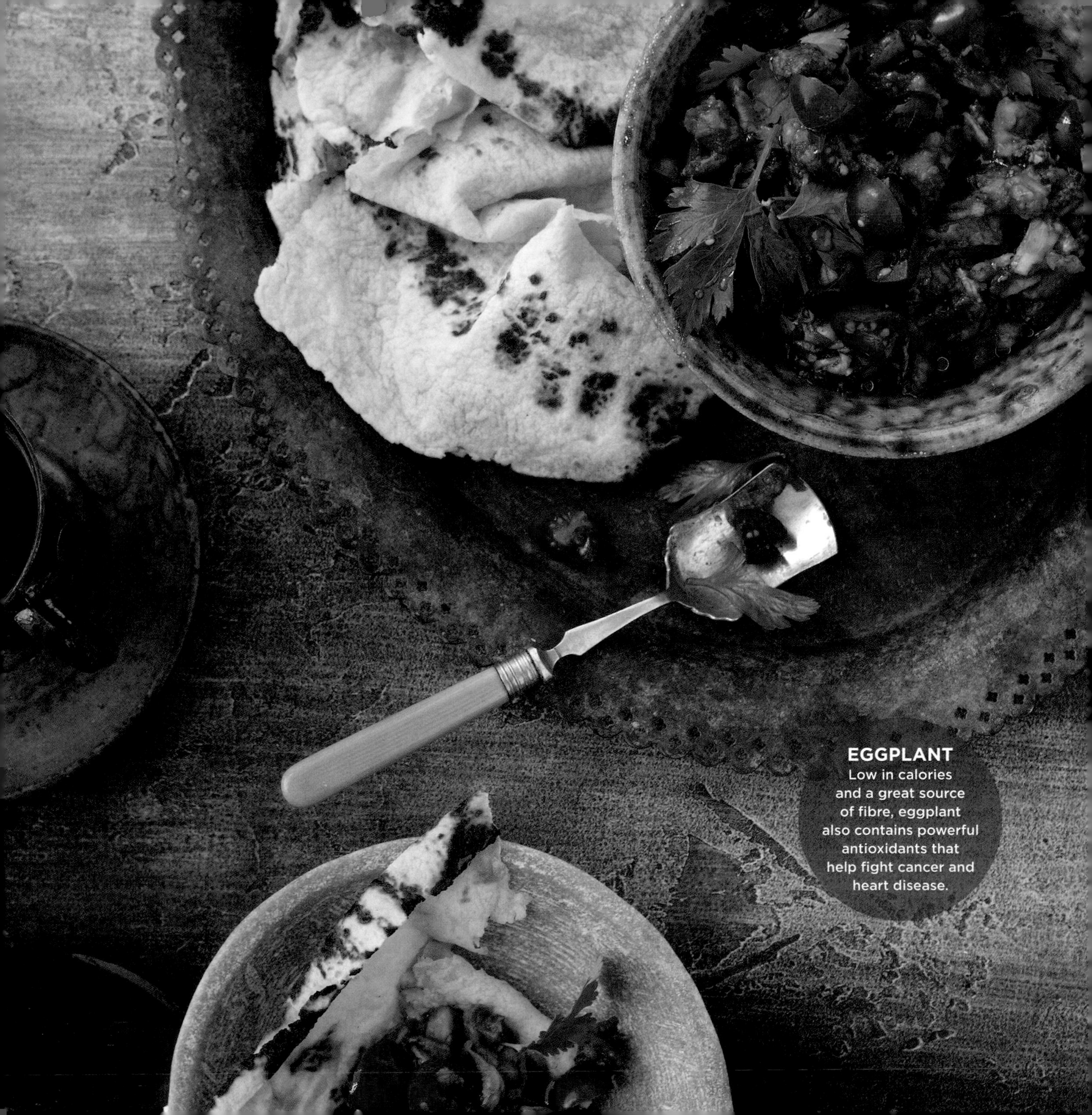

EGGPLANT
Low in calories and a great source of fibre, eggplant also contains powerful antioxidants that help fight cancer and heart disease.

EGGPLANT & TOMATO SALAD

SERVES 4

This richly flavoured salad can be served as an appetizer with flatbread, or as a side dish with grilled meat or fish.

2 small eggplants
¼ cup extra-virgin olive oil
2 garlic cloves, peeled and chopped
4 medium tomatoes, chopped
½ tsp paprika
1 tsp ground cumin
1 tbsp fresh lemon juice
8 cherry tomatoes, cut into quarters
1 handful each parsley and cilantro, chopped
10 black or green olives, pitted and chopped

1 Preheat oven to 425°F (220°C). Place whole eggplants on baking tray and bake for 30 minutes, or until wrinkly all over and very soft to touch. Remove from oven and place in a colander.

2 When cool enough to handle, peel off skin and, using of kitchen scissors, cut flesh into small pieces. With back of spoon, press flesh into colander to get rid of excess liquid.

3 Heat oil in medium saucepan over low heat and add garlic, chopped medium tomatoes, paprika and cumin. Cook about 20 minutes, remove and allow to cool.

4 Add lemon juice to cooked tomato mixture and season to taste with sea salt and freshly ground black pepper. Stir eggplant into tomato mixture, then spoon into a wide dish and top with cherry tomatoes, fresh herbs and olives.

PER SERVING: 218 calories, 4 g protein, 15 g total fat, 2 g saturated fat, 21 g carbohydrates, 10 g fibre, 0 mg cholesterol, 82 mg sodium.

SPINACH, GRAPEFRUIT AND AVOCADO SALAD

SERVES 4

Juicy grapefruit contrasts beautifully with buttery avocado and crisp spinach.

2 pink grapefruit
1 tbsp white wine vinegar or rice vinegar
¼ cup finely chopped shallot
2 tsp poppy seeds
1 tsp each, honey and Dijon mustard
3 tbsp extra-virgin olive oil
Salt and freshly ground pepper to taste
8 cups baby spinach, rinsed and dried
1 cup sliced radishes (1 bunch)
2 avocados, peeled, pitted, and sliced

1 Place sieve over medium bowl. Using sharp knife, remove skin and white pith from grapefruit. Working over sieve, cut grapefruit segments from membrane, letting segments collect in sieve and juices collect in bowl. When all segments are removed, squeeze membrane to extract as much juice as possible.

2 Place ¼ cup grapefruit juice in small bowl. Add vinegar, shallot, poppy seeds, honey, mustard, oil, salt and pepper. Whisk to blend.

3 Just before serving, place spinach and radishes in large bowl. Toss with half of grapefruit juice dressing. Divide salad among 4 plates. Strew avocado slices and grapefruit segments over salads and drizzle with remaining dressing. One serving is 2 cups.

PER SERVING: 326 calories, 4 g protein, 29 g carbohydrates, 10 g fibre, 25 g total fat, 3 g saturated fat, 0 mg cholesterol, 416 mg sodium.

3 more avocado ideas

- **Serve avocado slices with underripe mango cut into matchsticks, a lime and olive oil dressing, and half a finely sliced chili.**
- **Spread half an avocado over 2 slices of whole-wheat toast, and top with canned sardines—weird but delicious!**
- **Avocado and smoked salmon: perfect. They balance each other nicely in a salad or on a sandwich.**

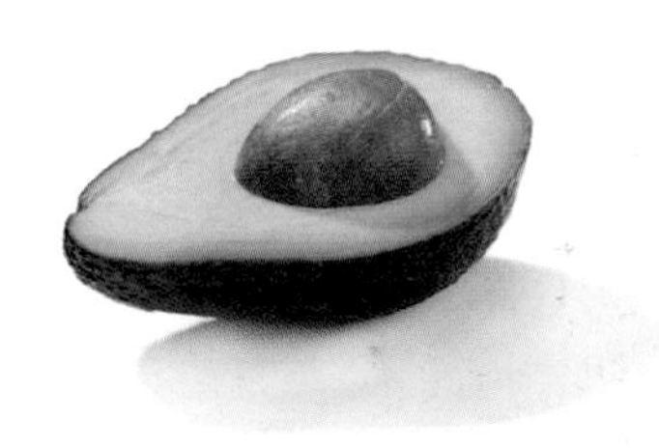

SHOPPING

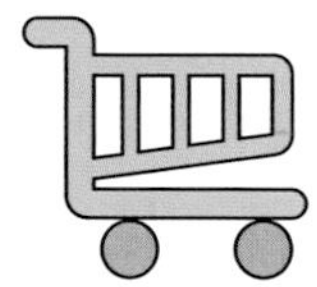

How to shop for feta

Greek feta, Canadian feta—what's the difference? The main divide is between cheese made with goat or sheep milk (or a combination of the two), and that made with cow milk. Purists insist that only Greek feta made with sheep or goat milk is any good, but that can be pricey. Canadian feta is still delicious—just try to find one that isn't made with cow's milk, for the most authentic flavour.

SUGAR SNAP PEAS WITH GRAPES AND FETA

SERVES 4

The sweet flavour of sugar snap peas goes well with the juicy taste of grapes and the salty feta in this salad. Sugar snaps are packed with vitamins, and are both heart-healthy and good for your bones.

Grated zest and juice of 1 small lemon
½ tsp superfine sugar
½ tsp Dijon mustard
Salt and freshly ground black pepper
1 tbsp extra-virgin olive oil
300 g sugar snap peas
250 g seedless black grapes, halved
250 g feta, thinly sliced
50 g arugula, shredded
175 g baby spinach leaves

1 Place lemon zest, juice, sugar, mustard and generous seasoning of salt and pepper in serving bowl. Whisk until sugar and salt have dissolved completely. Whisk in oil.

2 Cut sugar snap peas in half crosswise, leaving small ones whole. Bring large saucepan of water to boil. Add peas and bring water back to boil. Drain peas immediately and refresh under cold running water. Add to serving bowl. Turn to coat with dressing.

3 Add grapes, feta, arugula and spinach. Mix again gently to coat with dressing.

PER SERVING: 303 calories, 15 g protein, 21 g total fat, 10 g saturated fat, 43 mg cholesterol, 15 g carbohydrates, 3 g fibre.

TASTE TEST
Fond of stronger tasting lettuce? If so, feel free to use only arugula, or even add vibrant radicchio for an extra flavour and colour boost.

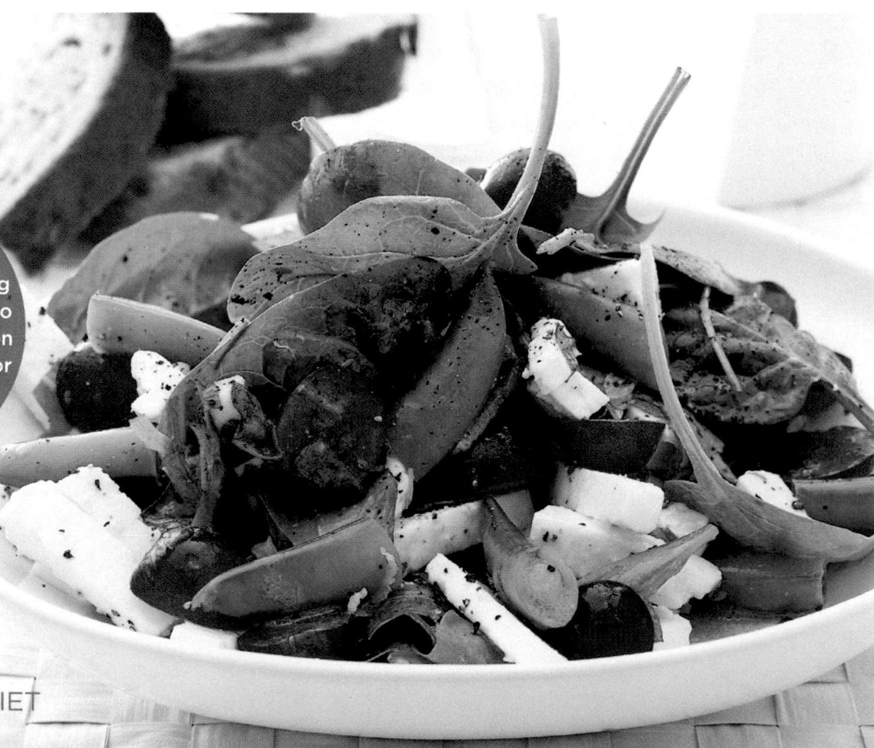

RICE SALAD WITH GINGER SOY DRESSING

SERVES 4

Basmati rice is named after a Hindu word meaning "fragrant." Its tasty nut-like flavour provides a delicious base for this zesty salad.

SALAD
$\frac{3}{4}$ cup basmati or other fragrant rice
$\frac{1}{2}$ tsp salt
125 g fresh baby corn (about 10)
150 g snow peas
1 medium red bell pepper
3 scallions, finely chopped
1 can (190 g) bamboo shoots, drained
4 tbsp roasted cashews

DRESSING
1 tbsp finely grated fresh ginger
3 tbsp rice vinegar
2 tbsp soy sauce
2 tbsp sunflower or peanut oil
1 tbsp medium-hot mango chutney

1 Combine rice, 1 cup water and salt in saucepan and bring to boil. Half-cover rice and cook over low heat 20 to 25 minutes. Remove from heat. Leave to cool. Loosen rice occasionally with fork.

2 Bring pan of lightly salted water to boil. Blanch corn 3 minutes and snow peas 1 minute. Plunge into iced water to stop cooking. Drain, then leave to cool.

3 Halve red pepper and cut into narrow strips. Cut snow peas and corn in half. Mix rice and all salad vegetables in a large bowl.

4 To make ginger-soy dressing, combine ginger, vinegar, soy sauce, oil and chutney in bowl. (If chutney contains large pieces of mango, break up with fork before adding.) Stir to combine.

5 Stir dressing into rice salad. Arrange salad on serving plates and sprinkle with cashews.

PER SERVING: 331 calories, 8 g protein, 16 g total fat, 2 g saturated fat, 0 mg cholesterol, 39 g carbohydrates, 4 g fibre.

VARIATION

For an extra-healthy take on this salad, swap basmati rice for brown rice. It's more wholesome than white rice, but because it takes a long time to prepare, you'll need to plan ahead—factor in around 45 minutes for the rice to cook completely.

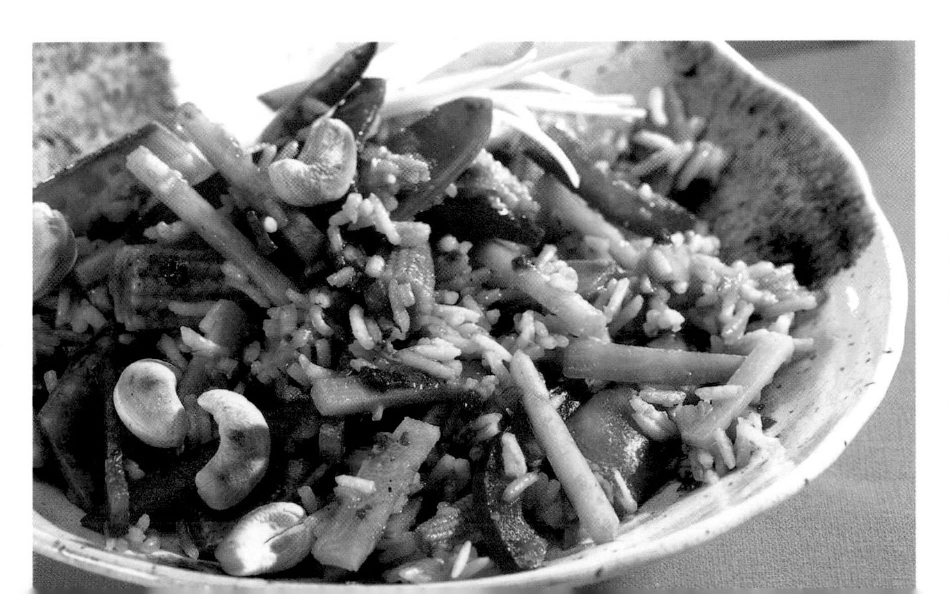

SWITCH IT UP
Love rice salads? They're easy to customize. Throw in whatever fresh vegetables you have handy, plus nuts or cooked chickpeas.

COUSCOUS SALAD WITH CHICKPEAS

SERVES 4

This salad is easy and quick to prepare—especially when you use instant couscous. This salad makes the best of juicy plum tomatoes, filling sausage and chickpeas.

SALAD
1 1/3 cups instant couscous
1/2 tsp salt
4 plum tomatoes
2 scallions
1/2 cup finely chopped fresh flat-leaf parsley
1 can (540 mL) chickpeas, rinsed and drained
200 g garlic sausage, sliced into small cubes

VINAIGRETTE
4 tbsp extra-virgin olive oil
1 tbsp red wine vinegar
3 tbsp lemon juice
1 clove garlic, crushed
1 tsp ground cumin
1 tsp ground sweet paprika
Salt and freshly ground black pepper

1 Bring 1 cup water to boil in a medium saucepan. Remove from heat. Stir in couscous and salt and leave to absorb liquid 20 minutes. Leave to cool.

2 Halve and core tomatoes and dice. Slice scallions into rings.

3 Vinaigrette: Whisk oil, vinegar, 2 tbsp lemon juice, garlic, cumin and paprika in large bowl. Add salt and pepper to taste. Stir parsley, couscous, chickpeas, tomatoes and scallions into vinaigrette.

4 Just before serving, taste salad and season with salt, pepper and remaining 1 tbsp lemon juice. Stir in cubes of sausage.

PER SERVING: 420 calories, 13 g protein, 32 g total fat, 8 g saturated fat, 22 mg cholesterol, 20 g carbohydrates, 4 g fibre.

Try this:

COUSCOUS SALAD WITH TUNA

1 Prepare 1 1/3 cups couscous as in main recipe. Halve 2 green peppers and cut into strips. Finely dice 1 red onion. Cut 2 zucchini into thin strips. Mix all ingredients in a bowl.

2 Whisk 3 tbsp olive oil, 3 tbsp lemon juice, 1 clove garlic (crushed), 1/2 tsp ground sweet paprika and salt and pepper to taste. Stir into couscous salad. Add 1 tbsp chopped fresh mint leaves. Stir in a drained can of flaked tuna.

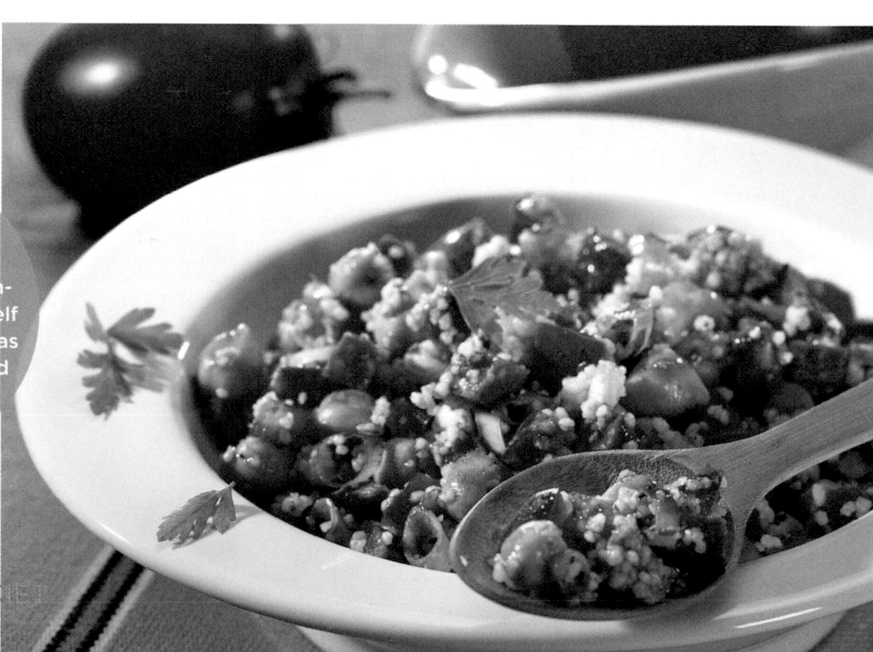

VEGGIE SWAP
Don't eat meat? This salad is still great without it—just help yourself to a few more chickpeas for added protein, and you're good to go.

TABBOULEH WITH ROMAINE

SERVES 4

This is a variation on the classic colourful Lebanese salad. For added health benefits, use twice the amount of parsley in place of the lettuce strips.

1 cup instant bulgur or couscous
2 medium tomatoes, finely diced
3 small Lebanese cucumbers, finely diced
4 scallions, sliced
2 cups finely chopped fresh flat-leaf parsley
1 1/2 cups finely chopped fresh mint
4 tbsp extra-virgin olive oil
6 tbsp lemon juice
Salt and freshly ground black pepper
Romaine lettuce leaves, for serving
1 heart of Romaine lettuce, cut into strips
Mint and cilantro sprigs, for garnish
1 large tomato, cut into wedges, for garnish

1 Place bulgur in pan with 2 cups water. Bring to boil. Remove from heat; leave 20 minutes to absorb liquid. Fluff with a fork.

2 Combine bulgur, tomatoes, cucumbers, scallions, parsley and mint in bowl. Whisk oil and 4 tbsp lemon juice, then add salt and pepper to taste. Pour over salad and toss to combine. Let sit 30 minutes.

3 Arrange lettuce leaves on large platter. Season salad to taste with salt and remaining 2 tbsp lemon juice, and fold in lettuce strips. Arrange on lettuce leaves. Garnish with herb sprigs and tomato wedges.

PER SERVING: 355 calories, 9 g protein, 20 g total fat, 3 g saturated fat, 0 mg cholesterol, 34 g carbohydrates, 12 g fibre.

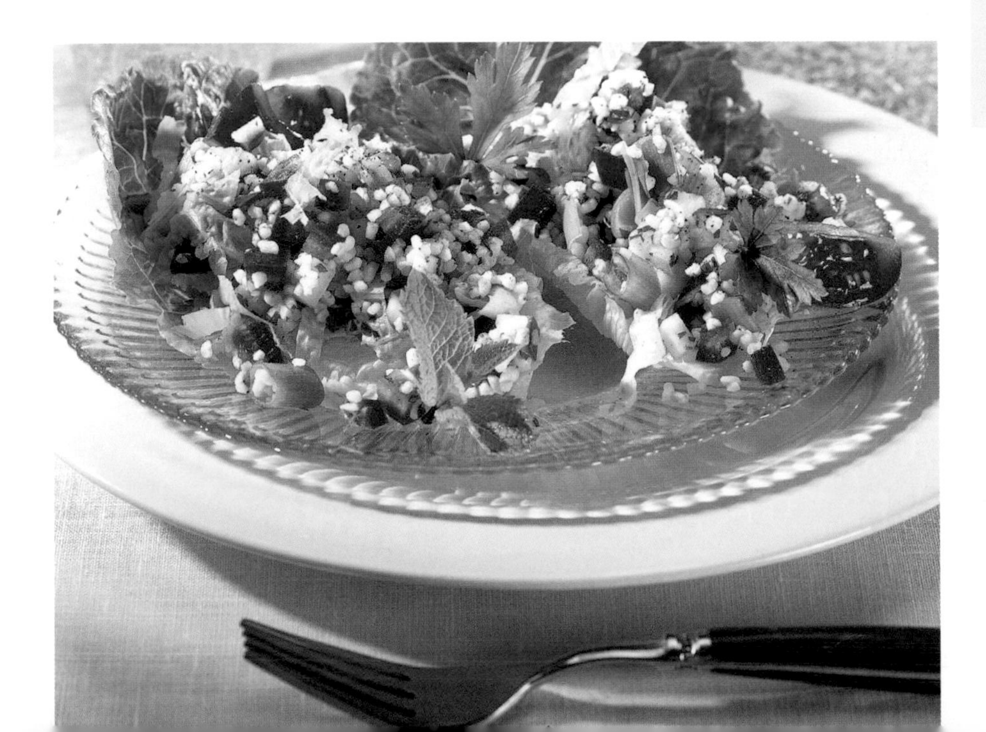

GOOD NEWS:

This is an ultra-nutritious salad, containing plenty of fibre. Consumed in portions of at least 30 g, fresh parsley contains useful amounts of vitamin C, iron and calcium.

Additional Recipes dinners

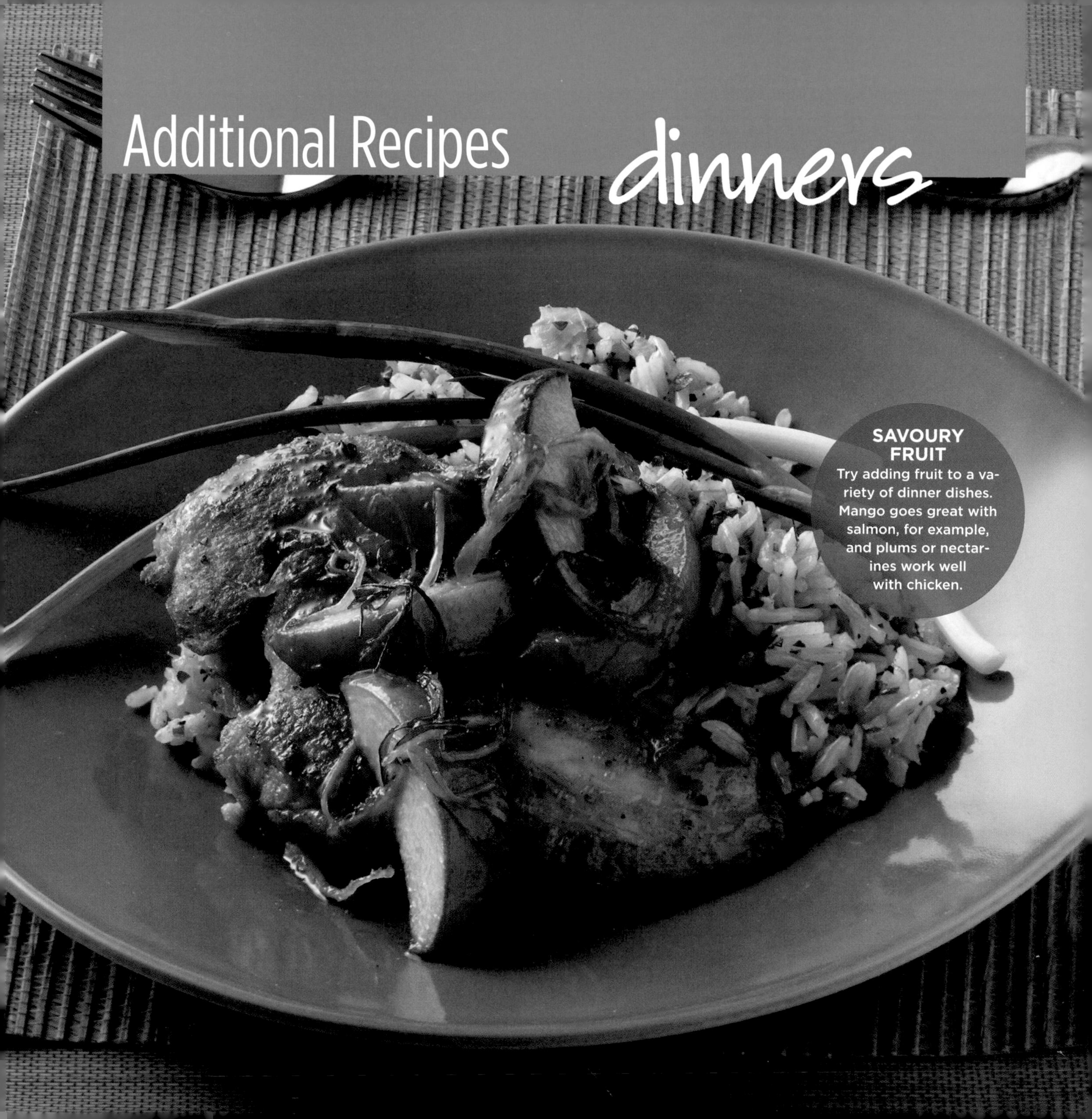

SAVOURY FRUIT

Try adding fruit to a variety of dinner dishes. Mango goes great with salmon, for example, and plums or nectarines work well with chicken.

CHICKEN BREASTS WITH PEACHES AND GINGER SERVES 4

Squeezing more fruit into your diet couldn't be simpler or more delicious. Here, sweet peaches accented with fresh ginger dress up chicken breasts. The vinegar in the sauce balances the flavours. In winter, you can substitute 1 cup frozen peaches for the fresh peach.

1 bunch scallions, trimmed
450 g boneless skinless chicken breast halves, trimmed
¼ tsp salt, or to taste
Freshly ground black pepper to taste
2 tsp canola oil
3 tbsp apple cider vinegar
2 tbsp sugar
½ cup no-sugar-added peach juice or nectar, or apple juice
2 tbsp grated fresh ginger
1 ¼ cups low-sodium chicken stock
1 large peach, peeled and sliced into 1 cm wedges
2 tsp cornstarch
2 tsp water

1 Chop scallions, reserving white portions and ¼ cup of green portions separately.

2 If chicken pieces are large, cut in half lengthwise so that you have at least four pieces. Place chicken between two pieces of plastic wrap and pound with rolling pin or meat mallet into 1 cm thickness. Season with salt and pepper.

3 Heat the oil in a large non-stick skillet over medium-high heat. Add chicken and cook until browned and no longer pink in centre, 3 to 3 ½ minutes per side. Transfer to plate.

4 Add vinegar and sugar to skillet. Stir to dissolve sugar. Cook, swirling skillet, until syrup turns dark amber, 30 to 60 seconds. Add scallion whites, peach juice and ginger. Bring to a boil, stirring to scrape up caramelized bits in skillet. Cook for 1 minute.

5 Add stock and peaches. Return to boil. Cook, turning peaches from time to time, until tender, or about 2 to 4 minutes. Mix cornstarch and water. Add to sauce. Cook, stirring, until slightly thickened, about 30 seconds.

6 Reduce heat to low and return chicken and any accumulated juices to skillet. Simmer gently until chicken is heated through, about 1 minute. Garnish with reserved scallion greens.

PER SERVING: 223 calories, 28 g protein, 17 g carbohydrates, 1 g fibre, 4 g total fat, 1 g saturated fat, 67 mg cholesterol, 275 mg sodium.

COOKING TIP:

● **PREPARING CHICKEN:**
Pounding chicken breasts to make them thinner ensures quick, even cooking. And, by cutting super-size chicken breasts in half, then pounding them, you can ensure appropriate portion sizes. If you purchase thin-cut chicken breasts, you can skip this step.

● **HOW TO PEEL PEACHES:**
Dip peaches in boiling water for 20 to 30 seconds to loosen skins. Remove with a slotted spoon and let cool slightly. Slip off skins with a paring knife.

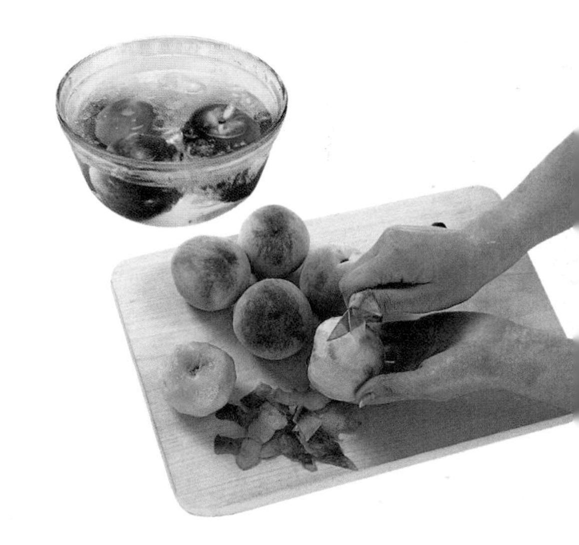

TURKEY AND BEAN CHILI WITH AVOCADO SALSA SERVES 8

Beans, with their wallop of soluble fibre, should always be on your weekly menu, and this full-flavoured chili's a great way to enjoy them. We lightened up the typical chili by using turkey instead of beef and gave it a boost with avocado salsa, full of good fat. Offer a selection of garnishes, such as chopped scallions, lime wedges, hot sauce, light sour cream and grated low-fat cheese, so your family and guests can personalize their chili bowls.

Perfect leftovers

Chili makes an ideal leftover, since its flavours will get richer and even more delicious with time. Set aside an extra cup of chili to eat as lunch the next day, alongside a quick green salad.

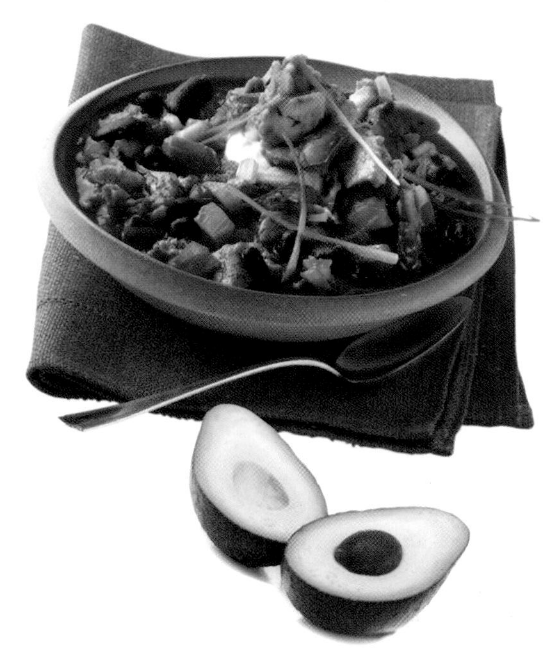

CHILI

340 g lean ground turkey breast
¼ cup chili powder
1 tbsp ground cumin
1 ½ tsp dried oregano
2 tsp canola oil
2 cups chopped onion
4 garlic cloves, minced
2 cans (127 mL each) chopped green chili peppers
1 can (796 mL) diced tomatoes, undrained
1 can (398 mL) low-sodium chicken stock
1 can (540 mL) black beans, drained and rinsed
1 can (540 mL) red kidney beans, drained and rinsed

AVOCADO SALSA

2 medium avocados, diced
⅔ cup diced, seeded fresh tomato
¼ cup finely diced white or red onion
2 tbsp minced seeded jalapeño pepper
2 tbsp chopped fresh cilantro
2 tbsp lime juice
¼ tsp salt, or to taste

1 Cook ground turkey with chili powder, cumin and oregano in large non-stick skillet over medium-high heat, breaking up meat and mixing in spices with a wooden spoon, until browned, 4 to 5 minutes. Remove from heat and set aside.

2 Heat oil in Dutch oven over medium heat. Add onion and cook, stirring often, until softened, 3 to 5 minutes. Add garlic and chili peppers. Cook, stirring, until fragrant, 1 to 2 minutes. Add tomatoes, stock and browned ground turkey. Bring to simmer. Reduce heat to low. Cover and simmer, stirring occasionally, for 45 minutes.

3 Stir in black beans and kidney beans. Return to simmer. Cover and simmer over low heat until flavours have blended, 15 to 20 minutes.

4 To make avocado salsa: Combine avocado, tomato, onion, jalapeño, cilantro, lime juice and salt in medium bowl. Toss gently to mix.

5 Spoon 2 tbsp of salsa onto each serving of chili. Covered, the chili will keep in the refrigerator for up to 2 days, or in the freezer in an airtight container for up to 3 months.

PER SERVING (1 ¼ CUPS CHILI AND 2 TBSP SALSA): 327 calories, 23 g protein, 38 g carbohydrates, 12 g fibre, 11 g total fat, 1 g saturated fat, 17 mg cholesterol, 748 mg sodium.

SHRIMP AND ORZO CASSEROLE

SERVES 6

This easy, heart-healthy shrimp recipe is prepared with tomatoes, orzo pasta cooked just until al dente and tangy low-fat feta cheese. Convenient canned artichokes are a surprisingly good source of fibre.

2 tsp olive oil
2 garlic cloves, minced
½ tsp dried oregano
Pinch of crushed red pepper
1 can (398 mL) diced tomatoes, undrained
1 can (398 mL) low-sodium chicken stock
1 cup orzo
1 can (398 mL) artichoke hearts, drained, rinsed, and quartered
1 tsp freshly grated lemon zest
Freshly ground pepper to taste
450 g cooked medium shrimp, tails removed
2 tbsp chopped fresh parsley
1 cup crumbled low-fat feta cheese

1 Preheat oven to 425°F (220°C). Coat 20-by-30 cm baking dish with cooking spray.

2 Heat oil in large saucepan over medium heat. Add garlic, oregano and red pepper. Cook, stirring, until fragrant but not coloured, 30 to 60 seconds. Add tomatoes and mash with potato masher. Add stock and bring to simmer. Stir in orzo, artichoke hearts, lemon zest and pepper. Transfer to baking dish. Cover tightly with aluminum foil.

3 Bake casserole for 15 minutes. Stir ingredients in casserole, then stir in shrimp. Sprinkle with parsley, then feta. Bake, uncovered, until orzo is firm-tender and feta starts to melt, or 5 to 10 minutes longer.

PER SERVING (1 CUP): 273 calories, 27 g protein, 33 g carbohydrates, 6 g fibre, 4 g total fat, 2 g saturated fat, 154 mg cholesterol, 544 mg sodium.

COOKING TIP:

To cook shrimp, place in a large saucepan of lightly salted boiling water. Cook until shrimp turn pink, or 2 to 3 minutes, then drain. You can also use frozen cooked shrimp, which you should always thaw before using.

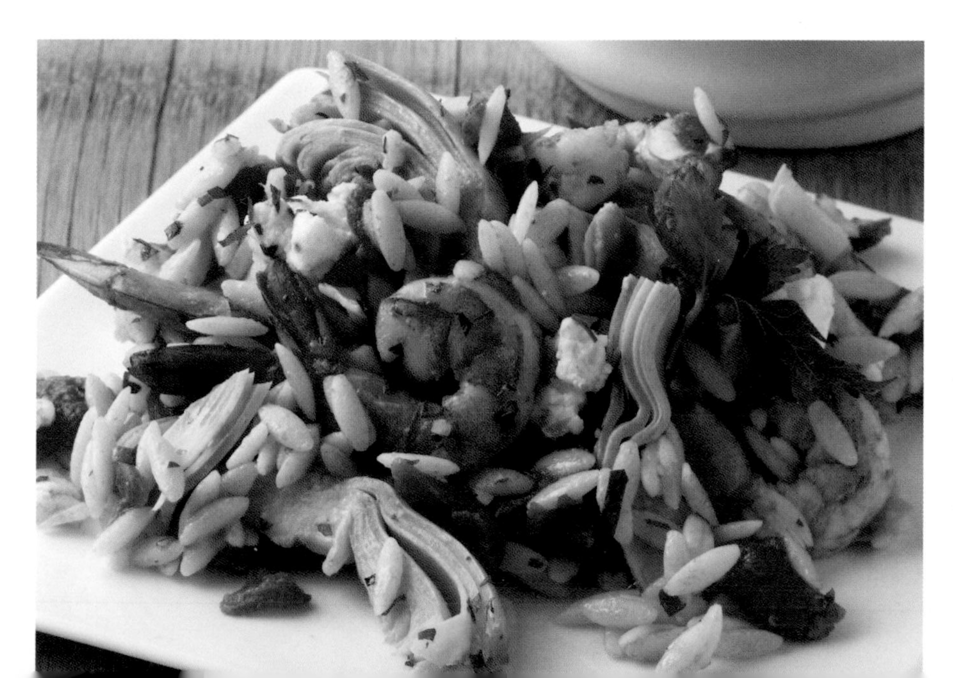

INGREDIENT NOTE:
If possible, use **whole-wheat orzo** for extra fibre and whole-grain goodness. It's available in most health food stores.

SEARED FISH STEAKS WITH TOMATO-OLIVE SAUCE SERVES 4

Firm fish like swordfish and halibut benefit from the easy two-step technique of first browning the steaks on one side before finishing by cooking them in the oven (cooking the fish entirely in the skillet can make the outside tough and requires more fat). The spicy tomato sauce sets off the succulent fish steaks beautifully.

1 tbsp lime juice
4 tsp olive oil, divided
Salt to taste
Freshly ground pepper to taste
4 x 2.5 cm thick halibut steaks (125 g each) or swordfish steaks (170 g each)
½ cup chopped onion
1 garlic clove, minced
½ tsp ground cumin
Pinch of crushed red pepper
1 can (398 mL) diced tomatoes with green chili peppers
⅓ cup water
1 tbsp chopped pitted green olives
2 tsp drained capers, rinsed
Lime wedges

1 Preheat oven to 425°F (220°C). Coat baking sheet with cooking spray.

2 Mix lime juice, 1 tsp oil, salt and pepper in a shallow glass dish. Add fish steaks and turn to coat. Cover and marinate in refrigerator for 10 to 20 minutes.

3 Meanwhile, heat 2 tsp oil in medium saucepan over medium heat. Add onion and cook, stirring often, until softened, 3 to 4 minutes. Add garlic, cumin and red pepper. Cook, stirring, for 30 seconds. Add tomatoes and water. Bring to simmer. Cook over medium heat, stirring occasionally, until thickened, about 10 minutes.

4 While sauce is simmering, cook fish. Heat remaining 1 tsp oil in large non-stick skillet over medium-high heat. Add fish and cook until browned on one side, 2 to 3 minutes. Transfer fish to baking sheet, browned side up. Bake until fish is opaque in centre, or 8 to 10 minutes.

5 Stir olives and capers into tomato sauce. Season with black pepper. Top each fish steak with sauce and serve with lime wedges.

PER SERVING (1 FISH STEAK AND ¼ CUP SAUCE): 198 calories, 22 g protein, 6 g carbohydrates, 1 g fibre, 10 g total fat, 2 g saturated fat, 41 mg cholesterol, 551 mg sodium.

SHOPPING

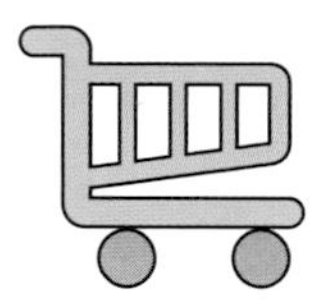

How to choose the freshest fish

When buying halibut, look for firm, white meat that is almost transluscent. It shouldn't be dull, yellowish or blotchy.

When buying swordfish, look for firm meat with a whorled texture. The steak's coloured patches should be very red, not brown.

For any fish, avoid anything that smells too fishy—it should have a fairly neutral smell.

TIP: The tomato-olive sauce is also delicious over grilled, boneless, skinless chicken breasts.

MUSHROOM AND HERB PIZZA

SERVES 4

Yes, pizza can be part of your **Swap & Drop** eating plan—especially when you make your own, with a thin, whole-grain crust, topped with lots of vegetables and a moderate amount of cheese.

340 g premade whole-wheat pizza dough
Cornmeal for dusting
1 tbsp olive oil, divided
3 cups baby bella or cremini mushrooms, stem ends trimmed, wiped clean and sliced
2 garlic cloves, minced
Pinch of salt
Freshly ground pepper to taste
2 tbsp chopped fresh parsley
2/3 cup prepared marinara sauce
2 tbsp chopped fresh marjoram or oregano
1/8 tsp crushed red pepper
1 cup shredded part-skim mozzarella cheese
1/2 cup diced red onion
1/4 cup grated parmesan cheese

1 Place baking stone or inverted baking sheet on lowest rack of oven. Preheat oven to 500°F (260°C) or highest setting. Coat 32 cm pizza pan with cooking spray. Dust with cornmeal.

2 Heat 2 tsp of oil in large non-stick skillet over medium-high heat. Add mushrooms and cook, stirring or shaking skillet from time to time, until tender and lightly browned, 3 to 4 minutes. Add garlic and cook, stirring, for 30 seconds longer. Remove from heat and stir in parsley, salt and pepper.

3 Mix marinara sauce, marjoram or oregano and red pepper in a small bowl.

4 On lightly floured surface, roll dough into 33 cm circle. Transfer to pizza pan. Turn edges under to make slight rim around outside edge. Brush remaining 1 tsp oil over rim. Spread marinara sauce over crust, leaving 1 cm border. Sprinkle mozzarella over sauce. Scatter mushrooms over mozzarella. Sprinkle with onion. Top with parmesan cheese.

5 Place pizza pan on heated baking stone (or baking sheet) and bake until bottom crust is crisp and golden, 10 to 14 minutes.

PER SERVING 1/4 OF A 30 CM PIZZA): 368 calories, 18 g protein, 45 g carbohydrates, 6 g fibre, 14 g total fat, 5 g saturated fat, 22 mg cholesterol, 916 mg sodium.

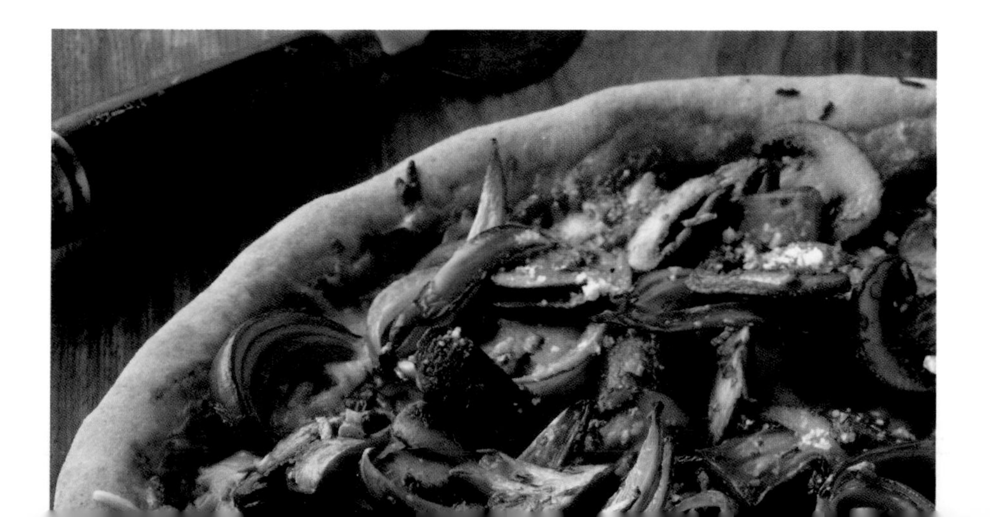

Try this

WHOLE-WHEAT PIZZA WITH BROCCOLI AND OLIVES

In Step 2, steam 2 cups broccoli florets (2 cm pieces) until crisp-tender, for 2 to 3 minutes. In Step 3, mix 2/3 cup prepared marinara sauce with 1 tsp dried oregano and 1/8 tsp crushed red pepper. In Step 4, spread the marinara sauce over the crust. Sprinkle 1 cup shredded part-skim mozzarella cheese over the sauce. Scatter the broccoli, 1/2 cup diced red onion and 1/4 cup coarsely chopped, pitted kalamata olives over top. Spritz the top lightly with olive oil cooking spray. Bake the pizza as directed in Step 5.

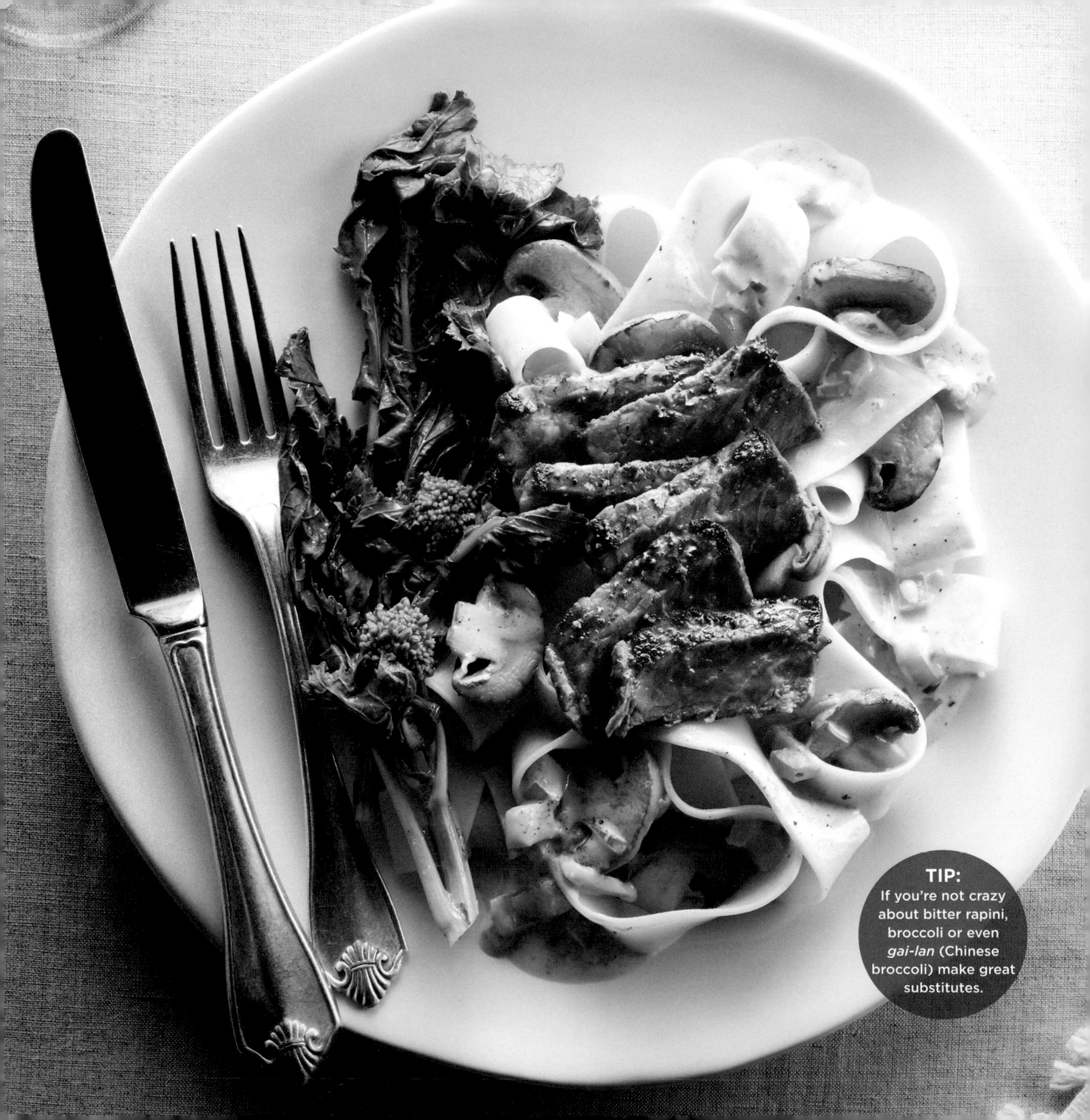

TIP:
If you're not crazy about bitter rapini, broccoli or even *gai-lan* (Chinese broccoli) make great substitutes.

SPEEDY STEAK STROGANOFF

SERVES 4

This tasty version of a comfort-food classic is lighter and faster than the original, and gets a great veggie boost from the rapini.

1 bunch rapini
½ cup light sour cream or yogourt
170 g wide egg noodles, uncooked
300–350 g steak, fat trimmed
1 tbsp olive oil, divided
1 small onion, diced
1 cup low-sodium beef stock
2 cups sliced mushrooms

1 Bring large pot of water to a boil and cook noodles according to package directions.

2 Meanwhile, pour 1 tsp oil into large skillet over medium-high heat. Add steak and cook, turning occasionally, about 5 minutes for medium-rare. Remove from skillet and let stand.

3 Pour remaining oil into skillet. Add onion and sauté until soft, 2 to 3 minutes. Then add mushrooms and cook until browned, 3 to 5 minutes.

4 Stir in stock. Simmer, uncovered, for 5 minutes and remove from heat. Drain cooked noodles, then stir them and sour cream into skillet. Steam rapini until tender-crisp.

5 Divide noodle mixture among 4 plates, slice steak and place overtop. Serve rapini on the side.

PER SERVING: 408 calories, 25 g protein, 20 g total fat, 8 g saturated fat, 33 g carbohydrates, 3 g fibre, 83 mg cholesterol, 80 mg sodium.

3 more ideas

- **Swap the low-sodium beef stock for homemade vegetable or mushroom stock.**
- **Use shiitake mushrooms instead of the standard buttons for an extra-mouthwatering flavour.**
- **Follow Speedy Steak Stroganoff with a fresh and fruity dessert—Moroccan Fruit Salad (page 181), for instance.**

MOROCCAN SPICED CARROTS

SERVES 4

It is hard to believe that humble carrots can be transformed into such a rich-tasting yet low-calorie dish. The secret is the Moroccan spice blend, which includes a subtle hint of cinnamon. And, of course, we use extra-virgin olive oil instead of butter.

700 g carrots (8–10 medium), peeled and cut into 6 cm-by-1 cm sticks (4 cups)
1 tbsp extra-virgin olive oil
1 garlic clove, minced
¾ tsp paprika
½ tsp ground cumin
⅛ tsp cinnamon
Pinch of cayenne pepper
3 tbsp lemon juice
2 tbsp chopped fresh parsley or cilantro
¼ tsp salt, or to taste

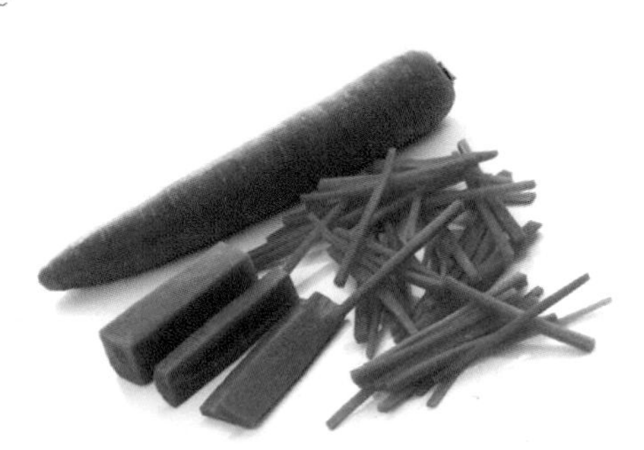

1 Steam carrots until crisp-tender, or 4 to 6 minutes.

2 Heat oil in large non-stick skillet over medium-low heat. Add garlic, paprika, cumin, cinnamon and cayenne. Cook, stirring, until fragrant, 1 to 2 minutes.

3 Add carrots, lemon juice, parsley (or cilantro) and salt. Stir to coat carrots with spice mixture.

PER SERVING (¾ CUP): 107 calories, 2 g protein, 18 g carbohydrates, 5 g fibre, 4 g total fat, 1 g saturated fat, 0 mg cholesterol, 265 mg sodium.

DAHL WITH SPINACH

SERVES 6

Dahl turns up frequently in Indian cooking and it is one of those confusing terms that refer to both a preparation and an ingredient. As an ingredient, dahl encompasses a wide variety of dried legumes, including lentils and split peas, both of which are valuable sources of soluble fibre and vegetable protein. Dahl as a preparation is a dish like this one, made with seasoned stewed legumes. We've squeezed three healthy seasonings—turmeric, fenugreek and garlic—into this spicy stew.

Pairing up

Dahl makes a great accompaniment to a variety of meals. Try a ½ cup alongside super-fresh dishes such as Radish and Cucumber Salad (page 140) or Radicchio and Fennel Salad with Oranges (page 141).

It can even make a great spread—just smoothe a little bit over toasted whole-wheat bread when you're putting together a sandwich.

DAHL

1 cup yellow split peas or chana dahl (split chickpeas), sorted and rinsed
3 cups water
½ tsp turmeric
1 tbsp canola oil
1 tsp cumin seeds
1 cup chopped onion
1 tbsp grated fresh ginger or 1 tsp ground ginger
3 garlic cloves, minced
1 tsp ground fenugreek (optional)
¼ tsp cayenne pepper
1 can (398 mL) diced tomatoes, undrained
1 package (300 g) frozen chopped spinach
½ tsp salt, or to taste

RAITA

1 cup low-fat plain yogourt
4 tsp lime juice
1 tsp ground cumin
⅛ tsp salt, or to taste

1 Dahl: Combine split peas or chana dahl, water and turmeric in large saucepan. Bring to simmer. Partially cover, reduce heat to medium-low, and cook until split peas are tender, or 40 to 45 minutes.

2 Meanwhile, heat oil in large non-stick skillet over medium heat. Add cumin seeds and cook, stirring, until fragrant, 10 to 20 seconds. Add onion and cook, stirring often, until softened, 2 to 3 minutes. Add ginger, garlic, fenugreek (if using) and cayenne. Cook, stirring, until fragrant, 20 to 30 seconds. Add tomatoes and cook until most of liquid has evaporated, or 5 to 10 minutes.

3 Cook spinach according to package directions. Drain, pressing out excess moisture.

4 When split peas are tender, stir them (and any remaining cooking liquid) into the tomato mixture, along with the spinach. Cook for 2 to 3 minutes to blend flavours. Season with salt.

5 Raita: Mix raita ingredients in small bowl. Serve dahl with raita. Leftover dahl will keep, covered, in refrigerator for up to 2 days. Reheat on stovetop or in microwave, adding additional water if too dry.

PER SERVING (¾ CUP DAHL AND 2 ½ TBSP RAITA): 199 calories, 12 g protein, 33 g carbohydrates, 12 g fibre, 4 g total fat, 0 g saturated fat, 0 mg cholesterol, 412 mg sodium.

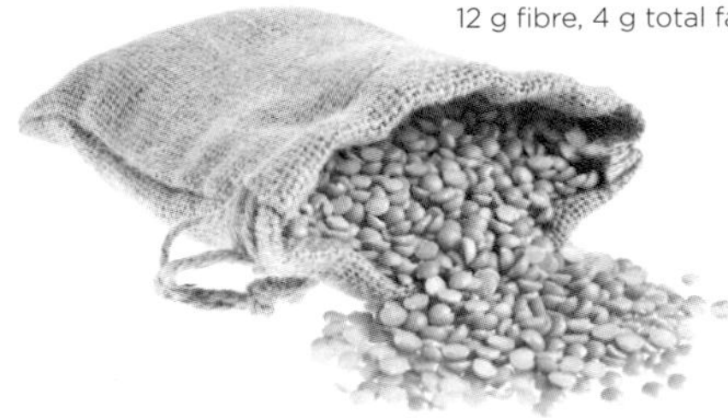

GREEK-STYLE SHRIMP SKILLET

SERVES 4

This quick dish is packed with vitamin C—thanks to the tomatoes and bell peppers—and protein from the shrimp. Rinse the black olives before adding them if you're watching your sodium intake.

500 g medium shrimp, peeled and de-veined
3 cloves garlic, minced
1 medium onion, chopped
1 can (396 mL) low-sodium diced tomatoes
1 tsp dried oregano
12 black olives, halved and pitted
1 large yellow or green pepper, diced
Small handful fresh parsley, chopped
½ cup crumbled feta
1 tbsp olive oil

1 Pour olive oil into large skillet over medium-high heat. Stir-fry onion and pepper until tender-crisp, about 2 to 3 minutes. Add garlic, and stir for 1 more minute.

2 Add tomatoes, oregano and olives, and mix thoroughly. Bring to a boil, reduce heat, cover and simmer for 5 minutes.

3 Add shrimp and cook, uncovered, until done, about 3 to 5 minutes. Divide equally among 4 bowls. Sprinkle feta and parsley overtop and garnish with a lemon slice, if desired. Serve with a crusty whole-grain or multi-grain bread or dinner roll.

PER SERVING: 276 calories, 30 g protein, 11 g total fat, 4 g saturated fat, 13 g carbohydrates, 2 g fibre, 207 mg cholesterol, 526 mg sodium.

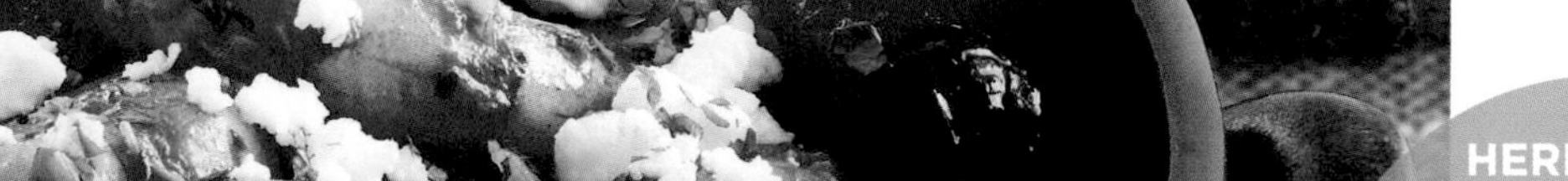

SHOPPING

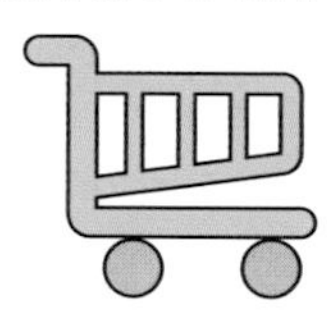

How to choose the best olives

Mediterranean delis often have a wide selection of olives. Which kind should you buy? Green olives, which are picked before they're ripe, tend to be denser and more bitter than black olives. Big, meaty kalamatas are great in salads; manzanillas are often stuffed; niçoise are small but intensely flavoured. Ask a deli employee to help you choose the right flavour for your purposes.

HERB SWAP

If you like the taste, try swapping out the parsley in this recipe for fresh cilantro—it'll add a nice kick—or use half and half. Don't be afraid to experiment with fresh herbs. It's a healthy way to add something special to a dinner dish.

BLACK BEAN AND SWEET POTATO BURRITOS

SERVES 8

Sweet potatoes and fibre-rich beans join forces in this flavour-packed vegetarian meal. If you are cooking for just one or two, make the sweet potato–bean filling (through Step 2) and store, covered, in the refrigerator for up to 2 days. For a quick pick-up meal, just heat leftover filling and individual tortillas in the microwave.

3 more ideas

- Omit a little of the cilantro and add some fresh mint and chives for a unique flavour.
- Use spinach tortillas instead of whole-wheat. They're green, so they look great, too.
- Try topping your burrito with plain fat-free yogourt—it's even lighter than sour cream, and will still add a mild tanginess.

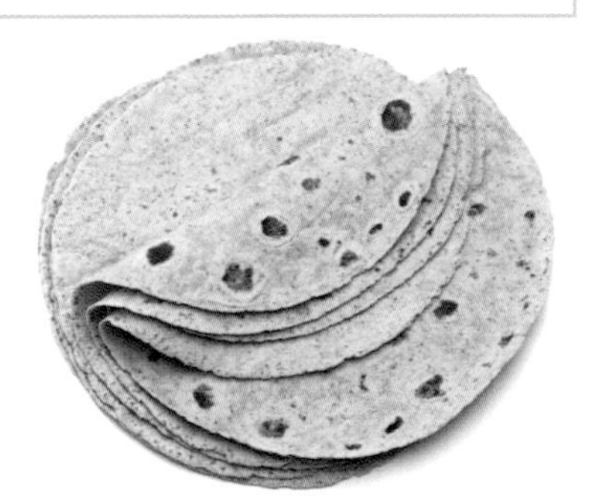

2 tsp canola oil
1 cup chopped onion
2 garlic cloves, minced
4 tsp ground cumin
½ tsp dried oregano
¾ cup vegetable stock or low-sodium chicken stock
1 medium sweet potato, peeled and diced
1 can (398 mL) diced tomatoes with green chili peppers, undrained
1 can (398 mL) black beans, drained and rinsed
¾ cup frozen corn
¼ cup chopped fresh cilantro
1 tbsp fresh lime juice
⅛ tsp freshly ground pepper
8 x 20 cm whole-wheat wraps or tortillas
1 cup shredded Monterey Jack cheese
½ cup light sour cream

1 Preheat oven to 325°F (160°C).

2 Heat oil in large non-stick skillet over medium heat. Add onion and cook, stirring often, until softened, or 2 to 3 minutes. Add garlic, cumin and oregano. Cook, stirring, until fragrant, 10 to 20 seconds. Add stock and sweet potato. Bring to a simmer. Cover and cook for 5 minutes. Add tomatoes, beans and corn. Return to a simmer. Cover and cook until sweet potatoes are tender, 5 to 10 minutes longer. Mash about ¼ of the vegetable mixture with potato masher. Stir mashed and unmashed portions together. Stir in lime juice, cilantro and pepper.

3 Meanwhile, enclose wraps or tortillas in aluminum foil and heat in oven for 10 to 15 minutes.

4 To serve, spoon about ⅔ cup of sweet potato filling down centre of each tortilla. Sprinkle with about 2 tbsp cheese. Fold in edges of wrap, then fold 1 side over filling and wrap up burrito. Serve with sour cream for dipping.

PER SERVING (1 WRAP): 262 calories, 14 g protein, 35 g carbohydrates, 15 g fibre, 10 g total fat, 4 g saturated fat, 21 g cholesterol, 784 mg sodium.

TIP:
Look for sweet potatoes without too many bruises or cuts on their outsides, and make sure they're nice and firm.

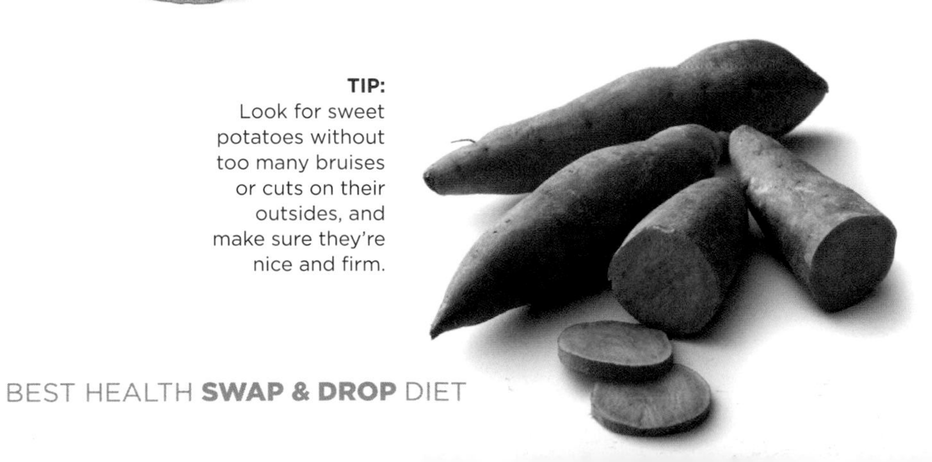

ORANGE BEEF STIR-FRY WITH BROCCOLI AND RED PEPPER

SERVES 4

Recipes for beef and broccoli stir-fries may be commonplace, but this one stands out. Stir-frying orange zest with fresh ginger gives the sauce extraordinary fragrance and flavour. This dish provides a generous quantity of vegetables balanced with lean protein, providing excellent nutritional value for the calories.

½ cup orange juice
2 tbsp low-sodium soy sauce
1 tbsp oyster sauce
1 tbsp rice vinegar
1 ½ tsp chili-garlic sauce or hot red pepper sauce
1 ½ tsp cornstarch
1 tbsp canola oil
340 g flank steak, trimmed, halved lengthwise and cut into 5 mm-thick slices
1 tbsp minced fresh ginger
2 tsp freshly grated orange zest
3 garlic cloves, minced
1 cup sliced onion
450 g broccoli crowns, cut into 2.5 cm florets (about 4 cups)
1 red or yellow bell pepper, cut into 5 cm-by-5 mm slivers

1 In small bowl, whisk together orange juice, soy sauce, oyster sauce, vinegar, chili-garlic sauce (or hot sauce) and cornstarch; set aside.

2 Heat 1 tsp oil in large non-stick skillet or stir-fry pan over high heat. Add half of steak and cook, without stirring or turning, until browned on underside, about 1 minute. Stir and turn slices, then cook just until browned on other side, about 30 seconds. Transfer to plate. Add another 1 tsp oil, repeat with remaining steak and transfer to plate.

3 Add remaining 1 tsp oil to skillet, then add ginger, orange zest and garlic and stir-fry until fragrant, 10 to 20 seconds. Add onion and stir-fry for 1 minute. Add broccoli and bell pepper and stir-fry for 30 seconds. Add ¼ cup water, cover and cook just until crisp-tender, about 1 ½ minutes. Push vegetables to outside of pan. Stir reserved sauce, pour into centre of pan, and cook, stirring, until glossy and thickened, about 1 minute. Stir vegetables into sauce, return steak to skillet and turn to coat. Serve with brown rice.

PER SERVING (1 ½ CUPS): 247 calories, 25 g protein, 17 g carbohydrates, 3 g fibre, 9 g total fat, 3 g saturated fat, 34 mg cholesterol, 655 mg sodium.

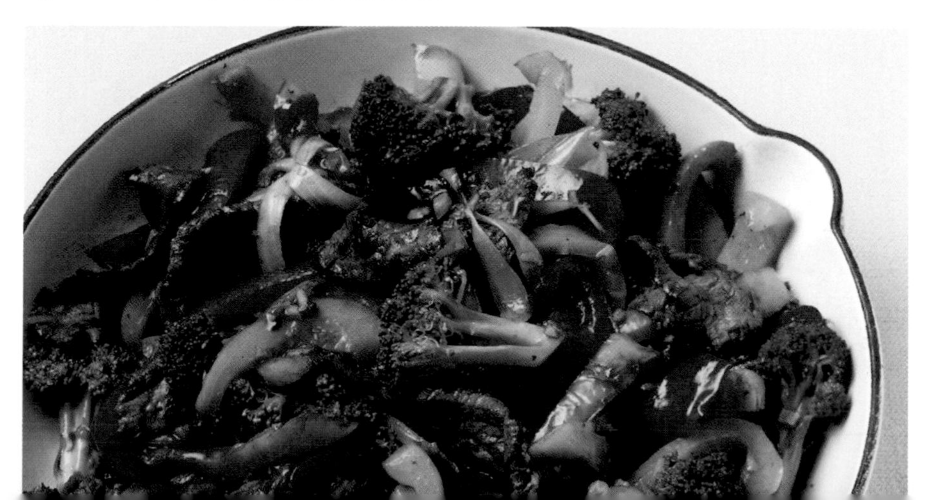

COOKING TIP: ZESTING CITRUS

A zester is the easiest way to remove zest from oranges and lemons. If you don't have one, use a vegetable peeler and mince the peels.

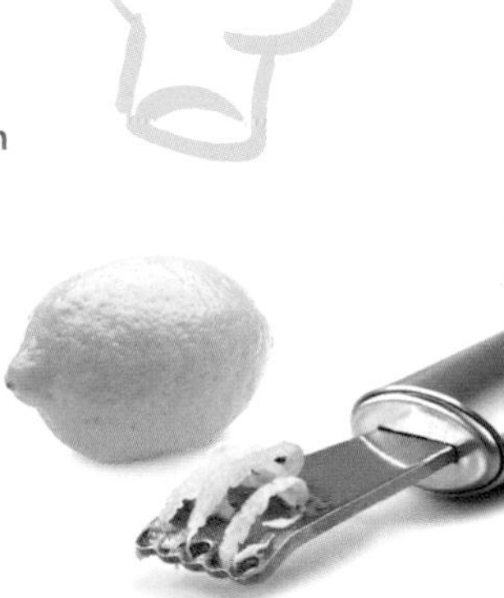

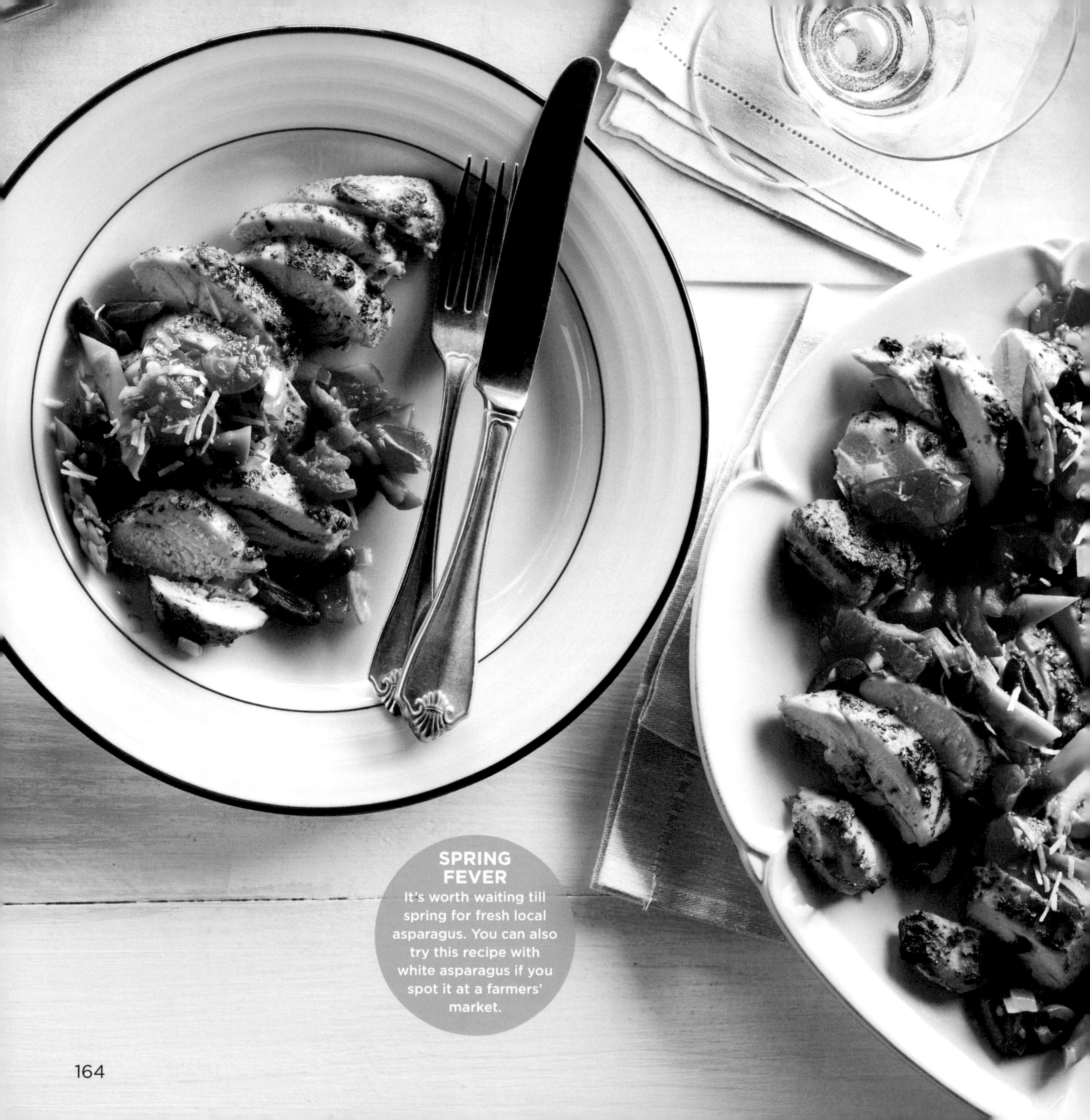

SPRING FEVER

It's worth waiting till spring for fresh local asparagus. You can also try this recipe with white asparagus if you spot it at a farmers' market.

PESTO-STUFFED CHICKEN BREASTS WITH ASPARAGUS RAGOUT

SERVES 4

The pesto in this recipe is simple to make with either a mortar and pestle or an electric hand mixer. If you want, you can double the amount of pesto and freeze the extra. Fresh local asparagus needs hardly any cooking and is deliciously crisp. For this recipe, choose thin stalks; if you use thicker ones, you will need to blanch them for a couple of minutes to soften.

Large handful fresh basil, minced (reserve some for garnish)
4 cloves garlic, minced (divided)
3 tbsp extra virgin olive oil (divided)
Salt and pepper to taste
4 boneless chicken breasts
1 large red onion, diced
2 large tomatoes, diced
16 asparagus stalks, cut into quarters
16 kalamata olives, pitted and chopped
2 tbsp lemon zest
¼ cup parmesan, grated

1 Preheat oven to 375°F (190°C), then make pesto: Place basil, two cloves of minced garlic, 2 tbsp of olive oil and pinch of salt and pepper in small bowl, and mix until it forms a paste.

2 Using sharp knife, make lengthwise split on side of each chicken breast to form deep pocket. Stuff chicken breasts evenly with pesto, rubbing some on outsides as well.

3 Place chicken on lightly oiled baking pan in oven until cooked through, for about 20 minutes.

4 While chicken is cooking, make ragout. In sauté pan, add 1 tbsp olive oil, plus onion and remaining garlic. Sauté until onion is translucent.

5 Add tomatoes, asparagus and olives, and continue cooking 5 minutes. Add lemon zest and season to taste with salt and pepper.

6 Slice chicken breasts into 1 cm slices and divide evenly among four plates. Top with vegetable ragout. Garnish with parmesan cheese and fresh basil before serving.

PER SERVING: 324 calories, 31 g protein, 17 g total fat, 3 g saturated fat, 13 g carbohydrates, 3 g fibre, 71 mg cholesterol, 349 mg sodium.

3 more ideas

- **Swap half the basil for arugula to try a different take on pesto. (You can still garnish with basil at the end.)**
- **Have you ever tried romano cheese? It's tastes like a more intense parmesan, and you need very little of it. (Great for dieters!)**
- **Substitute a couple handfuls of cherry tomatoes for the large tomatoes for a sweeter flavour.**

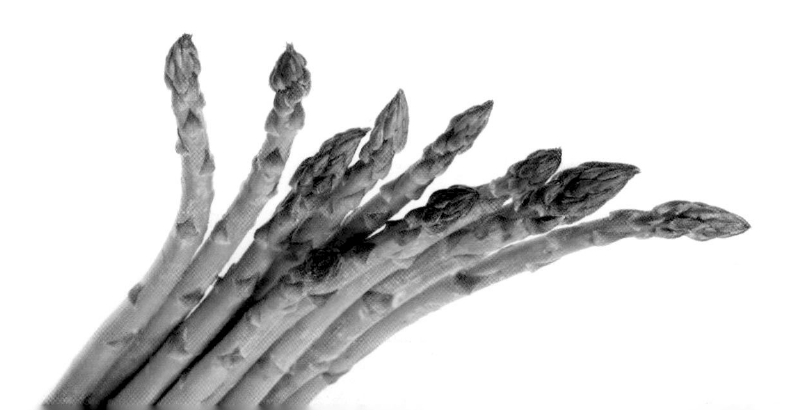

CHICKEN FAJITA POCKETS

SERVES 4

You can replace the chicken with any other meat. And if you want, you can swap the pita pockets for whole-grain wraps—delicious!

- 1 tsp chili powder
- 1 tsp cumin
- Juice of 1/2 a lime
- 2 tbsp and 1 tsp extra-virgin olive oil, divided
- Pinch each salt and pepper
- 230 g boneless, skinless chicken breast, thinly sliced
- 1/2 avocado, peeled and mashed
- 1/4 cup light sour cream
- 1/4 bell pepper (any colour), julienned
- 1/4 medium red onion, julienned
- 8 shiitake mushrooms, stems removed, julienned
- 1 small clove garlic, minced
- 8 cherry tomatoes, quartered
- 1/2 cup fresh cilantro
- 2 whole-wheat pitas, halved
- Small handful arugula or baby spinach

1 Put chili powder, cumin, lime juice, 1 tsp extra-virgin olive oil, salt and pepper into small bowl. Stir to blend. Add chicken strips and mix till well coated. Set aside.

2 Stir together avocado and sour cream. Place in the fridge.

3 Add 1 tbsp olive oil and the chicken to sauté pan and sauté on high heat until chicken is cooked through, about 2 minutes. Remove chicken from pan, add 1 tbsp olive oil and peppers, onions, mushrooms and garlic. Sauté until onions and peppers soften, about three minutes.

4 Remove from heat and return chicken to pan along with tomato and cilantro. Stir to mix. Season with salt and pepper.

5 Inside each pita half, spread 1/4 of avocado mixture, then add 1/4 of arugula or spinach. Divide chicken and vegetable mixture among four pita pocket halves. Garnish with sliced cucumber, if desired.

PER SERVING: 313 calories, 19 g protein, 15 g total fat, 3 g saturated fat, 30 g carbohydrates, 6 g fibre, 35 mg cholesterol, 226 mg sodium.

SHOPPING

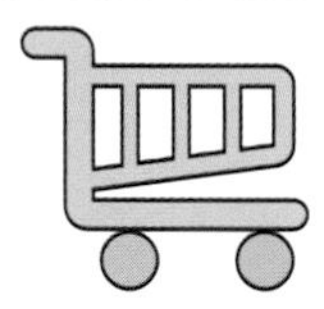

The best way to buy shiitakes

Make a trip to an Asian supermarket to buy dried shiitake mushrooms. They're cheaper, and the water you use to rehydrate them takes on their rich, mouthwatering flavour—great for using in stews. To rehydrate, soak the mushrooms in hot water for around 20 minutes or until soft. Drain and discard stems before cooking.

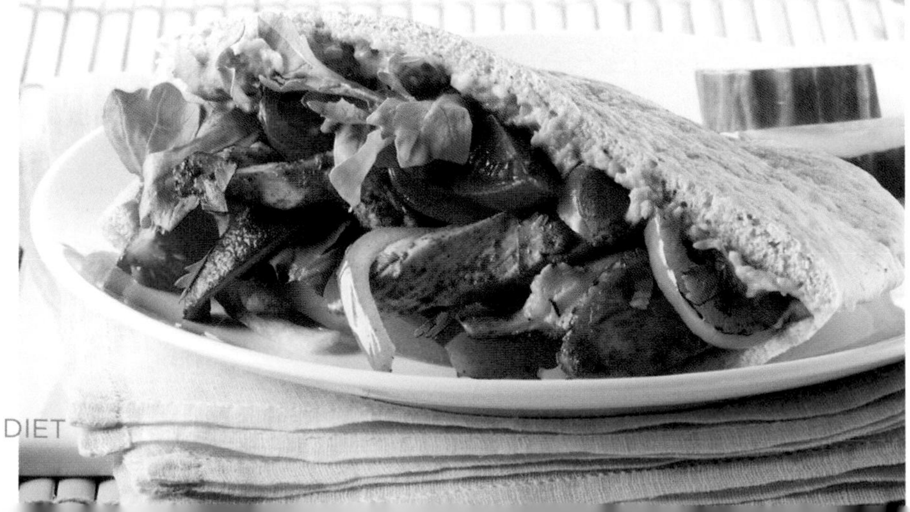

BULGUR WITH GINGER AND ORANGE

SERVES 4

Instead of cooking a side of rice or potatoes, reach for a bag of bulgur. It cooks in about the same time as white rice but is also rich in soluble fibre.

2 oranges, scrubbed
2 tsp canola oil
2 tbsp minced fresh ginger
2 garlic cloves minced
1 cup bulgur, rinsed
2 tsp firmly packed brown sugar
¼ tsp salt, or to taste
⅔ cup chopped scallions
1 tbsp low-sodium soy sauce
⅓ cup slivered almonds, toasted (see tip)

1 Grate orange peels to make 1 tbsp zest. Juice oranges and add enough water to measure 1 ½ cups.

2 Heat oil in large, heavy saucepan over medium-high heat. Add ginger and garlic. Cook, stirring, until fragrant, about 30 seconds. Add bulgur and stir to coat. Add diluted orange juice, sugar and salt. Bring to a simmer. Reduce heat to low, cover and simmer until bulgur is tender and most of liquid has been absorbed, 15 to 20 minutes.

3 Add scallions, soy sauce and reserved orange zest to bulgur. Mix gently and fluff with fork. Sprinkle with almonds. Leftovers will keep, covered, in the refrigerator for up to 2 days. Reheat in the microwave.

PER SERVING (¾ CUP): 234 calories, 7 g protein, 38 g carbohydrates, 8 g fibre, 7 g total fat, 1 g saturated fat, 0 mg cholesterol, 295 mg sodium.

COOKING TIP:

● **HOW TO TOAST ALMONDS:** Put the nuts in a small dry skillet over medium-low heat, stirring constantly, until light golden and fragrant, about 2 to 3 minutes. Transfer to a plate and let cool.

Another idea

● ● ● BULGUR WITH CARROT JUICE AND SESAME SEEDS

For a change, swap carrot juice for the orange juice and toasted sesame seeds for almonds.

SAUTEED SPINACH WITH GINGER AND SOY SAUCE

SERVES 2

This simple side dish features aromatic toasted sesame oil, which has an appealing nutty flavour.

300 g fresh spinach, stems trimmed, washed
1 tbsp low-sodium soy sauce
2 tsp rice vinegar
1 tsp toasted sesame oil
¼ tsp firmly packed brown sugar
2 tsp canola oil
1 garlic clove, minced
1 ½ tsp minced fresh ginger
Dash of crushed red pepper
1 tbsp sesame seeds, toasted

1 Wash spinach and cook in large, wide pot over medium-high heat just until wilted, 3 to 5 minutes. Drain, refresh under cold running water and press out excess moisture.

2 Mix soy, vinegar, sesame oil and sugar in a bowl. Heat oil in non-stick pan over medium-high heat. Add garlic, ginger and red pepper. Stir-fry until fragrant not browned, about 10 seconds.

3 Add spinach and cook, stirring often, until heated, through 2 to 3 minutes. Stir in soy sauce mixture and toss to coat well. Sprinkle with sesame seeds.

PER SERVING (¾ CUP): 119 calories, 4 g protein, 7 g carbohydrates, 3 g fibre, 10 g total fat, 2 g saturated fat, 0 mg cholesterol, 348 mg sodium.

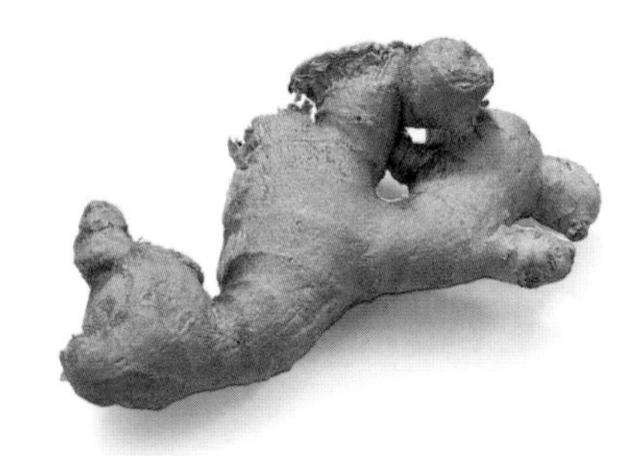

Try this:

While you've got the barbecue going, try throwing some kale on there! This leafy green is hardy enough to take the heat. Dunk large pieces of de-stemmed kale in coconut milk, sprinkle with cayenne and black pepper, and place carefully on the grill. It's done when the leaf becomes tender and its edges blacken.

SHANGHAI TOFU "STEAKS" ON KALE

SERVES 4

Firm tofu takes on a delicious smoky flavour when it's marinated and grilled on the barbecue. Serve with nutritious kale for an antioxidant boost.

425 g block firm tofu
3 tbsp low-sodium soy sauce
8 cups kale, stems discarded, leaves chopped
2 tsp canola oil, divided
1 tsp sesame oil
1 medium red pepper, thinly sliced
1 medium yellow zucchini, cut into 10 cm sticks
1 tbsp honey
2 tsp each, minced fresh ginger and garlic

1 Cut tofu into four 1 cm-thick oblong "steaks." Wrap in paper towel and top with a baking sheet weighted down for 5 minutes.

2 For marinade, combine soy sauce, sesame oil, honey, ginger, garlic and 1 tsp canola oil. Place tofu in dish and pour marinade overtop. Let stand 10 minutes.

3 Drain and reserve marinade. Oil barbecue grate and heat to medium. Cook tofu until grill marks form, 3 to 5 minutes per side.

4 Meanwhile, pour remaining 1 tsp canola oil into a large skillet over medium heat. Add zucchini and red pepper, and sauté 3 minutes. Stir in kale, marinade and a splash of water. Stir-fry until kale wilts. Divide among 4 plates. Top with grilled tofu.

PER SERVING: 293 calories, 23 g protein, 14 g fat (2 g saturated fat), 27 g carbohydrates, 6 g fibre, 0 mg cholesterol, 479 mg sodium.

COTTAGE PIE

SERVES 4

This "pie"—actually a turkey-and-veggie bake, topped with mashed, vitamin-rich sweet potatoes—is perfect for eating on a frigid evening. It's healthy comfort food.

¼ cup extra-virgin olive oil
500 g ground raw turkey or chicken
½ cup onion, diced
2 cloves garlic, diced
1 tbsp thyme, fresh or dried
1 cup mushrooms, diced
2 tbsp parsley, chopped
½ cup chicken stock
Salt and pepper to taste
1 large sweet potato, peeled, diced and boiled
¼ cup low-fat yogourt

1 Preheat oven to 350°F (180°C). In medium sauté pan, add olive oil, ground turkey, onion, garlic and thyme. Sauté until turkey is cooked through and onions soften.

2 Add mushrooms, parsley and chicken stock. Season with salt and pepper to taste. Pour into 20 cm-by-20 cm baking dish. Set aside.

3 In medium bowl, mash sweet potatoes and add yogourt. Season to taste. Top turkey mixture with mashed sweet potatoes, and use spatula to smooth. Bake for 40 minutes.

PER SERVING: 356 calories, 23 g protein, 24 g fat (5 g saturated fat), 12 g carbohydrates, 2 g fibre, 91 mg cholesterol, 181 mg sodium.

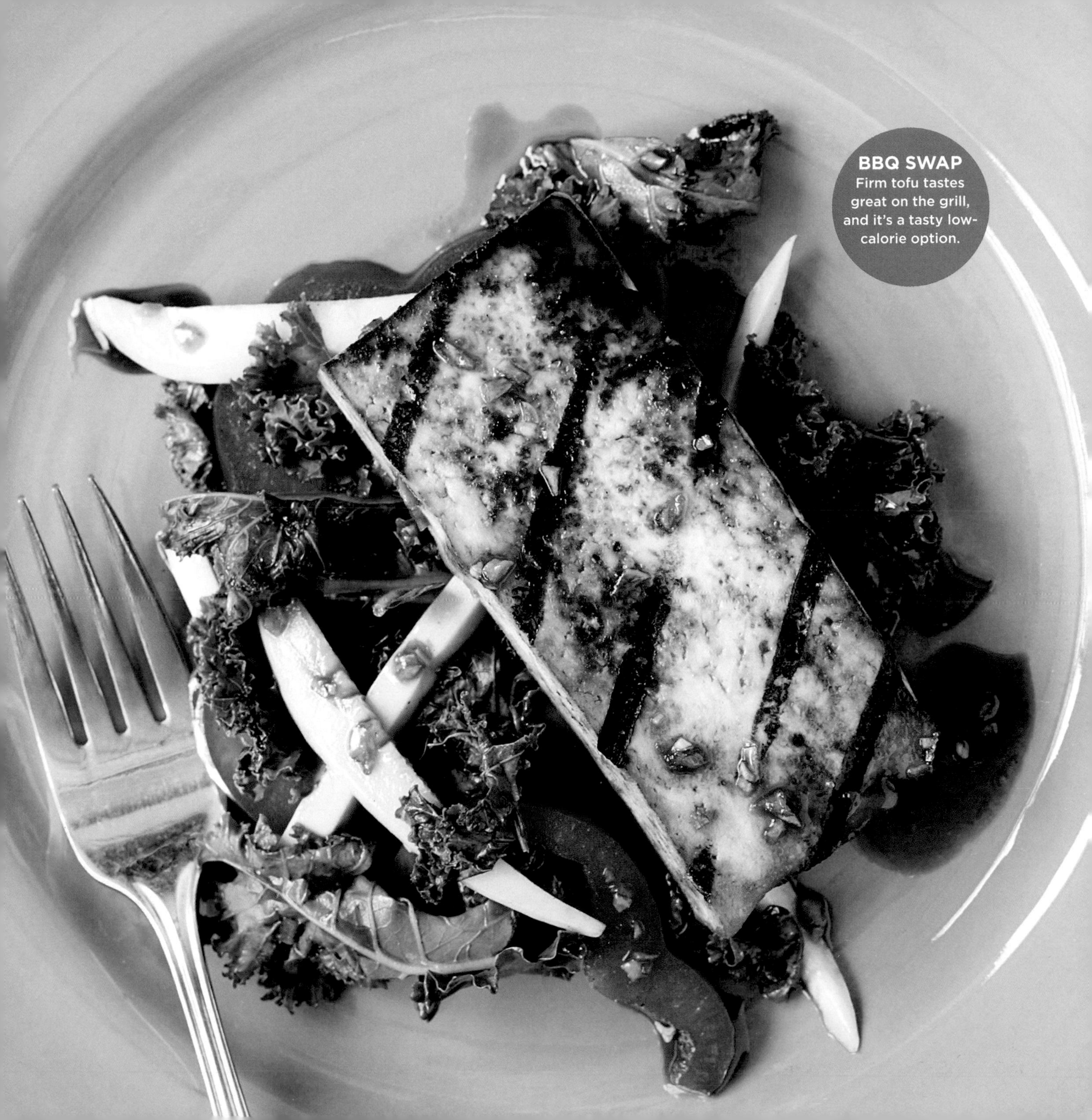

BBQ SWAP
Firm tofu tastes great on the grill, and it's a tasty low-calorie option.

Additional Recipes

snacks & desserts

VANILLA ANGEL FOOD CAKE

SERVES 12

Virtually fat-free, this light sponge cake really could be the food of angels. It is made using egg whites only, and develops a delicious golden crust during baking that hides the tender white interior. Here it is served with creamy low-fat yogourt and summer berries, but it is just as tempting with juicy peaches, mangoes or apricots.

CAKE

1 cup sifted cake flour
⅓ cup sugar
8 large egg whites, at room temperature
1 tsp cream of tartar
½ cup sugar
¼ tsp salt
1 tsp vanilla extract

GARNISH

1 cup strawberries, cut into quarters
1 cup raspberries
1 cup blueberries
250 g low-fat vanilla yogourt

1 Preheat oven to 350°F (180°C). Sift flour and ⅓ cup sugar onto large plate and set aside.

2 Place egg whites and cream of tartar into large bowl and whisk until frothy. Combine ½ cup sugar and salt, and add to whites, while whisking, in slow, steady stream. Add vanilla extract and keep whisking until mixture forms stiff peaks.

3 Sift flour mixture over egg whites and fold in very gently with large metal spoon until well-blended.

4 Spoon mixture into ungreased 25 cm tube pan, gently smoothing top. Bake until golden brown and cake springs back when lightly touched in centre, or about 35 minutes.

5 Invert cake, still in pan, onto wire rack and leave to cool completely. Once cool, slide long knife around side of pan to loosen cake, then invert onto serving plate. (Cake can be kept, wrapped in plastic or stored in airtight container, for 1 to 2 days.)

6 Just before serving, mix together strawberries, raspberries and blueberries. Spoon fruit into hollow in centre of cake. Serve each slice with dollop of vanilla yogourt.

PER SERVING: 195 calories, 6 g protein, 1 g total fat, 0 g saturated fat, 0 mg cholesterol, 42 g carbohydrates, 3 g fibre, 23 g sugar.

VARIATIONS

- **Lemon-Lime Angel Food Cake:** Add the finely grated zest of 1 lemon and 1 lime to the beaten egg whites with the sifted flour and sugar. While the cake is cooling, peel a cantaloupe and remove the seeds. Cut the melon into small chunks and place in a bowl. Squeeze the juice from the lemon and lime, sprinkle it over the melon and toss to coat well. Serve the cake with the melon pieces piled up in the centre.

- **Chocolate Angel Food Cake:** Sift 2 tbsp cocoa powder with the flour and sugar. Decorate the cake by dusting it with a mixture of 1 tbsp cocoa powder and 1 tbsp icing sugar, sifted together.

- **Coffee Angel Food Cake:** Sift 1 tbsp instant coffee powder (not granules) with the flour and sugar. Garnish with sifted icing sugar.

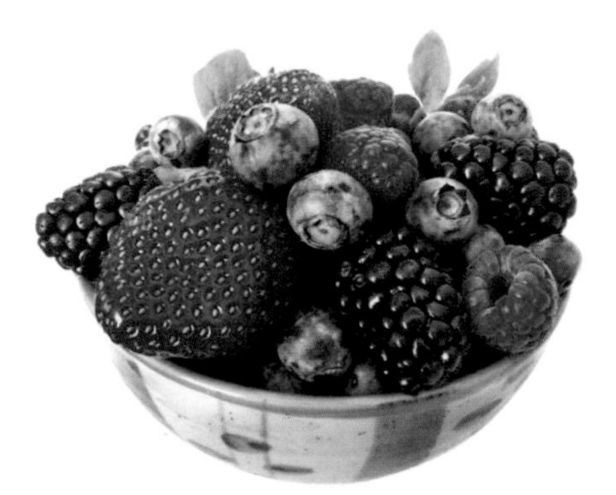

LEMONY BLUEBERRY CHEESECAKE BARS

MAKE 24 BARS

If you love cheesecake (and who doesn't?), you'll enjoy these wholesome bars. We've used blueberries to stretch the creamy filling and swapped the traditional buttery crust for whole-wheat.

CRUST

- 1 ½ cups whole-wheat pastry flour
- ¼ tsp baking powder
- ¼ tsp baking soda
- ¼ tsp salt
- 2 tbsp unsalted butter, softened
- 2 tbsp canola oil
- ½ cup sugar
- 1 large egg, lightly beaten
- 1 tsp vanilla extract

CREAM CHEESE FILLING

- 340 g reduced-fat cream cheese (or Neufchâtel cheese)
- ½ cup sugar
- 1 tbsp cornstarch
- 2 large eggs, lightly beaten
- 4 tsp freshly grated lemon zest
- 1 ½ tsp vanilla extract
- 3 cups fresh (or partially thawed frozen) blueberries

1 Preheat oven to 350°F (180°C). Coat a 23-by-33 cm baking dish with cooking spray.

2 To make crust: Whisk flour, baking powder, baking soda and salt in medium bowl. Beat butter, oil and sugar with electric mixer in mixing bowl until smooth. Add egg and vanilla. Beat until smooth. Add dry ingredients and mix with rubber spatula just until dry ingredients are moistened. Transfer dough to prepared baking dish. Use plastic wrap to press dough into even layer.

3 Bake crust, uncovered, until puffed and starting to brown around edges, about 20 minutes.

4 To make filling: Blend cream cheese, sugar and cornstarch with electric mixer or in food processor until smooth. Add eggs, lemon zest and vanilla. Beat or process until smooth. Spread blueberries over crust. Pour cream cheese batter over the blueberries, spreading evenly.

5 Bake bars until filling has set, or 35 to 40 minutes. Let cool in pan on wire rack. Cut into 24 bars with knife coated with cooking spray. Bars will keep, covered, in refrigerator for up to 4 days, or in freezer for up to 1 month.

PER SERVING (1 BAR): 140 calories, 3 g protein, 17 g carbohydrates, 1 g fibre, 6 g total fat, 3 g saturated fat, 40 mg cholesterol, 105 mg sodium.

SHOPPING

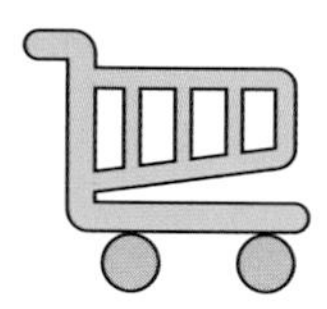

Neufchâtel vs. cream cheese

The original Neufchâtel cheese is French, but Canadian or American Neufchâtel is quite different. Created by an American who was attempting to replicate the French cheese, it's actually a lot more like cream cheese. It is, however, lower in fat: 23% milk fat to cream cheese's 33.

While fat-free cream cheese is still the least calorific option of all, if you're only using a little, why not try Neufchâtel instead?

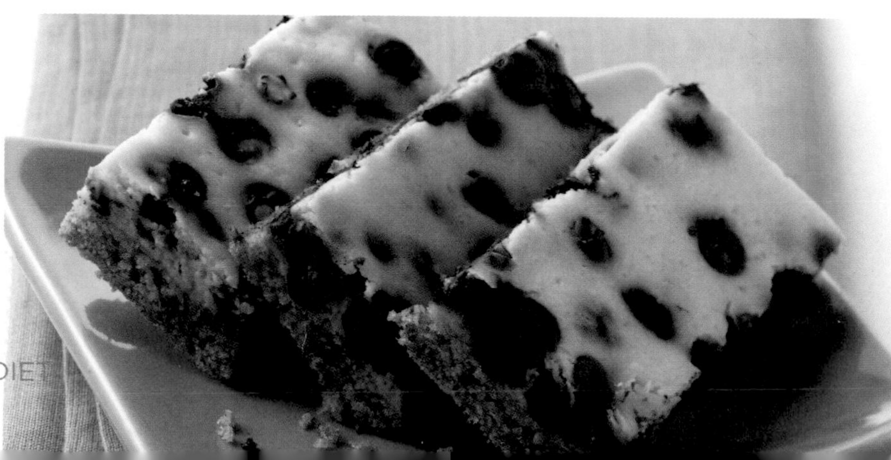

BERRY SWAP
Fresh out of blueberries? These bars would be equally delicious with fresh or frozen blackberries or raspberries.

PEACH AND BLACKBERRY PHYLLO PIZZAS

SERVES 6

For this impressive dessert, layers of light and flaky phyllo make crisp, elegant "pizza" crusts. The phyllo bases are sprinkled with almonds and then topped with an arrangement of sliced peaches and blackberries.

5 sheets phyllo pastry (36 by 46 cm)
Butter-flavoured cooking spray
2 tbsp ground almonds
3 large ripe peaches
1 cup fresh blackberries
5 tsp sugar

TO SERVE (optional):
1 cup light sour cream
1 tbsp light brown sugar

1 Preheat oven to 400°F (200°C) and coat baking sheet with cooking spray. Lay out 5 phyllo sheets and immediately cover with plastic wrap, then cover with damp towel (phyllo dries out in a couple of minutes if left uncovered). Work fast!

2 Place sheet of phyllo on work surface and spray with cooking spray. Layer 4 more phyllo sheets, spraying with cooking spray each time, and finally spray top sheet with cooking spray. Using 13 cm saucer as guide, cut out 6 circles from layered phyllo. Transfer each layered circle to baking sheet and sprinkle with ground almonds.

3 To decorate, cut peaches in half (do not peel), twist apart and remove pits. Slice peaches very thin. Place peach slices on phyllo pastry circles in pinwheel design. Divide blackberries among pizzas. Sprinkle 1 tsp sugar onto each pizza.

4 Bake pizzas until golden brown and peaches are tender and light brown, about 15 minutes. These pizzas are best served within 15 minutes, as the pastry can lose its crispness quickly if the fruit is juicy. If desired, serve with sour cream sweetened with brown sugar.

PER SERVING (ONE PIZZA): 107 calories, 2 g protein, 22 g carbohydrates, 3 g fibre, 2 g total fat, 0 g saturated fat, 0 mg cholesterol, 13 g sugar.

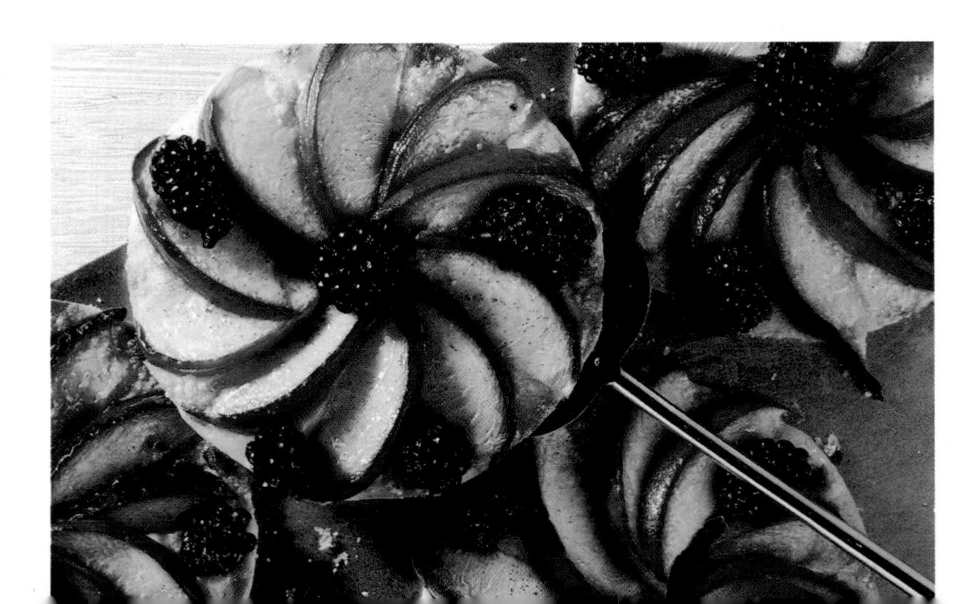

VARIATIONS

- **Pear and Raspberry Phyllo Pizzas:** Substitute 500 g ripe pears (preferably Bartlett) for the peaches; core the pears (do not peel) and cut into slices 3 mm thick. Use 1 cup fresh raspberries instead of blackberries. If you wish, drizzle the pizzas with a little brandy after decorating and before sprinkling them with the sugar.

- **Nectarine and Raspberry Phyllo Pizzas:** Substitute 500 g ripe, unpeeled nectarines for the peaches and 1 cup fresh blueberries for the blackberries. Toss the sugar with pinch of cinnamon before sprinkling over the pizzas.

- **Quick Brandied Peach Pizzas:** Substitute frozen, defrosted (or well-drained, canned) peach slices with brandy for the fresh peaches.

- **Plum and Raspberry Phyllo Pizzas:** Use 2 cups pitted, unpeeled plums instead of peaches. Slice 3 mm thick. Replace the blackberries with 1 cup raspberries.

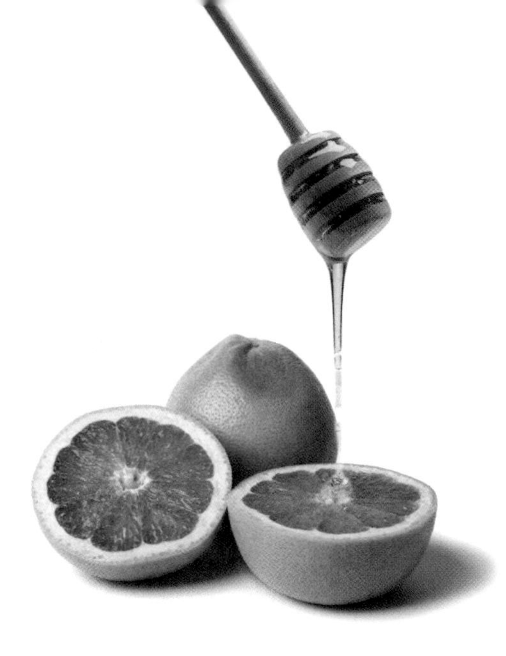

PINK GRAPEFRUIT BRÛLÉE

SERVES 2

Chilled fresh grapefruit is always a refreshing breakfast treat, but when caramelized with a cinnamon-scented honey drizzle and warmed, it becomes a simple and satisfying winter dessert.

1 pink grapefruit
2 tsp honey
Pinch of cinnamon

1 Preheat broiler. Line small baking sheet with aluminum foil (caramelized drippings can be hard to clean up). Cut grapefruit in half crosswise. Use paring knife or grapefruit knife to separate flesh from rind and membrane.

2 Drizzle 1 tsp honey over each grapefruit half and spread evenly. Sprinkle with cinnamon. Set grapefruit halves on baking sheet and broil until grapefruit skin is lightly browned in places and grapefruit is warmed through, or about 5 to 7 minutes. One serving is half a grapefruit.

PER SERVING: 59 calories, 1 g protein, 15 g carbohydrates, 1 g fibre, 0 g total fat, 0 g saturated fat, 0 mg cholesterol, 0 mg sodium.

OATMEAL-PEANUT BUTTER TRAIL BARS

MAKES 24 BARS

Peanut butter stands in for butter in these treats, reducing the saturated fat and boosting protein. These bars make ideal snacks—throw one in your bag before you head out the door.

½ cup whole-wheat flour
1 tsp cinnamon
½ tsp baking soda
⅛ tsp salt
½ cup unsalted smooth peanut butter
½ cup firmly packed brown sugar
⅓ cup honey
1 large egg
2 large egg whites
2 tbsp canola oil
2 tsp vanilla extract
2 cups old-fashioned rolled oats
1 cup dried cranberries or raisins
½ cup coarsely chopped walnuts or almonds
½ cup bittersweet or semisweet chocolate chips

1 Preheat oven to 350°F (180°C). Coat a 23-by-33 cm baking pan with cooking spray.

2 Whisk flour, cinnamon, baking soda and salt in medium bowl. Beat peanut butter, sugar and honey in another bowl with electric mixer until blended. Separately, blend egg and egg whites with fork. Add to peanut butter mixture, along with oil and vanilla. Beat until smooth. Add reserved flour mixture and mix with rubber spatula. Mix in oats, dried cranberries or raisins, walnuts or almonds and chocolate chips. Scrape batter into prepared baking dish. Use plastic wrap to spread batter into even layer.

3 Bake bars until lightly browned and firm, or 20 to 25 minutes. Let cool completely in pan on rack before cutting into 24 bars. One serving is one 5 cm-by-5 cm bar.

PER SERVING: 175 calories, 4 g protein, 24 g carbohydrates, 2 g fibre, 8 g total fat, 1 g saturated fat, 9 mg cholesterol, 68 mg sodium.

Notes on ingredients

If you're allergic to peanut butter, you can substitute soy-nut butter or sunflower-seed butter in the Trail Bars. You can also replace the nuts with unsalted roasted pumpkin seeds or sunflower seeds—look for unsalted seeds in the bulk bins of health food stores.

To avoid wasting egg yolks in recipes that only call for whites, use reconstituted dried egg whites, which are available in the baking or natural foods sections of most large supermarkets.

PUMPKIN CUSTARDS

SERVES 6

Think of these custards as the best part of a pumpkin pie. They're also low in calories and easy to make. A good pumpkin filling is distinguished by its seasoning, and this one has lots of cinnamon—a spice which may help lower your cholesterol. Vanilla soy milk makes exceptionally rich-tasting, low-fat custards, but if you don't have any, substitute 1% milk and increase the vanilla to 1 tsp.

- 2 large eggs
- 2 large egg whites
- 2/3 cup sugar
- 3/4 cup canned unseasoned pumpkin purée
- 1 1/2 tsp cinnamon
- 1/2 tsp ground nutmeg
- 1/4 tsp salt
- 1/2 tsp vanilla extract
- 1 1/2 cups vanilla soy milk
- 3 tbsp whipped cream or low-calorie whipped topping

1 Preheat oven to 325°F (160°C). Line roasting pan with folded kitchen towel to prevent custard cups from sliding around. Put kettle of water on to boil.

2 Whisk eggs, egg whites and sugar in large bowl until smooth. Add pumpkin purée, cinnamon, nutmeg, salt and vanilla. Whisk until blended. Gently whisk in soy milk.

3 Divide mixture among six custard cups (3/4 cup each). Skim foam from surface of custards. Set custard cups on towel in roasting pan. Pour enough boiling water into roasting pan to come halfway up sides of custard cups. Place roasting pan in oven and bake, uncovered, until custards are set, 50 to 55 minutes. Transfer custard cups to rack and let cool. Cover custards and refrigerate until chilled, at least 1 hour.

4 Just before serving, top each custard with dollop of whipped cream. One serving is 1 custard and 1/2 tbsp whipped cream.

PER SERVING: 166 calories, 5 g protein, 28 g carbohydrates, 1 g fibre, 4 g total fat, 1 g saturated fat, 75 mg cholesterol, 165 mg sodium.

LIL' PUMPKIN

For many of us, a slice of pumpkin pie is just the thing to top off a holiday dinner. But that can be a major indulgence: A single slice can have over 300 calories! Add that to an already-massive meal, and you've got calorie trouble.

This holiday season, why not surprise your family with these Pumpkin Custards instead? They're equally delicious, for half the calories of pie.

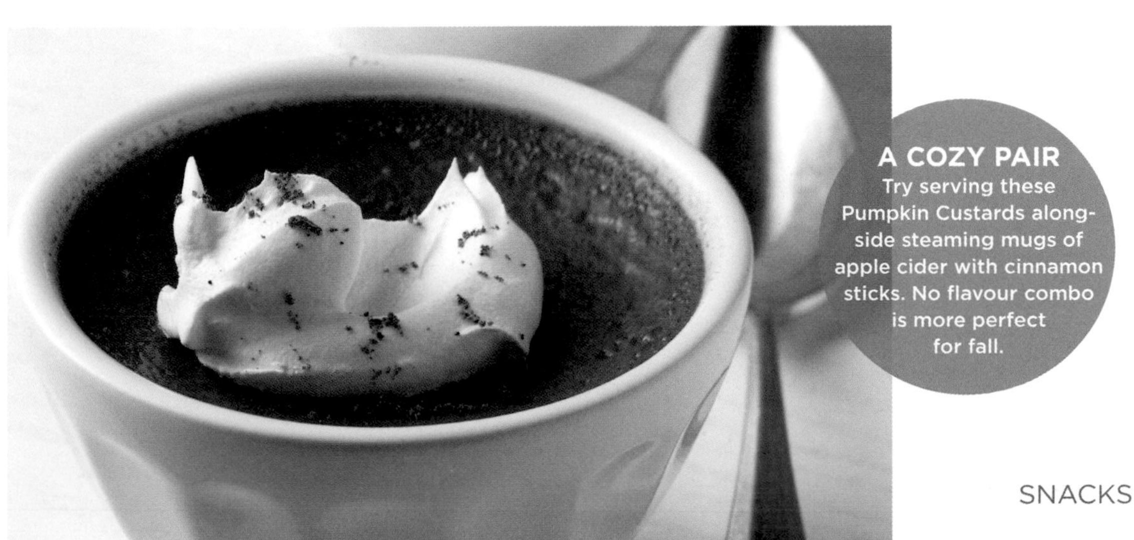

A COZY PAIR
Try serving these Pumpkin Custards alongside steaming mugs of apple cider with cinnamon sticks. No flavour combo is more perfect for fall.

SAFFRON AND VANILLA GRILLED FRUIT

SERVES 6

Pick a collection of luscious fruits, spice them elegantly with saffron and vanilla, then grill them until they are warm, fragrant and beginning to release their juices. Top with vanilla frozen yogourt for an exotic yet comforting treat.

MARINADE

1 small pinch of saffron threads, or ½ tsp ground saffron
¼ cup hot water
¼ cup fresh orange juice
1 tbsp Marsala wine or sweet sherry
1 tsp vanilla extract
1 tsp honey

SALAD

½ large papaya
1 large navel orange
1 large kiwi
1 large banana
½ cup seedless black or purple grapes

TO SERVE (optional):
6 small scoops sugar-free vanilla frozen yogourt

1 Marinade: Heat small, dry saucepan over high heat until hot, for about 1 minute. Add saffron and toast, stirring until fragrant or about 30 seconds. Remove saffron from heat and chop finely or crush with mortar and pestle. Place saffron in medium bowl and add hot water. Stir in orange juice, Marsala wine, vanilla and honey.

2 Prepare fruits, adding to marinade as you go. Peel papaya, remove seeds and cut into bite-sized chunks. Using serrated knife, peel orange, removing white pith; cut between membranes and lift out sections.

3 Peel kiwi, then cut lengthwise into 6 wedges. Peel banana, halve lengthwise and cut into bite-sized chunks. Add grapes. You will have about 4 cups of fruit. Stir gently to coat fruit with marinade. If time permits, let fruit marinate 1 hour before cooking.

4 Preheat broiler or heat grill pan on stovetop. Pour fruit and marinade into shallow ovenproof dish if using broiler. Spread out fruit in even layer. Broil until heated through, or about 5 minutes. If using grill pan, place fruit in even layer in pan and cook until heated through, for about 5 minutes (or sauté fruit in large skillet over medium-high heat for 5 minutes). Ladle fruit into 6 dessert dishes. Serve warm with scoop of frozen yogourt.

PER SERVING (WITHOUT FROZEN YOGOURT): 78 calories, 1 g protein, 2 g fibre, 0 g total fat , 0 g saturated fat, 0 mg cholesterol, 19 g carbohydrates, 14 g sugar.

Fruit benefits

- Kiwis are cultivated in California and New Zealand. Because these two places have opposite seasons, kiwis are available year-round. They can be kept in the refrigerator for up to 3 weeks and served as a healthy snack. Simply cut the fruit in half and scoop the flesh out with a spoon.
- The banana, kiwi and citrus fruit all provide potassium, which keeps body fluids and blood pressure in balance.

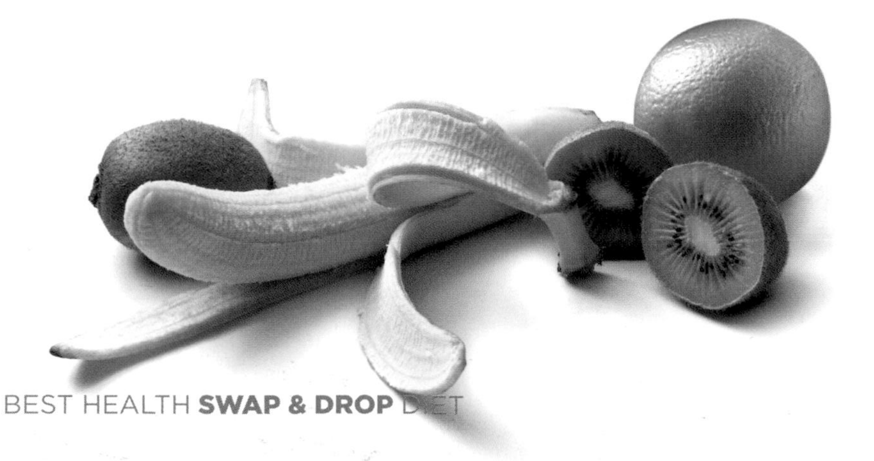

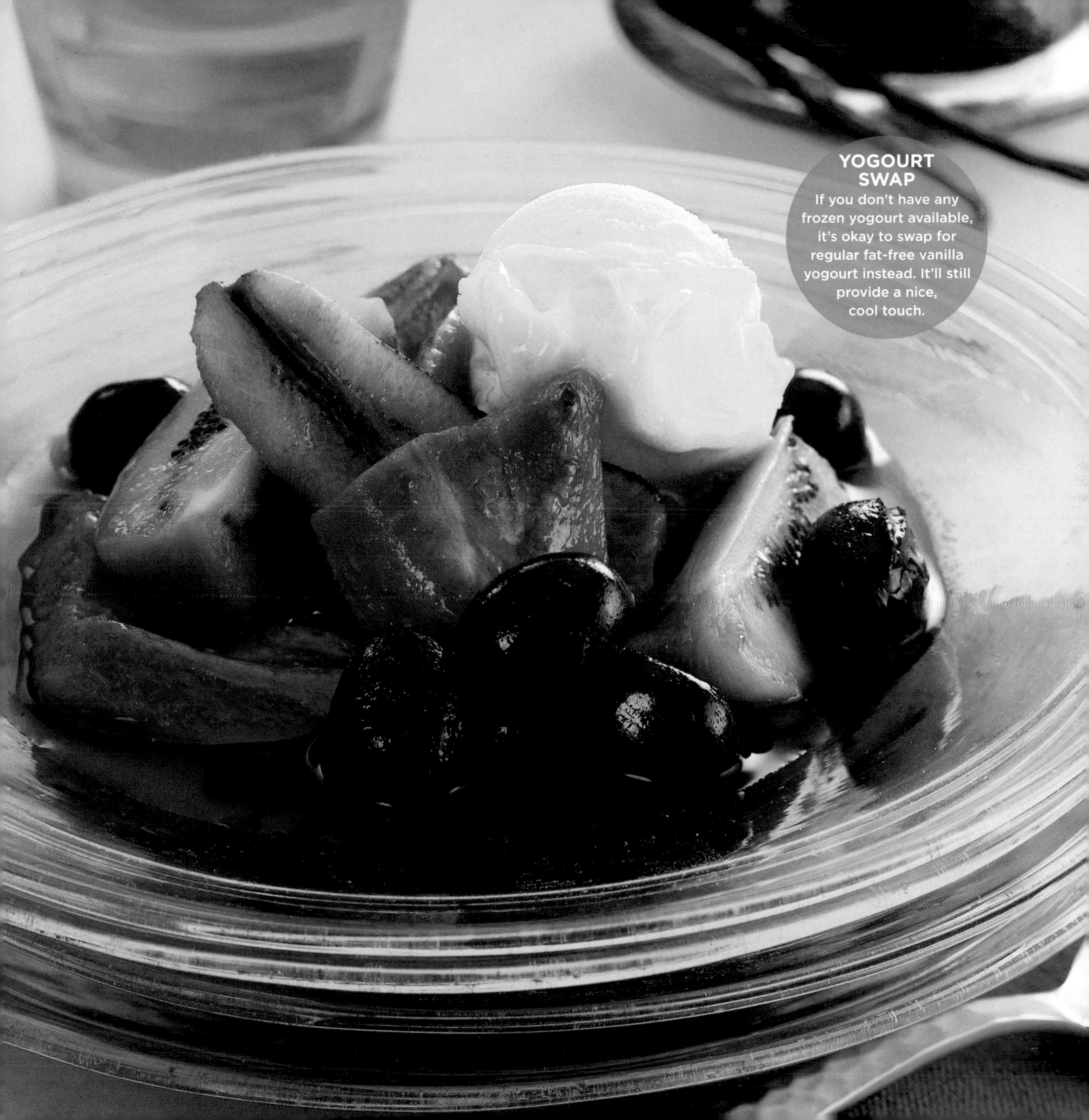

YOGOURT SWAP

If you don't have any frozen yogourt available, it's okay to swap for regular fat-free vanilla yogourt instead. It'll still provide a nice, cool touch.

Another idea

●●● **Mixed-Berry Almond Gratin:** In Step 4, substitute 3 cups mixed berries, such as raspberries, blackberries and blueberries (fresh or frozen and partially thawed), for the cherries.

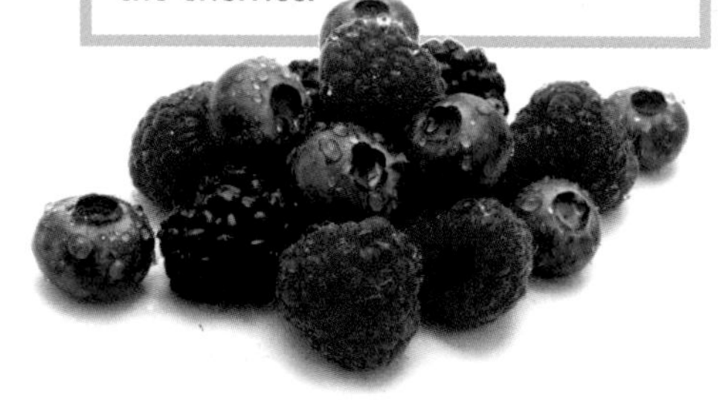

CHERRY-ALMOND GRATIN

SERVES 6

Fruit baked in a rich-tasting almond cream creates a special dessert. Tofu may seem like a surprising ingredient, but it makes a very healthy substitute for butter.

- **⅓ cup slivered almonds**
- **⅓ cup sugar**
- **1 tbsp all-purpose flour**
- **Pinch of salt**
- **1 large egg**
- **1 large egg white**
- **½ cup reduced-fat firm silken tofu**
- **1 tbsp unsalted butter, softened**
- **¼ tsp almond extract**
- **3 cups fresh or partially thawed frozen sweet cherries, pitted**
- **Icing sugar for dusting**

1 Preheat oven to 375°F (190°C). Coat 24 cm pie pan with cooking spray.

2 Spread almonds in small baking dish. Toast in oven until light golden and fragrant, or 4 to 6 minutes. Let cool.

3 Combine almonds, sugar, flour and salt in food processor. Process until almonds are ground. Add egg, egg white, tofu, butter and almond extract. Process until smooth.

4 Spread cherries in pie pan. Scrape tofu mixture evenly over cherries. Bake gratin until light golden and firm, 30 to 40 minutes. Let cool slightly. Dust with icing sugar. Serve warm.

PER SERVING: 168 calories, 5 g protein, 26 g carbohydrates, 2 g fibre, 6 g total fat, 2 g saturated fat, 40 mg cholesterol, 28 g sodium.

MAPLE-WALNUT ROASTED APPLES

SERVES 4

Our sophisticated yet simple baked apple features walnuts for a dose of protein and "good" fat. If possible, use Cortland apples—they're the best choice for baking.

- **⅓ cup maple syrup**
- **3 tbsp apple cider or apple juice**
- **2 tsp unsalted butter**
- **2 large apples, halved and cored, with skin**
- **2 tbsp chopped walnuts**
- **1 cup low-fat vanilla frozen yogourt**

1 Preheat oven to 400°F (200°C). Coat 20 cm square baking dish with cooking spray.

2 Combine maple syrup, apple cider and butter in small saucepan. Bring to a simmer, stirring. Remove from heat.

3 Place apples cut side up, in baking dish. Pour maple syrup mixture over apples. Cover with aluminum foil and bake for 20 minutes.

4 Baste apples with maple syrup mixture. Sprinkle with walnuts. Return to oven and bake, uncovered, until apples are tender and glazed, 10 to 20 minutes, basting once or twice. Let cool slightly. Place 1 apple half on each dish and drizzle with syrup. Serve with scoop of frozen yogourt.

PER SERVING (1 APPLE HALF, 2 TBSP SYRUP AND ¼ CUP ICE CREAM): 207 calories, 2 g protein, 38 g carbohydrates, 2 g fibre, 6 g total fat, 2 g saturated fat, 10 mg cholesterol, 29 mg sodium.

CHERRY CLAFOUTI

SERVES 8

When it comes to cherries, there are few better ways to use them than in a clafouti. This rustic French dessert, a cross between a custard and a baked pancake, is simple to make and oh-so-comforting. If you're using fresh cherries, use a cherry pitter to speed the pitting process. You can also use frozen cherries, which are already pitted.

2 tbsp plus ½ cup sugar, divided
½ cup all-purpose flour
2 large eggs
2 large egg whites
1 cup 1% milk
1 tbsp unsalted butter, melted
1 tsp vanilla extract
3 cups fresh or partially thawed frozen sweet cherries, pitted
Icing sugar for dusting

1 Preheat oven to 400°F (200°C). Coat a 24 cm pie pan with cooking spray. Sprinkle with 1 tbsp sugar and tilt to coat.

2 Place flour, eggs, egg whites, milk, butter, ½ cup sugar and vanilla in food processor or blender. Process until smooth.

3 Spread cherries in pie pan. Pour egg batter over cherries. Sprinkle with remaining 1 tbsp sugar. Bake clafouti until light brown and puffed, 35 to 40 minutes. Let cool slightly. (Clafouti will sink as it cools.) Dust with icing sugar and serve warm. Leftovers are also delicious chilled.

PER SERVING: 176 calories, 5 g protein, 33 g carbohydrates, 1 g fibre, 3 g total fat, 2 g saturated fat, 59 mg cholesterol, 48 mg sodium.

Another idea

Pear-Berry Clafouti: In Step 2, add 2 tsp grated lemon zest to the custard. In Step 3, substitute 2 sliced, peeled Anjou pears and 1 cup fresh or frozen raspberries for the cherries.

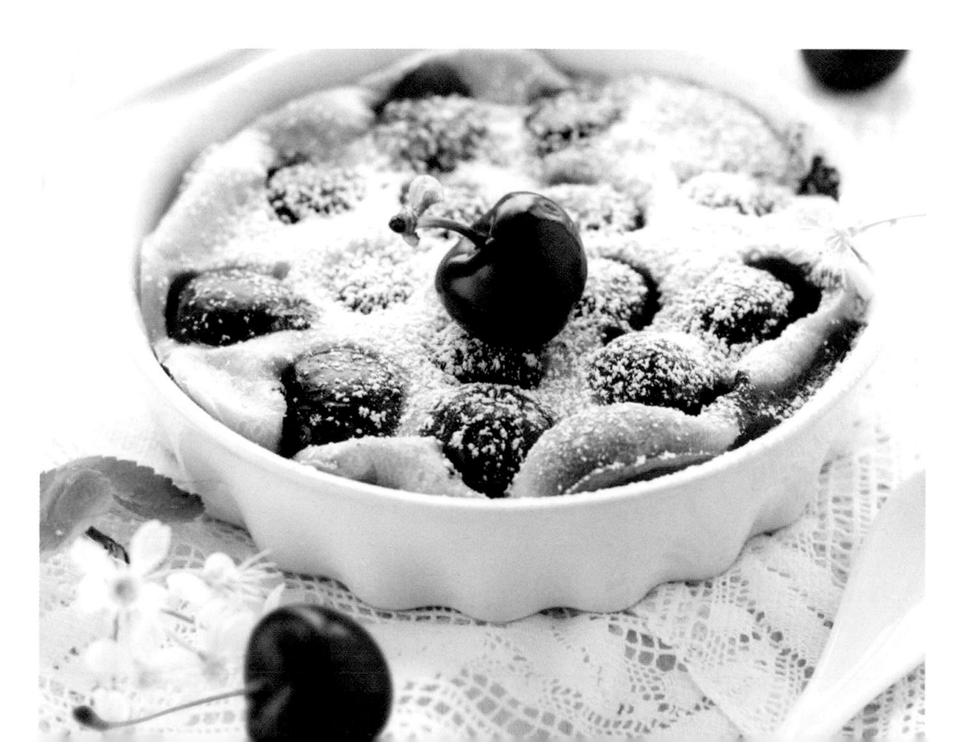

FRUIT FIX
Cherries not ripe? Try tossing them with a little sugar and lemon juice, then roasting them in the oven at 350°F (180°C) for 10 minutes.

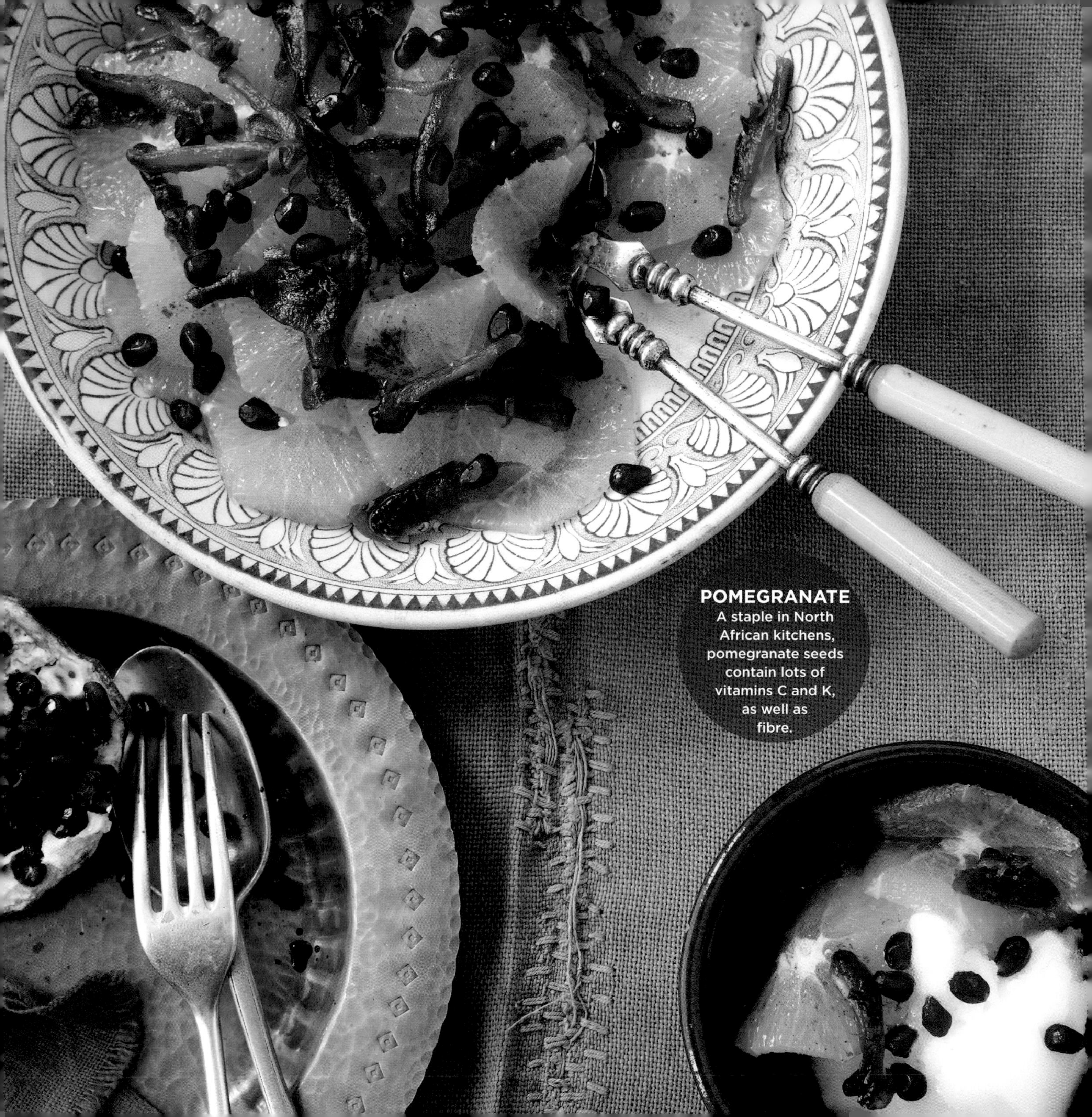

POMEGRANATE
A staple in North African kitchens, pomegranate seeds contain lots of vitamins C and K, as well as fibre.

MOROCCAN FRUIT SALAD

SERVES 6

The combined flavours of cinnamon, dates, pomegranate seeds and oranges make this simple dessert a healthy winner. Ruby-red pomegranate seeds add a beautiful and delicious touch.

5 medium oranges
8 fresh or semi-dried dates, pitted
1 tsp ground cinnamon
1 tsp honey
1 pomegranate, peeled

1 Peel and thinly slice four oranges and place in medium bowl. Thinly slice dates lengthwise and add to bowl.

2 Squeeze juice from remaining orange into small bowl, and stir in cinnamon and honey. Pour this liquid over fruit and garnish with lots of pomegranate seeds. Serve salad on its own for dessert, or as a topping with sorbet.

PER SERVING: 184 calories, 2 g protein, 1 g total fat, 0 g saturated fat, 47 g carbohydrates, 6 g fibre, 0 mg cholesterol, 3 mg sodium.

Top it off

- **For an especially Moroccan end to a meal, serve a pot of strong coffee flavoured with a few cardamom pods.**
- **Indulge in a macaron, a diminutive French pastry (below), alongside this juicy fruit salad.**

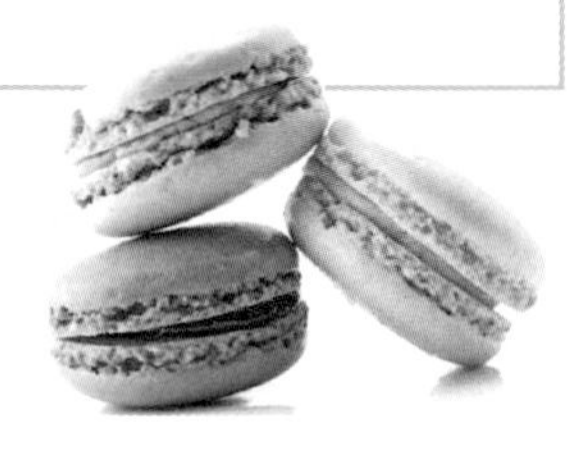

CANTALOUPE AND BLUEBERRY COMPOTE WITH GREEN TEA AND LIME

SERVES 6

Cantaloupe and blueberries are a natural pair. Here, a tart lime seasoning and light green-tea syrup give a distinctive and thoroughly refreshing finish to this low-calorie dessert. It also makes a tasty breakfast compote.

2 green tea bags
2/3 cup boiling water
2 tbsp sugar
1 tsp grated lime zest
2 tbsp lime juice
1/2 cantaloupe, cut into 4 cm cubes (about 3 cups)
2 cups blueberries, rinsed and dried

1 Place tea bags in boiling water and let steep for 3 to 4 minutes. Remove tea bags. Add sugar to tea and stir until dissolved. Stir in lime zest and lime juice. Let cool to room temperature.

2 Combine cantaloupe and blueberries in a large bowl. Pour green tea mixture over fruit and toss to coat well. Compote will keep, covered, in refrigerator for up to 2 days.

PER SERVING (2/3 CUP): 72 calories, 1 g protein, 18 g carbohydrates, 2 g fibre, 0 g total fat, 0 g saturated fat, 0 mg cholesterol, 13 mg sodium.

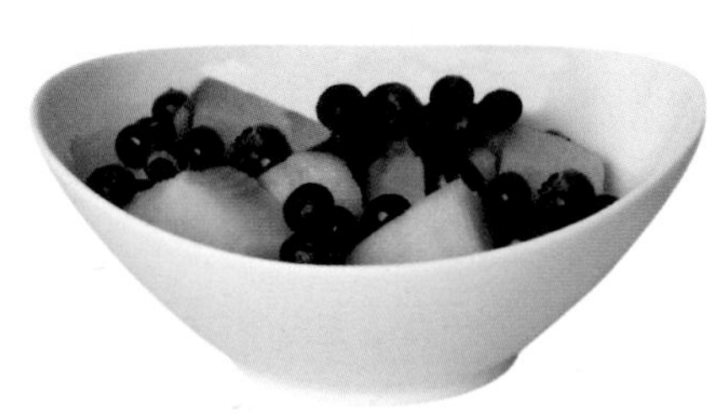

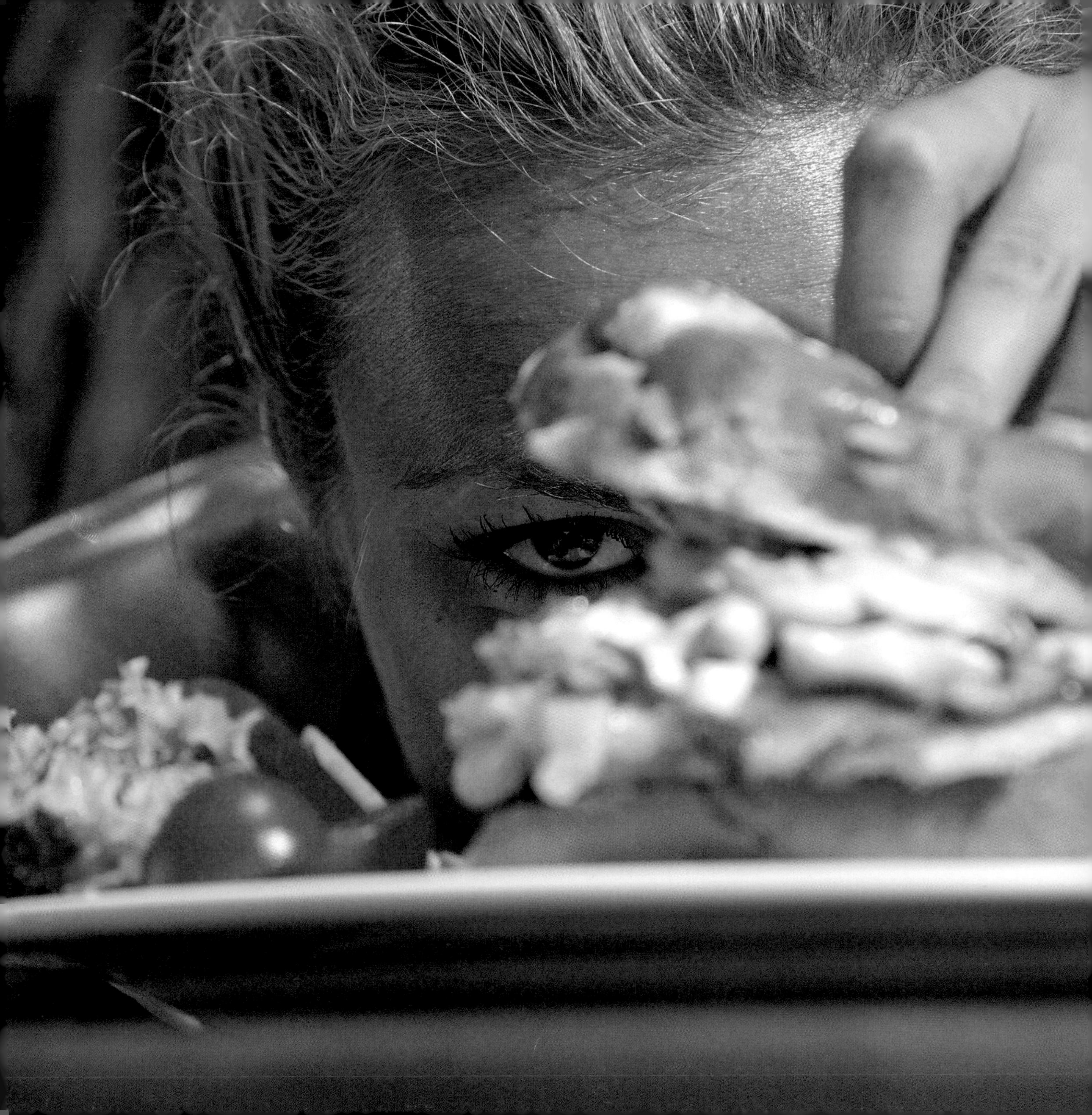

3

Swap & Drop

Eat in, dine out and grab a meal on the go!

I love dining out, to a fault. I have a very full, busy life, which allows me to justify eating out or picking up food on the run. I confess that I also often fail to keep my cupboards stocked with quick and healthy meal options. That said, I'm pleased to report that since reading Part 1 of this book, I have become a much more inspired and effective grocery shopper, have been cooking a lot more at home and have only dined out twice in the last few weeks!

This section of **Swap & Drop** *contains lots of fabulous tips to turn your favourite meals and snacks into healthier, smarter, less fattening versions. I've been sharing similar tips with patients, clients and readers for years: Add fruit and nuts to cereal and yogourt, use mustard instead of mayo and substitute or add in whole grains at every opportunity.*

I agree that it's time to say goodbye to white breads and rolls. I make a pact with virtually everyone I dine out with: No matter how much we'd love to say yes, when the server arrives with a tempting basket of breads, we steel ourselves and immediately say, "No, thank you!"

The information on restaurant dishes surprised me and will surely surprise you. For example, many people who are trying to lose weight order a large salad as their meal when dining out. Yet as you'll see, some innocent-looking salads are actually shockingly high in calories and fat.

The truth really can and will set you free. You'll see how effectively swapping for a better choice adds up to pounds lost over time. I think that you'll also find that once you know the true fat and calorie content of a favourite restaurant dish, with very little effort, you won't love or want it like you used to.

– Dr. Susan Biali, M.D.

BREAKFAST SWAP&DROPS

▼ SWAP THIS	▼ FOR THAT

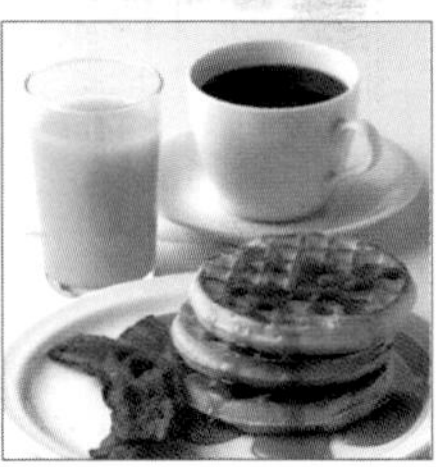

3 10 cm white-flour waffles with 3 tbsp maple syrup
2 slices regular bacon
250 mL orange juice
1 cup coffee
Total calories: 597

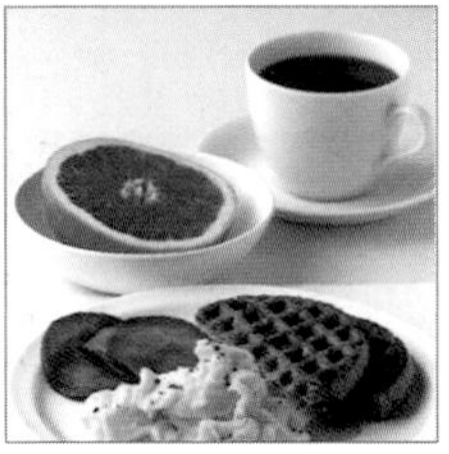

1 10 cm Multi-Grain Waffle with 1 tbsp syrup (recipe pg. 135)
2 large eggs, scrambled
2 slices Canadian back bacon
½ medium grapefruit
1 cup coffee or tea
Total calories: 337

Why it's a Good Swap

- Swapped white-flour waffles for the Multi-Grain Waffle, which has much more healthy fibre.
- Decreased the number of waffles from three to one.
- Added protein-rich eggs to replace the waffle calories.
- Decreased the amount of maple syrup for fewer calories.
- Substituted Canadian back bacon for regular bacon. It's much lower in saturated fat.
- Replaced the orange juice with half a grapefruit. Whole fruit has more fibre than juice does.

EVEN BETTER SWAP: Substitute a slice of rye or whole-grain toast for the waffle and maple syrup.

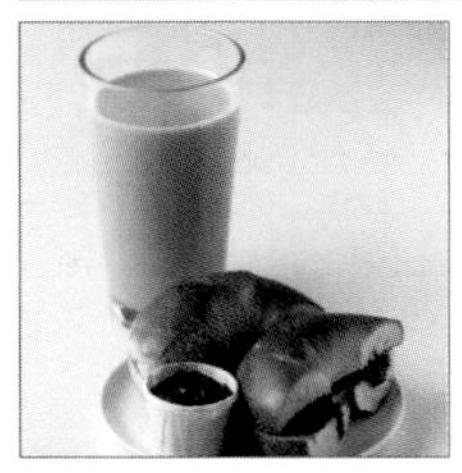

1 toasted large plain bagel with 2 tbsp jam or jelly
341 mL French vanilla coffee beverage
Total calories: 612

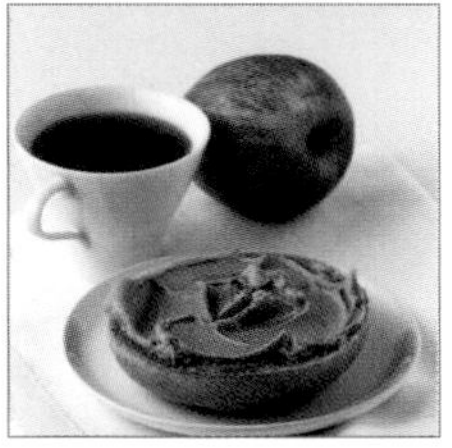

½ toasted large whole-wheat bagel, 1 tbsp peanut butter
1 medium apple
1 cup coffee or tea
Total calories: 275

Why it's a Good Swap

- Swapped the white-flour bagel for a whole-wheat bagel, which has more fibre.
- Cut the bagel portion in half to limit calories.
- Added peanut butter as a source of protein and "good" fat, to keep you fuller, longer.
- Replaced the high-calorie artificial coffee beverage with plain coffee or tea.

EVEN BETTER SWAP: Opt for two slices of whole-grain toast instead of a bagel.

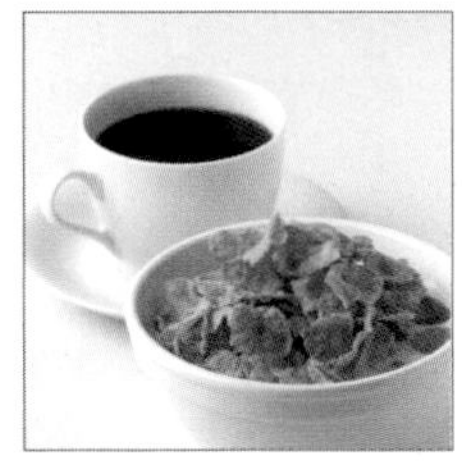

2 cups Corn Flakes with 1 cup 2% milk
1 cup coffee or tea
Total calories: 321

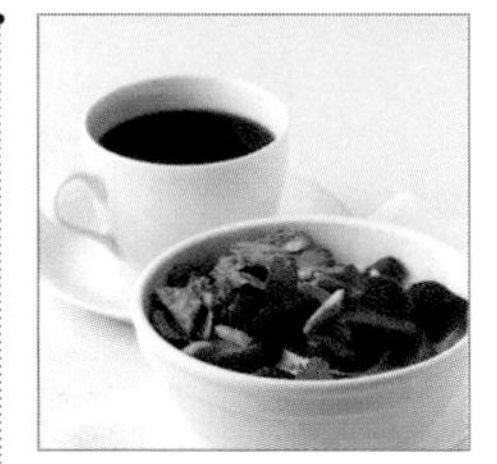

¾ cup Grape-Nuts Flakes, ½ cup skim milk, ½ cup strawberries, 14 g slivered almonds
1 cup coffee or tea
Total calories: 258

Why it's a Good Swap

- Swapped the cereal and decreased the serving.
- Cut calories and fat by switching from 2% milk to skim milk.
- Added fruit and nuts to the cereal to make up for the smaller portion. The fruit provides extra vitamins and phytochemicals, while the nuts, with their healthy fats, slow the digestion of the meal for a slower rise in blood sugar.

EVEN BETTER SWAP: Go for Fiber One cereal instead of Grape-Nuts Flakes—it has even more healthy fibre. (See page 35 for even more cereal suggestions.)

LUNCH SWAP&DROPS

▼ SWAP THIS	▼ FOR THAT

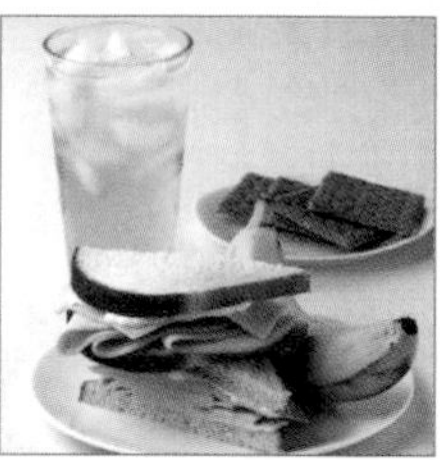

2 slices white bread with 2 slices roasted turkey, 2 slices cheese and mayo
1 medium banana
3 or 4 graham crackers
495 mL apple juice
Total calories: 891

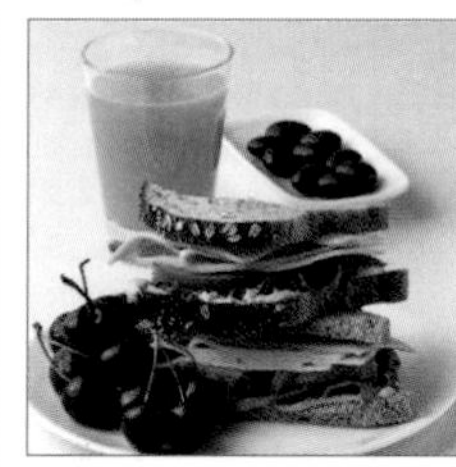

2 slices whole-grain bread with 2 slices turkey, 1 slice cheese, lettuce, tomato and mustard
12 cherries
9 chocolate almonds
180 mL grapefruit juice
Total calories: 452

Why it's a Good Swap

- Swapped white bread for whole-grain to boost fibre.
- Cut approximately 60 calories by switching from mayonnaise to mustard.
- Exchanged the apple juice for grapefruit juice (it has more vitamin C), and cut the quantity to reduce calories.
- Switched the banana for low-cal cherries.
- Included chocolate-covered almonds instead of graham crackers. The almonds offer protein, "good" fats, vitamins and fibre, while the graham crackers don't provide as much nutrition.

EVEN BETTER SWAP: If you're not hungry enough at lunchtime, skip the almonds or save them for a snack later in the day.

---

2 slices regular cheese pizza
730 mL pop
Total calories: 580

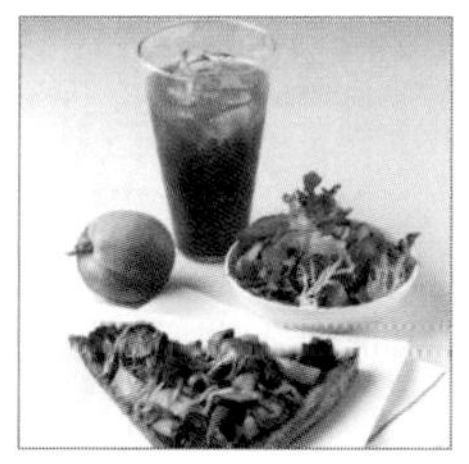

1 slice whole-wheat pizza with cheese and vegetables
1 cup side salad with 1 tbsp oil-vinegar dressing
1 medium peach
495 mL unsweetened iced tea
Total calories: 333

Why it's a Good Swap

- Cut carbs, fat and calories by limiting pizza to one slice.
- Boosted fibre by switching to whole-wheat crust and adding healthy vegetables.
- Made up for the slice you're not eating by adding a side salad made from mixed greens, tomato and cucumber, with oil and vinegar dressing, and a piece of fruit—much more nutritious foods than pizza.

EVEN BETTER SWAP: Make your own pizza at home by topping a whole-grain pita with 2 tbsp tomato sauce, 60 g part-skim mozzarella or other low-fat cheese, and plenty of veggies.

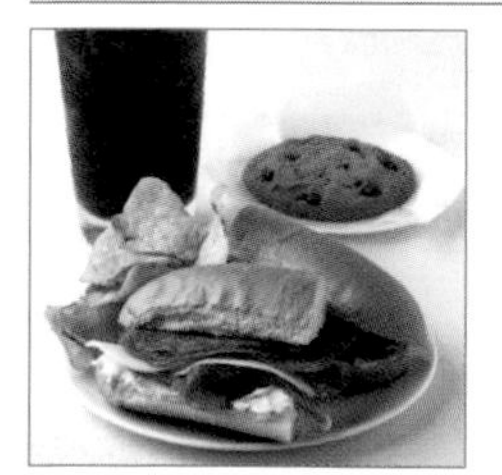

1 white roll, 4 slices each salami & prosciutto, 2 slices provolone cheese, 1 tbsp mayo
60 g bag potato chips
1 large chocolate chip cookie
730 mL pop
Total calories: 1,972

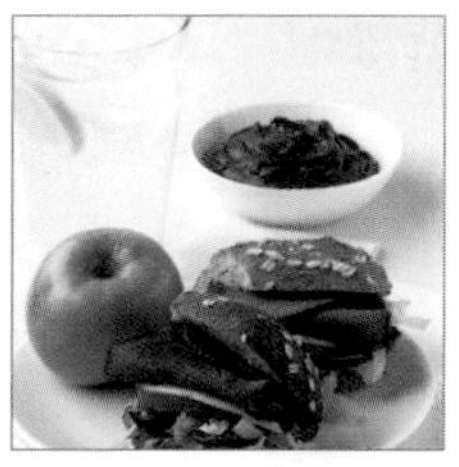

½ whole-grain roll, 2 slices lean roast beef, 1 slice provolone, lettuce, tomato, cucumber
125 mL low-fat chocolate pudding & 1 medium apple
Mineral water with lemon
Total calories: 588

Why it's a Good Swap

- Switched to a whole-grain roll, which has more fibre, and only used half to cut calories.
- Substituted leaner meat for meats high in saturated fat, reduced the quantity of meat and beefed up the sandwich with a generous helping of veggies.
- Replaced the chips with an apple for much less fat and many more nutrients.
- Cut saturated fat and calories by replacing the cookie with light pudding, which also provides some calcium.

EVEN BETTER SWAP: This is still fairly calorific. It would be best to skip dessert (it's just lunch, after all), and opt for a whole-grain salad with chickpeas and veggies instead of a sandwich.

DINNER SWAP&DROPS

▼ SWAP THIS ▼ FOR THAT

Swap This

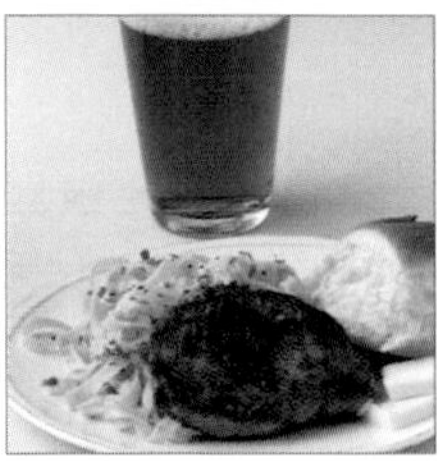

125 g pork chop
1½ cups cooked fettuccine with 1 tbsp butter, 1 tbsp parmesan, 1 tbsp parsley
1 white dinner roll with 1 tbsp butter
341 mL beer
Total calories: 942

For That

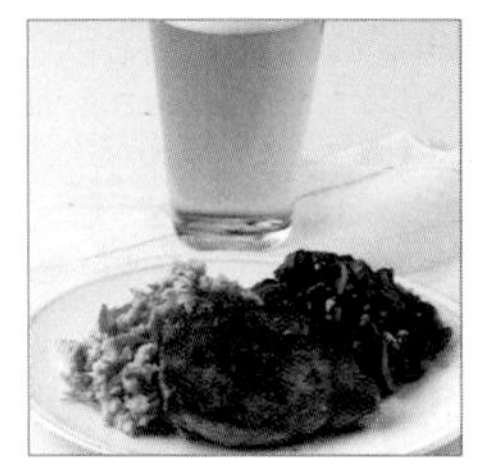

125 g pork chop
½ cup Bulgur with Ginger and Orange (recipe pg. 167)
Sautéed Spinach with Ginger and Soy Sauce (recipe pg. 167)
341 mL light beer
Total calories: 665

Why it's a Good Swap

- Swapped the fettuccine for bulgur, a better carbohydrate choice. Pasta's not bad for you, but bulgur has more fibre.
- Eliminated the white roll, which adds little but calories.
- Added sautéed spinach to replace the roll. Spinach is loaded with fibre and nutrients, and has far fewer calories.
- Changed the regular beer to light beer to reduce calories.

EVEN BETTER SWAP: Split the beer with your partner so you can both enjoy the taste without all the extra added calories. Or, even better, opt for an unsweetened iced tea or mineral water instead of alcohol.

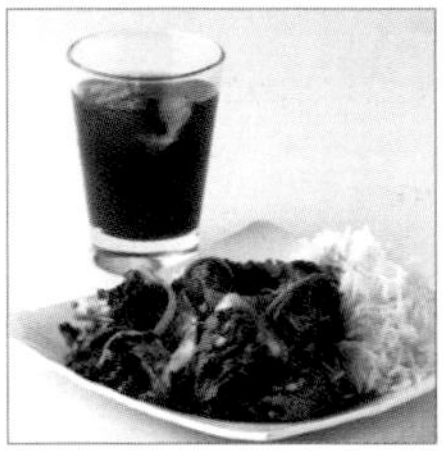

Swap This

1½ cups take-out beef and broccoli stir-fry
1 cup white rice
250 mL pop
Total calories: 1,223

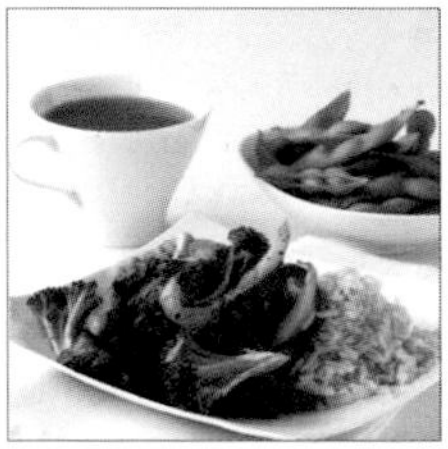

For That

1 cup unshelled edamame
1½ cups Orange Beef Stir-Fry (recipe pg. 163)
½ cup brown rice
Black or green tea
Total calories: 612

Why it's a Good Swap

- Made the stir-fry at home using leaner beef, less oil and more vegetables, including broccoli and red peppers. The result: fewer calories and less saturated fat, which clogs arteries.
- Substituted brown rice for white and cut the portion in half.
- Started the meal with edamame (steamed green soybeans) to fill you up on a fibre- and protein-rich food, so you won't miss the rest of the rice. Edamame also slows eating because it takes time to get the beans out of their shells.
- Replaced calorific pop with practically calorie-free tea.

EVEN BETTER SWAP: Eat slowly—you may not even need the entire serving of stir-fry. Pay attention to your hunger cues.

Swap This

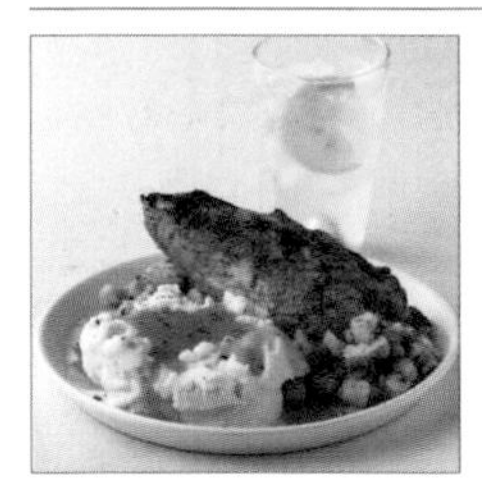

1 roasted chicken breast with skin
1 cup mashed potatoes
½ cup gravy
1 cup stuffing
Mineral water with lemon
Total calories: 1,053

For That

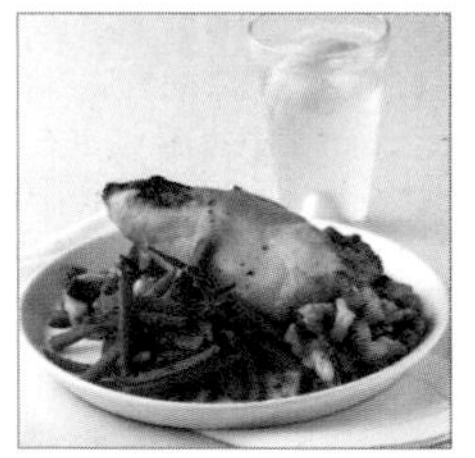

1 roasted chicken breast, no skin
⅓ cup gravy
1 cup apple-walnut stuffing
¾ cup Moroccan Spiced Carrots (recipe pg. 159)
Mineral water with lemon
Total calories: 760

Why it's a Good Swap

- Eliminated the chicken skin, a significant source of saturated fat and calories.
- Cut out the mashed potatoes and replaced them with Moroccan Spiced Carrots to increase fibre and vitamins.
- Added apples and walnuts to the stuffing—more apples and walnuts mean less bread. Nuts also add healthy fats.

EVEN BETTER SWAP: Don't overcook the chicken—if it stays tender and moist, you can easily skip the gravy.

DINNER SWAP&DROPS

▼ SWAP THIS **▼ FOR THAT**

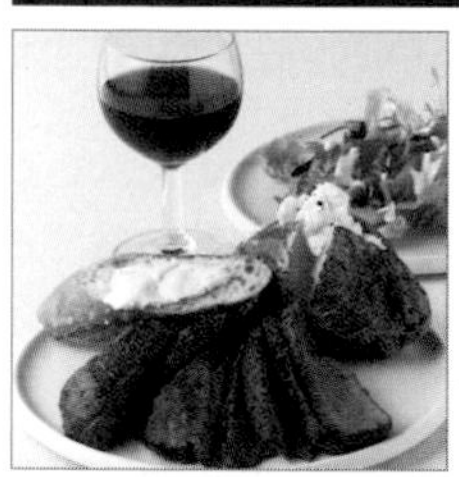

200 g grilled sirloin steak
1 medium baked potato, 1 tbsp butter
1 cup salad, 1 tbsp ranch dressing
1 slice crusty bread, 1 tbsp butter
125 mL red wine
Total calories: 1,003

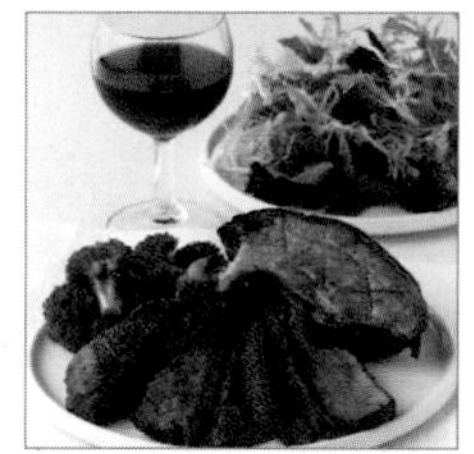

200 g grilled sirloin steak
½ baked medium sweet potato, ½ tbsp margarine, cinnamon
½ cup steamed broccoli
2 cups salad greens with bell peppers, 2 tbsp oil and vinegar
125 mL red wine
Total calories: 481

Why it's a Good Swap

- Replaced the white potato with half a sweet potato to increase the nutrient load. Sprinkle a little good-for-you nutmeg and cinnamon on top, and eat the skin for added fibre.
- Doubled the salad size. Salad is filling and full of vitamins.
- Changed the ranch dressing to oil and vinegar vinaigrette to decrease unhealthy saturated fat.
- Replaced the bread with broccoli to add vitamins and fibre.

EVEN BETTER SWAP: Replace the wine with a spritzer or sparkling water, and you'll cut the calories even more.

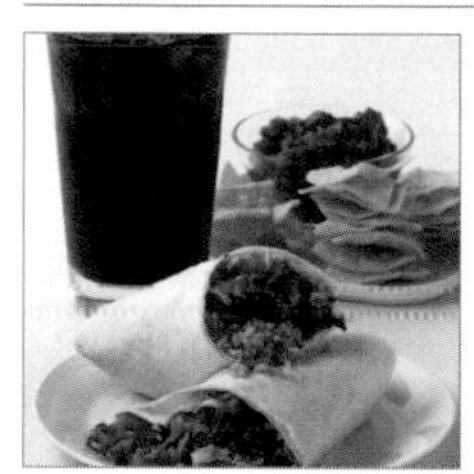

1 burrito (33 cm white tortilla, 1 cup white rice, 60 g beef filling, 30 g cheese, 2 tbsp salsa)
45 g tortilla chips, ¼ cup salsa
730 mL pop
Total calories: 1,422

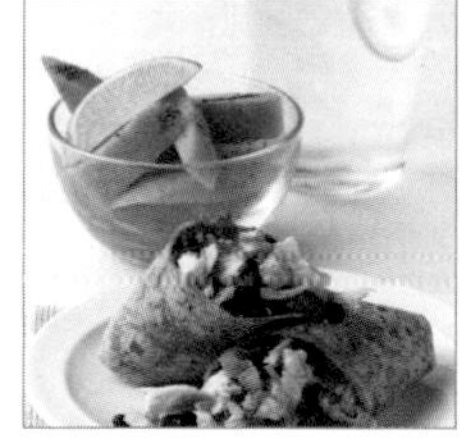

1 burrito (15 cm whole-wheat tortilla, ½ cup black beans, 42 g chicken, lettuce, tomato and salsa, 15 g cheese)
½ mango and a glass of water
Total calories: 519

Why it's a Good Swap

- Cut carbs by switching from a large white-flour tortilla to a smaller whole-wheat tortilla.
- Swapped the ground beef for grilled chicken.
- Made the filling significantly more healthy and added fibre by eliminating the white rice and including black beans instead.
- Added fruit instead of tortilla chips. Chips are full of empty calories, whereas fruit is packed with fibre and vitamins.

EVEN BETTER SWAP: Eat the grilled chicken with the black bean and salad filling, with no tortilla. Without the bread, it's called a "naked burrito" and is even healthier.

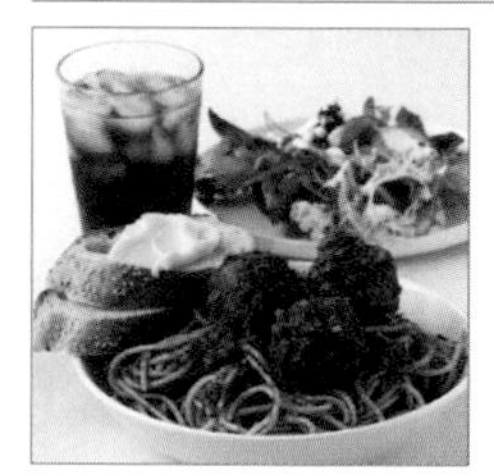

2 cups white pasta, 1 cup tomato sauce, 100 g beef meatballs
2 slices bread, 1 tbsp butter
1 cup salad, 1 tbsp blue cheese dressing
250 mL pop
Total calories: 1,770

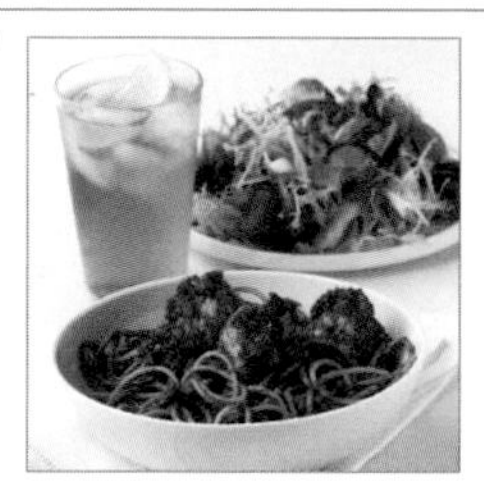

1 cup whole-wheat pasta, ½ cup tomato sauce, 100 g turkey meatballs
2 cups salad, 2 tbsp oil and vinegar dressing
250 mL unsweetened iced tea
Total calories: 550

Why it's a Good Swap

- Cut the pasta portion in half and switched to whole-wheat spaghetti to add fibre. You'll feel fuller longer.
- Eliminated the bread and doubled the size of the salad (just as filling as bread), thus swapping empty calories for added fibre and vitamins.
- Topped the salad with oil and vinegar dressing instead of blue cheese to cut saturated fat.

EVEN BETTER SWAP: Choose a pasta like Catelli Smart, which contains inulin. It has 2½ times the fibre of traditional white pasta and no added sodium.

DESSERT SWAP&DROP

▼ SWAP THIS | **▼ FOR THAT**

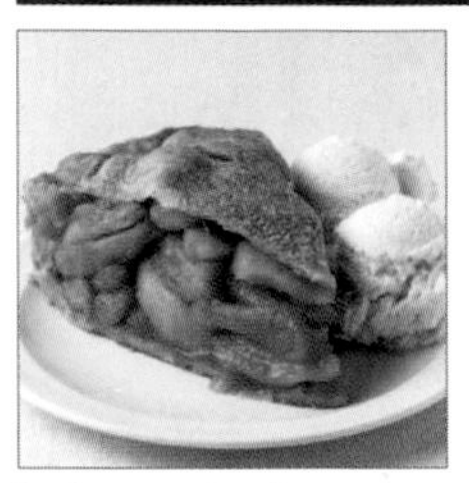

1 slice apple pie
with ½ cup ice cream
Total calories: 363

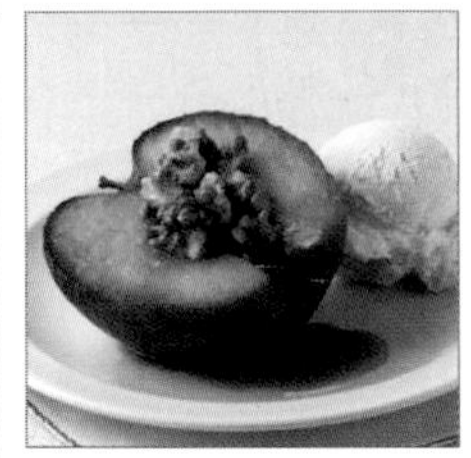

1 Maple-Walnut Roasted Apple with low-fat ice cream (recipe pg. 178)
Total calories: 207

Why it's a Good Swap

- Kept the apple, but got rid of the pie crust and extra sugar used for the filling. Both of these ingredients are responsible for increasing the calories in apple pie.
- Added walnuts for protein and "good" fat to help fill you up.
- Cut the ice cream down to one small scoop and switched to reduced-fat ice cream to lower the saturated fat.

EVEN BETTER SWAP: Substitute non-fat vanilla yogourt for the ice cream—it will still add a satisfyingly creamy touch.

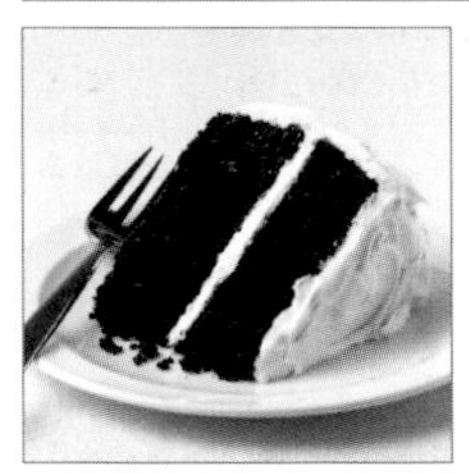

1 large piece chocolate cake with frosting
Total calories: 439

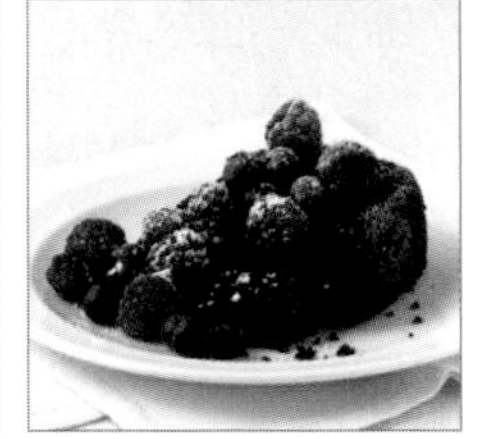

1 small piece unfrosted chocolate cake dusted with confectioner's sugar
½ cup mixed blueberries and raspberries
Total calories: 309

Why it's a Good Swap

- Decreased the portion size of the cake to cut refined carbohydrates and calories.
- Eliminated the frosting, which was full of calorific fat.
- Added berries to increase the nutritional value of the dessert and make the smaller portion of cake more satisfying.

EVEN BETTER SWAP: Split a slice of cake with a friend. Nothing beats bonding over a tasty dessert.

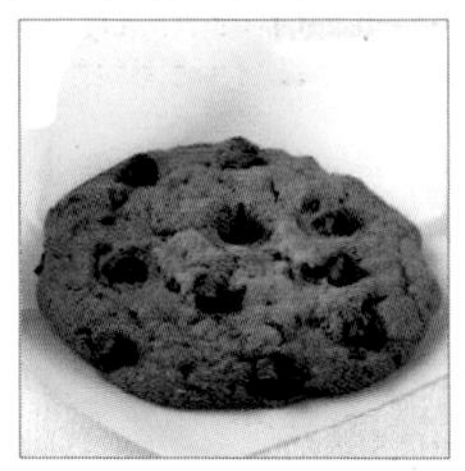

1 large chocolate chip cookie
Total calories: 196

1 Oatmeal-Peanut Butter Trail Bar (recipe pg. 174)
Total calories: 175

Why it's a Good Swap

- Swapped the cookie—made with sugar, butter and white flour—for an even more delicious trail bar made with whole grains (full of fibre) and peanut butter (with protein and "good" fat), to keep you fuller longer. The bar also provides extra nutrition from dried fruit.

EVEN BETTER SWAP: Eat half the trail bar now, and save the rest to nibble on later.

SNACK SWAP&DROPS

▼ SWAP THIS	▼ FOR THAT	▼ SWAP THIS	▼ FOR THAT

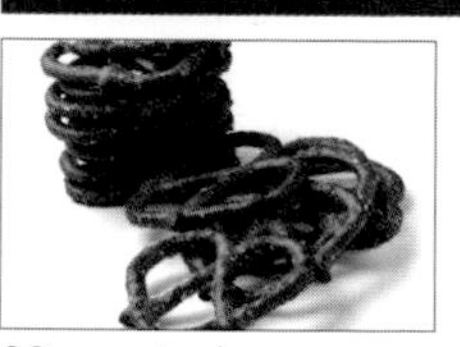

60 g pretzels
Total calories: 216

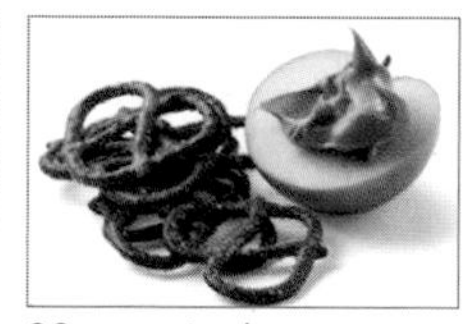

20 g pretzels
½ green apple with 1 tbsp peanut butter
Total calories: 208

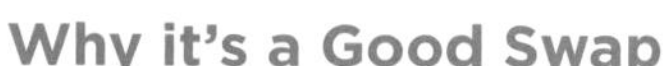

Why it's a Good Swap

- Decreased the number of pretzels by two thirds.
- Beefed up the snack with a filling piece of fruit and some peanut butter for staying power. This snack will help you stay full significantly longer than if you ate just the pretzels, and it contains less sodium.

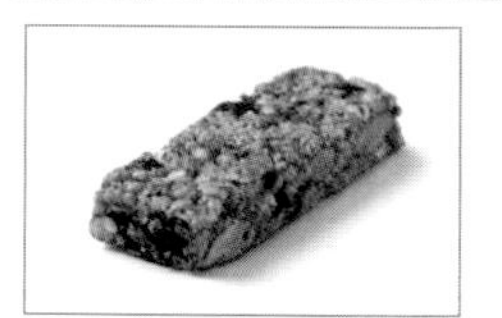

1 berry cereal bar
Total calories: 140

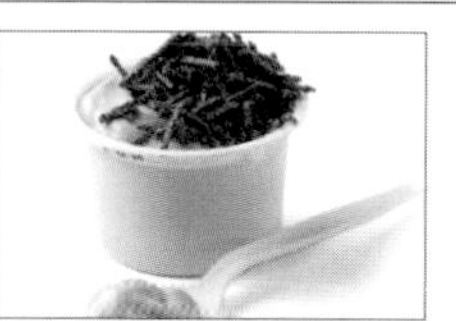

125 mL low-fat mixed-berry yogourt topped with 2 tbsp All-Bran cereal
Total calories: 148

Why it's a Good Swap

- Substituted yogourt for the cereal bar. These bars may contain cereal, but they're often lower in fibre and higher in sugar than their cereal counterparts.
- Added All-Bran cereal on top for whole grains and fibre.

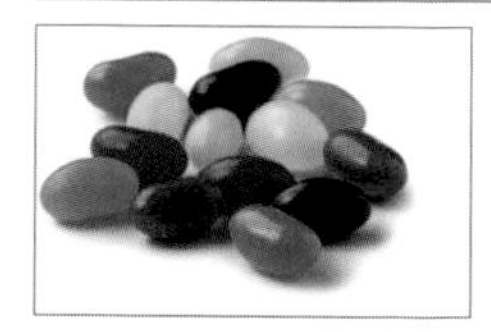

14 jelly beans
Total calories: 150

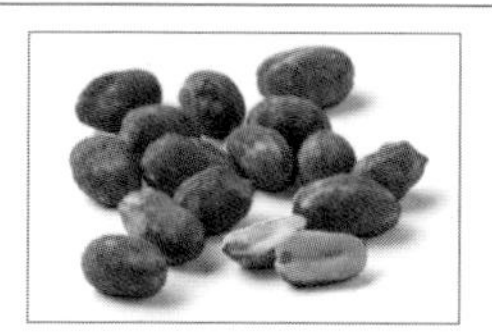

15 dry-roasted peanuts
Total calories: 84

Why it's a Good Swap

- Swapped jelly beans—which are full of nothing but calories—for peanuts, which are satisfying and full of protein, fibre and healthy fat.

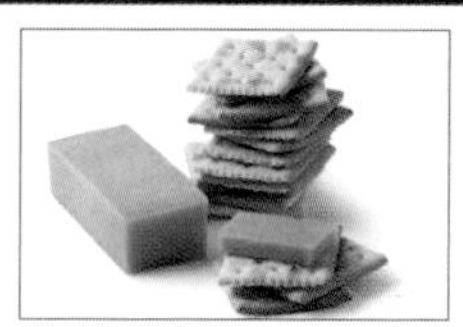

15 plain salted crackers
85 g cheddar cheese
Total calories: 525

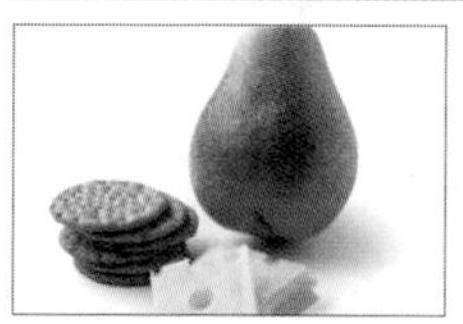

6 whole-wheat crackers
30 g Swiss cheese
1 small pear
Total calories: 299

Why it's a Good Swap

- Switched to whole-wheat crackers and cut the portion in half.
- Limited the cheese to decrease saturated fat.
- Added a piece of fruit to add some healthier calories. Because of its fibre and water, the pear will fill you up more than the crackers.

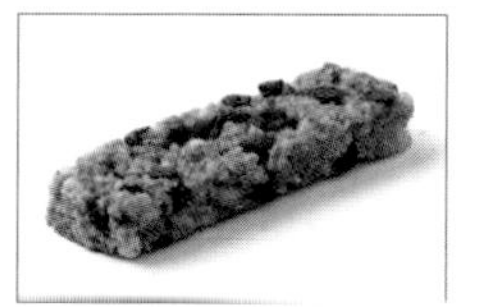

1 chocolate-chip granola bar
Total calories: 163

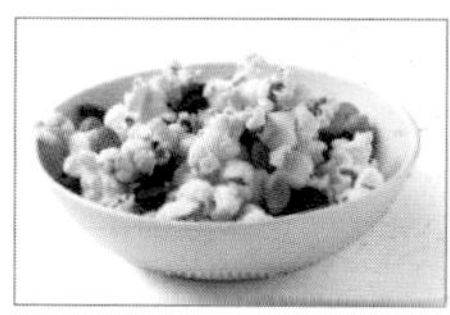

1 cup light popcorn mixed with 10 peanuts and 1 tbsp semi-sweet chocolate chips
Total calories: 160

Why it's a Good Swap

- Swapped the granola bar for popcorn (a high-fibre food).
- Added peanuts for a dose of protein and "good" fats that will help you stay fuller longer.
- Threw in some chocolate chips to satisfy your sweet tooth.

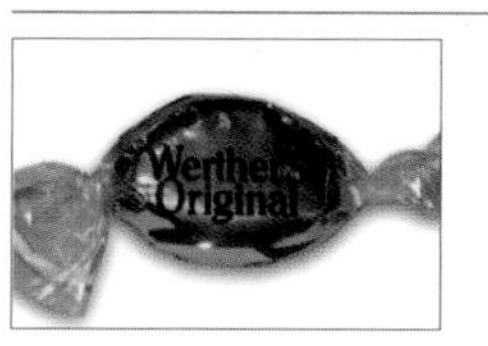

5 Werther's Original candies
Total calories: 100

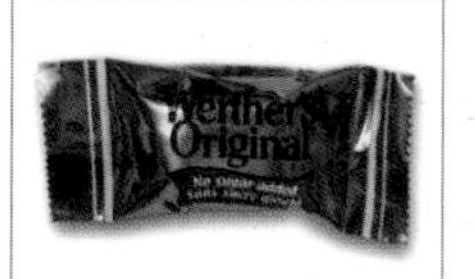

5 Werther's Original Sugar-Free
Total calories: 40

Why it's a Good Swap

- Swapped regular Werther's Original hard candies for the sugarless version. Most hard candies are full of nothing but calories, but sugar-free treats are just as satisfying.

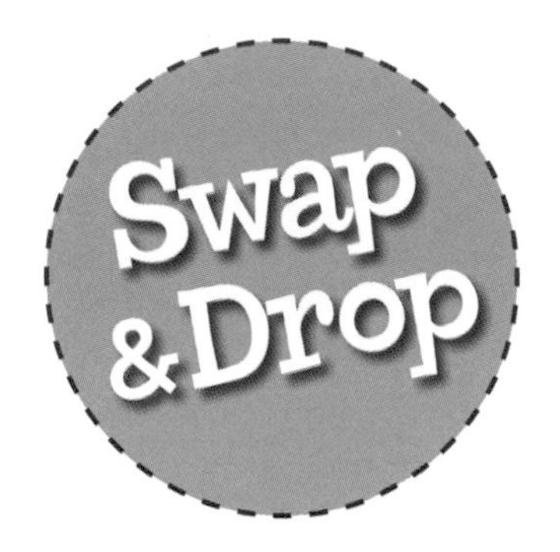

BOSTON PIZZA

This chain—which was actually founded in Edmonton—is a popular destination for birthdays and get-togethers. Here's how to turn a pizza party into a **Swap & Drop** party.

swap this | **or this**

▼ PIZZAS

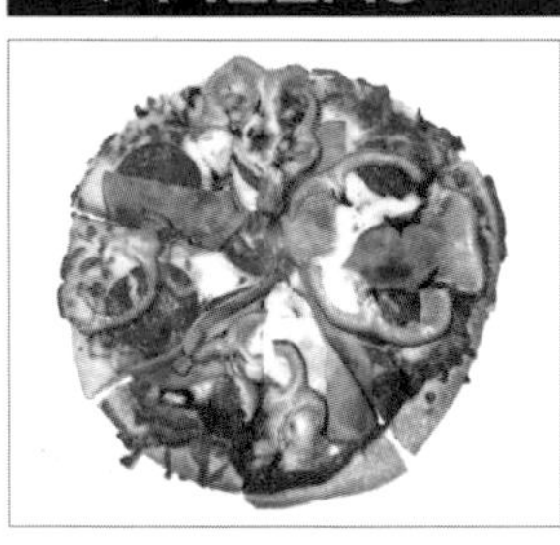

Classic Individual Deluxe Pizza

(sauce, mozzarella, ham, pepperoni, green pepper and mushrooms)

Calories: 850
Fat (g): 29
Saturated fat (g): 14
Sodium (mg): 2,690

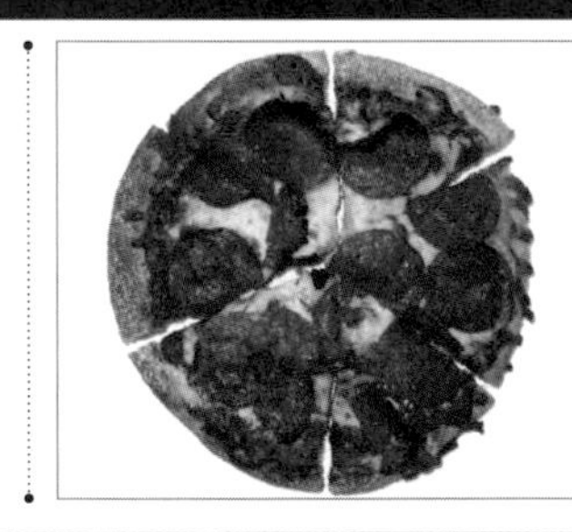

Individual Pepperoni Pizza

(sauce, mozzarella and pepperoni)

Calories: 750
Fat (g): 27
Saturated fat (g): 13
Sodium (mg): 1,460

▼ PASTAS

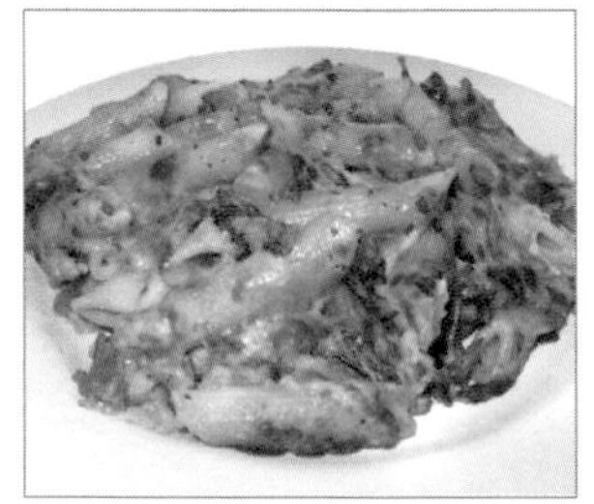

Baked Chipotle Bacon Penne

(penne in bacon and alfredo sauce with mushrooms, green onion, tomato, cheddar and pizza mozzarella)

Calories: 1,430
Fat (g): 88
Saturated fat (g): 40
Sodium (mg): 2,740

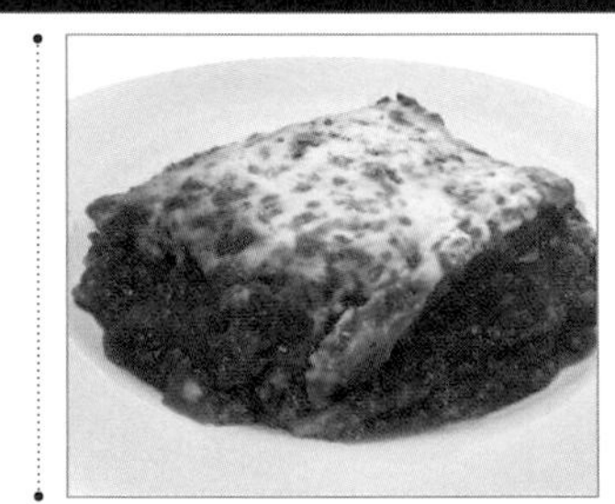

Homestyle Lasagna

(ricotta and parmesan cheese, Bolognese and Pomodoro sauces, ground beef, tomato, green pepper, onion, garlic and herbs)

Calories: 930
Fat (g): 48
Saturated fat (g): 22
Sodium (mg): 2,280

▼ SWEETS

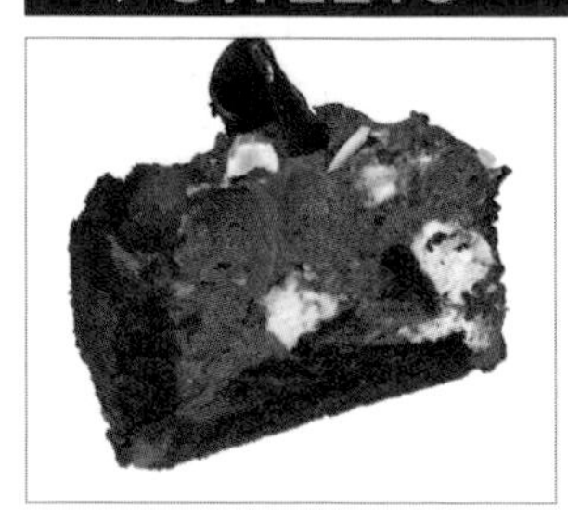

Chocolate Explosion

(chocolate mousse, cheesecake, caramel, toffee, pecans and almonds)

Calories: 870
Fat (g): 49
Saturated fat (g): 28
Sodium (mg): 530

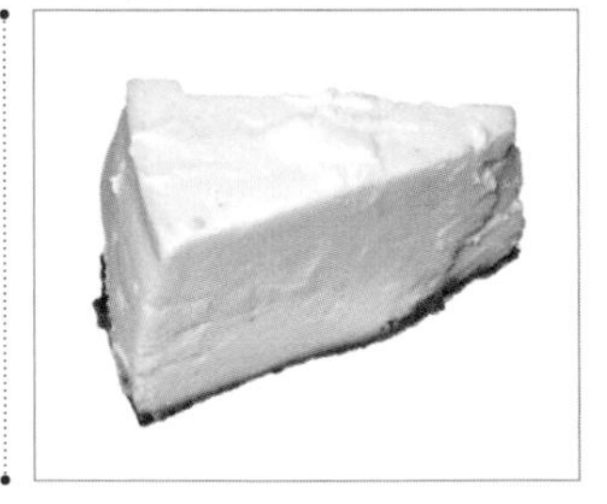

New York Cheesecake

(cheesecake on a graham-cracker crust)

Calories: 600
Fat (g): 32
Saturated fat (g): 16
Sodium (mg): 460

All menu information was accurate at time of writing according to the nutritional information made available by each restaurant.

DINE OUT • GRAB A MEAL ON THE GO

The menus of many Canadian eateries tempt you with high-calorie, fat-laden meals. But there are usually healthy—or at least lower-calorie—options available as well. Here are suggestions for swaps you can make at ten of Canada's most popular restaurant chains.

for that

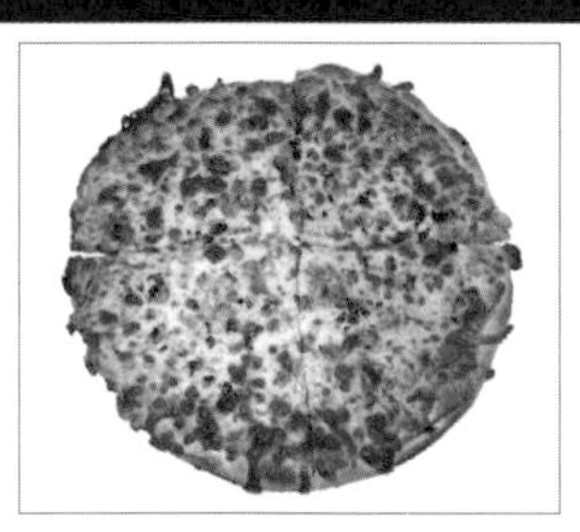

Small Baja Thin-Crust Pizza

(Pomodoro sauce, chipotle seasoning, mozzarella, corn, red and green peppers, red onion, parmesan and cilantro)

Calories: 580
Fat (g): 22
Saturated fat (g): 11
Sodium (mg): 1,160

Switching from the first swap to the third

once a month will save you 3,240 calories in a year—almost one pound.

- It's tough to find an individual pizza under 500 calories from the regular menu (you can always have just half, and save the other half for next day's lunch). But it's nice that Boston Pizza makes it possible to choose your own ingredients to build your pasta or pizza.

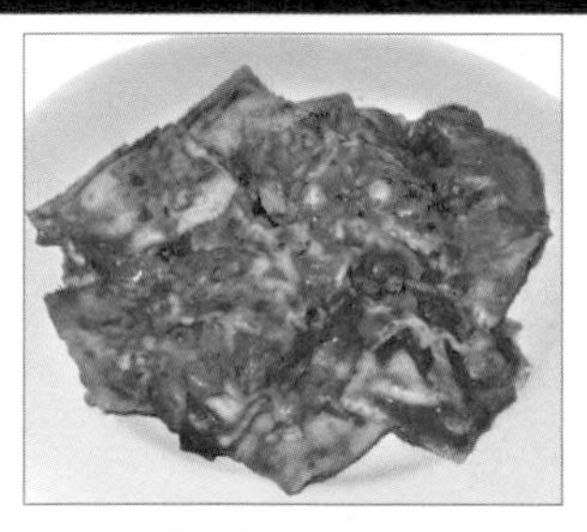

Baked Seven-Cheese Ravioli

(pasta, various cheeses and Bolognese or Pomodoro sauce)

Calories: 490
Fat (g): 26
Saturated fat (g): 15
Sodium (mg): 850

Switching from the first swap to the third

once a month will save you 11,280 calories in a year—more than three pounds.

- According to the Dietitians of Canada, in a diet that totals 2,000 calories a day, total fat intake should be only 20 to 35 percent of those calories. So be careful with even the best choice of pasta dishes here.

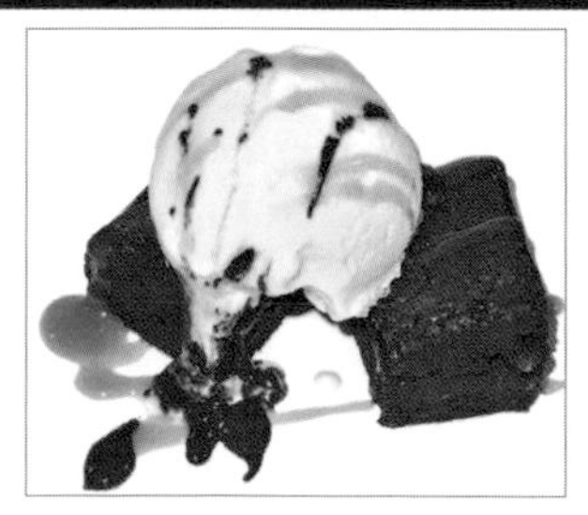

Bite-size Chocolate Brownie Addiction

(brownie, ice cream, caramel and chocolate sauce)

Calories: 250
Fat (g): 9
Saturated fat (g): 3
Sodium (mg): 130

Switching from the first swap to the third

once a month will save you 7,440 calories in a year—more than two pounds.

- You can save even more calories on the brownie choice by ordering it without ice cream.

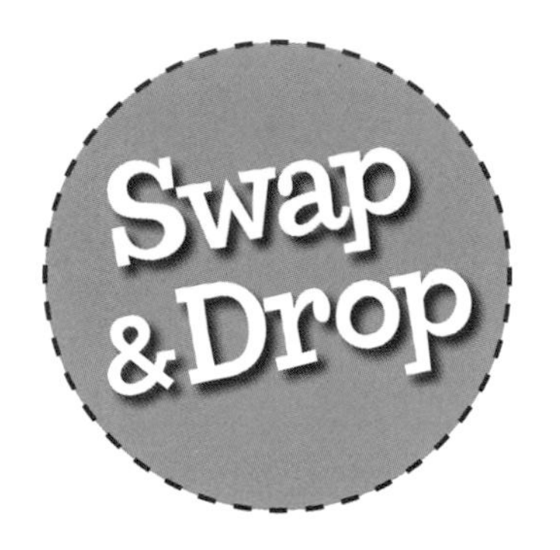

EAST SIDE MARIO'S

This Italian chain is big on the classic pasta and pizza combination. It can also be big on calories—all of the worst choices below have more than 1,000. But there is hope!

swap this | **or this**

▼ STARTERS

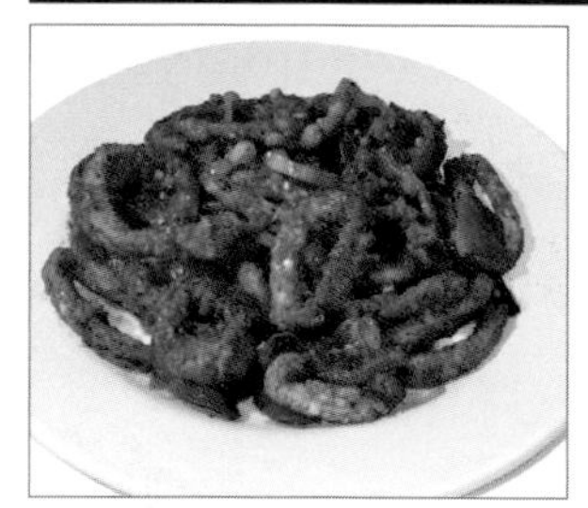

Sizzling Calamari al Diavolo

(flour-covered calamari with garlic, onions, bell peppers and chilies)

Calories: 1,010
Fat (g): 53
Saturated fat (g): 10
Sodium (mg): 3,420

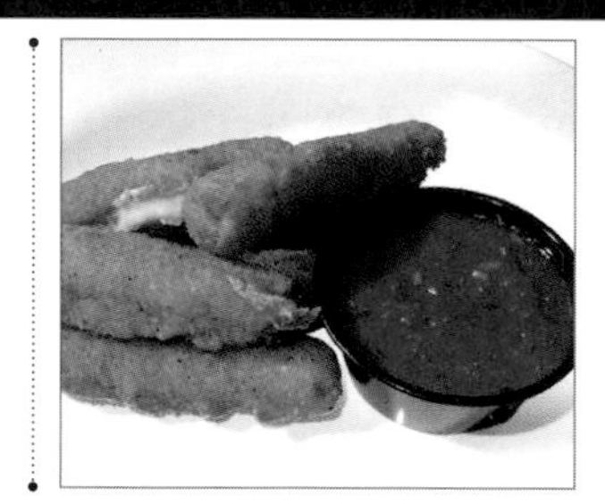

Cheese Sticks

(breadcrumb coating, cheddar cheese and Napolitana dipping sauce)

Calories: 470
Fat (g): 27
Saturated fat (g): 10
Sodium (mg): 1,630

▼ PASTAS

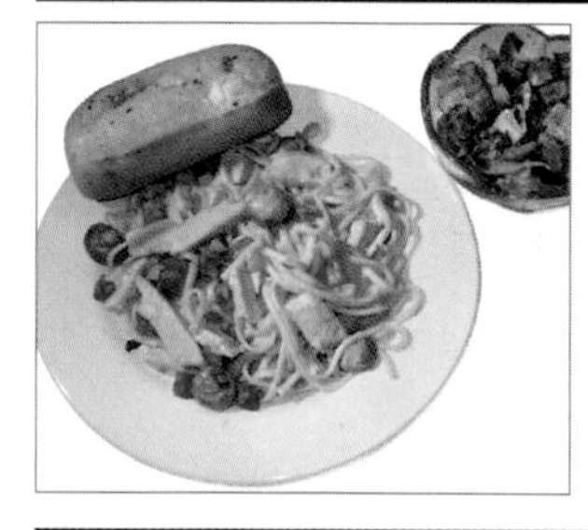

Linguine Chicken Tettrazini

(chicken breast, mushrooms, garlic and tomatoes in alfredo sauce, with side Caesar salad and garlic homeloaf)

Calories: 1,730
Fat (g): 98
Saturated fat (g): 18
Sodium (mg): 2,590

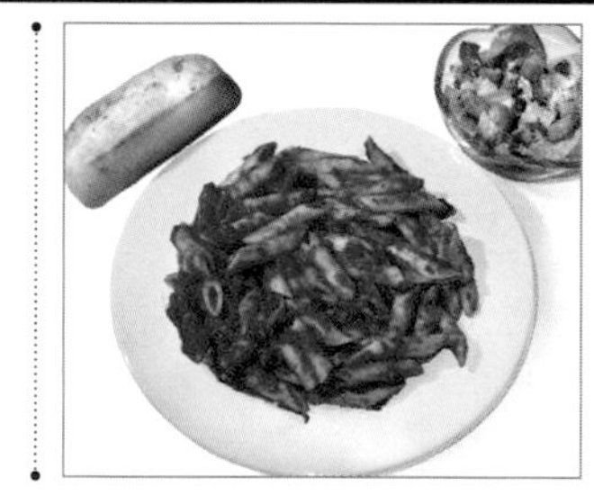

Penne Napolitana

(tomato sauce, with side Caesar and garlic homeloaf)

Calories: 1,260
Fat (g): 57
Saturated fat (g): 7
Sodium (mg): 2,340

▼ SWEETS

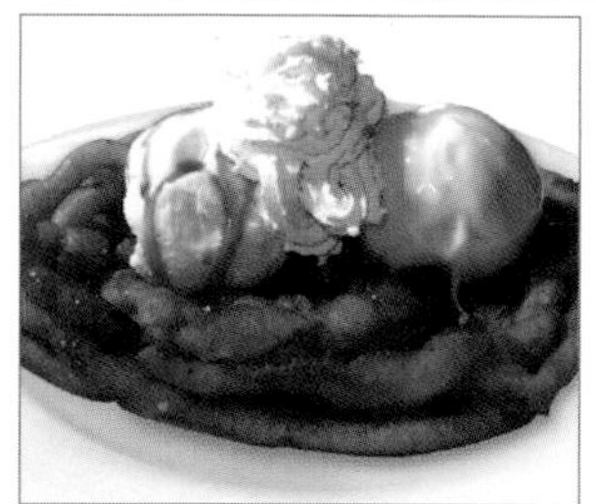

Funnel Cake

(fried funnel cake topped with vanilla ice cream and strawberry and caramel sauces)

Calories: 1,210
Fat (g): 55
Saturated fat (g): 24
Sodium (mg): 1,140

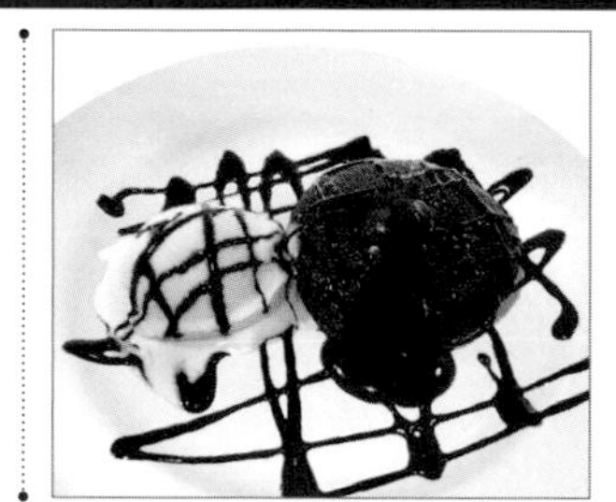

Chocolate Vesuvius

(cake with soft chocolate centre, served with ice cream and chocolate sauce)

Calories: 590
Fat (g): 34
Saturated fat (g): 19
Sodium (mg): 330

All menu information was accurate at time of writing according to the nutritional information made available by each restaurant.

for that

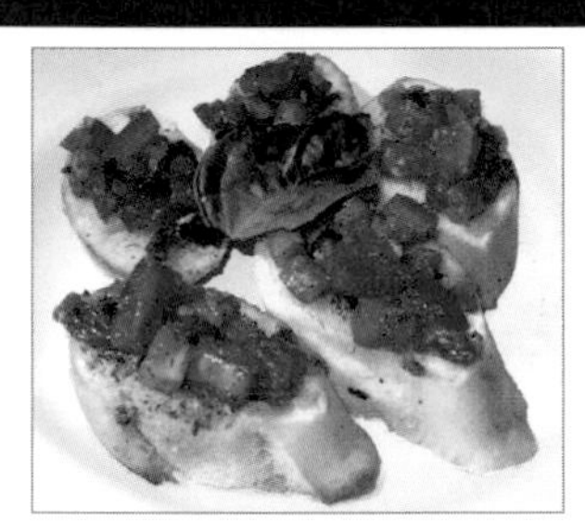

Bruschetta for One

(tomatoes, garlic and basil on crisp white bread)

Calories: 350
Fat (g): 19
Saturated fat (g): 4
Sodium (mg): 75

Switching from the first swap to the third

once a month will save you 7,920 calories in a year—more than two pounds.

- This bruschetta may be the best appetizer option, but with 350 calories and 19 grams of fat, you should still consider splitting it with a friend.

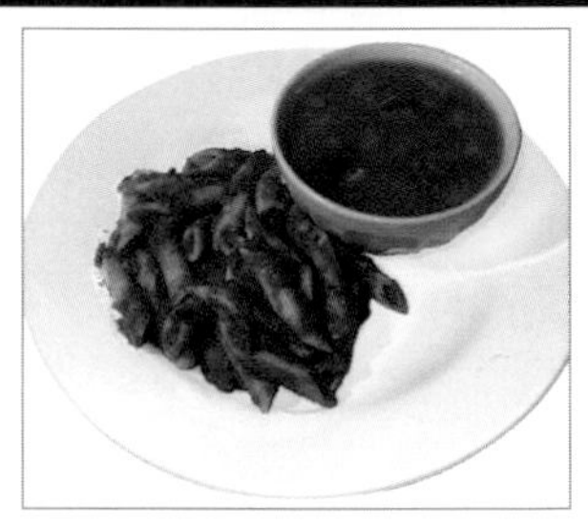

Side Serving of Pasta with Napolitana Sauce

(with side vegetable soup)

Calories: 440
Fat (g): 9
Saturated fat (g): 1
Sodium (mg): 1,360

Switching from the first swap to the third

once a month will save you 15,480 calories in a year—more than four pounds.

- East Side Mario's has the option of all-you-can-eat bread, soups and salads. But indulging will jack up those calorie counts faster than you can say bada-bing.

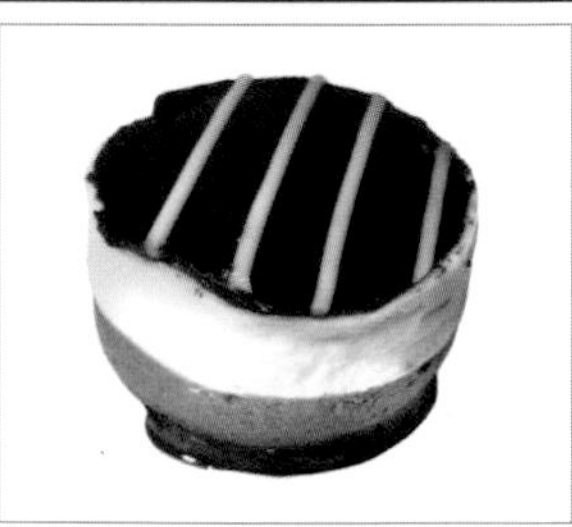

Black & White Mousse Cake

(cake topped with layers of mousse)

Calories: 290
Fat (g): 22
Saturated fat (g): 13
Sodium (mg): 75

Switching from the first swap to the third

once a month will save you 11,040 calories in a year—more than three pounds.

- Let's be honest with ourselves: No dessert at East Side Mario's is particularly healthy. But if that's where your family wants to go, allow yourself to split this slice of mousse cake with someone; it only takes a few bites to be satisfied.

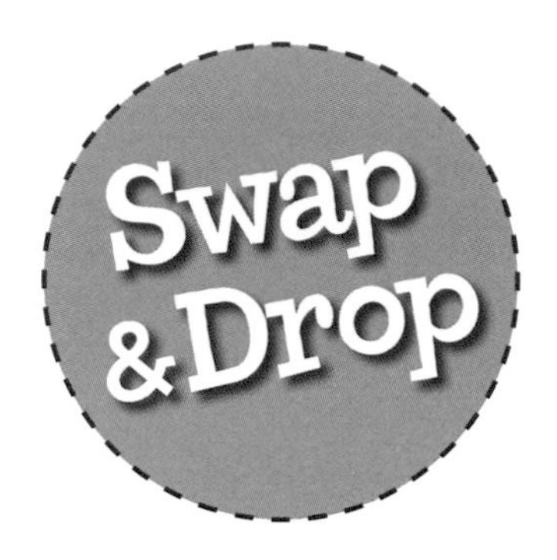

HARVEY'S

Harvey's is known for its charbroiled hamburgers and customizable toppings. Skip the heavy condiments and beef patties and go for a salad or veggie burger.

swap this / **or this**

▼ BURGERS

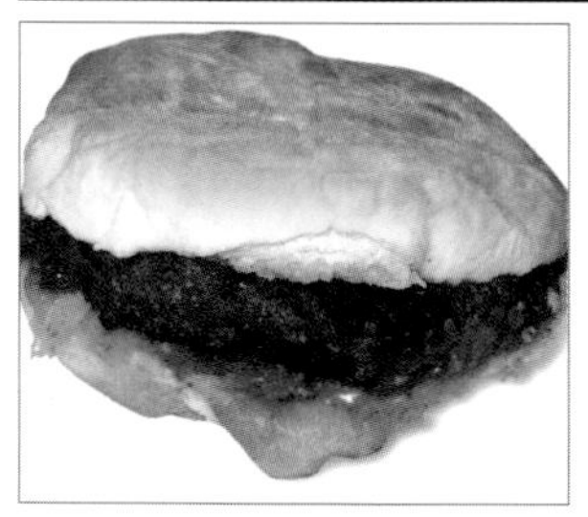

Great Canadian Burger with Cheese & Bacon
(charbroiled beef patty with cheese and bacon, no toppings, on white bun)
Calories: 690
Fat (g): 35
Saturated fat (g): 16
Sodium (mg): 1,430

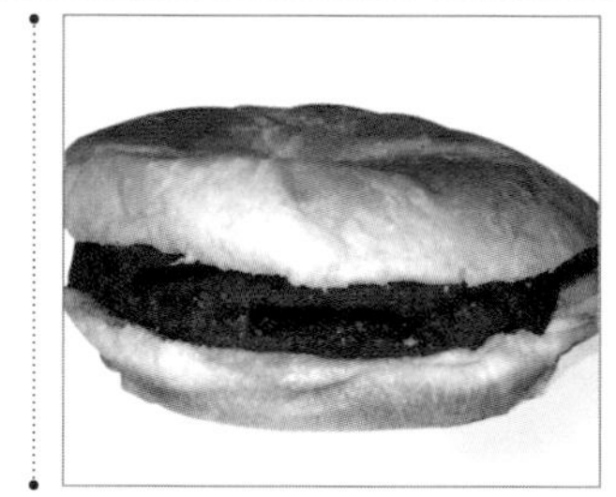

Original Hamburger
(charbroiled beef patty with no toppings, on white bun)
Calories: 380
Fat (g): 16
Saturated fat (g): 7
Sodium (mg): 980

▼ CHICKEN CHOICES

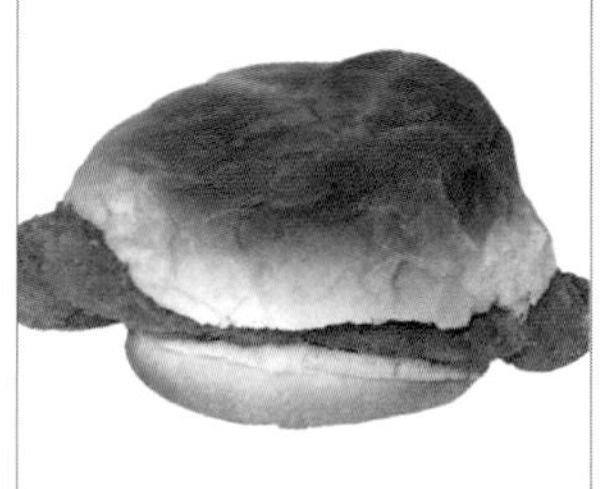

Crispy Chicken Sandwich
(breaded chicken with no toppings, on white bun)
Calories: 470
Fat (g): 16
Saturated fat (g): 2
Sodium (mg): 1,320

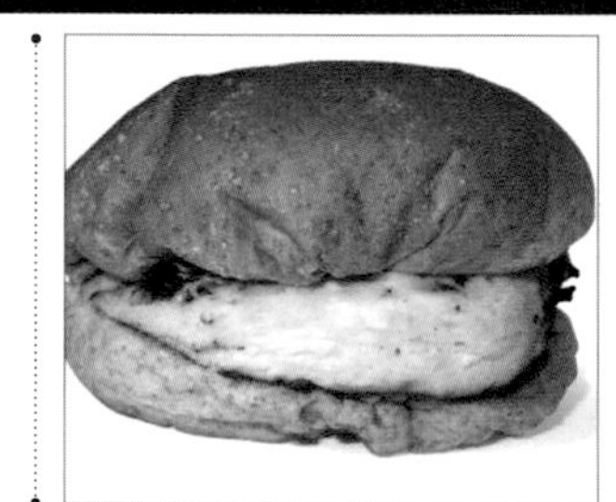

Grilled Chicken Sandwich
(grilled chicken with no toppings, on whole-wheat bun)
Calories: 290
Fat (g): 5
Saturated fat (g): 1.5
Sodium (mg): 810

▼ SIDES

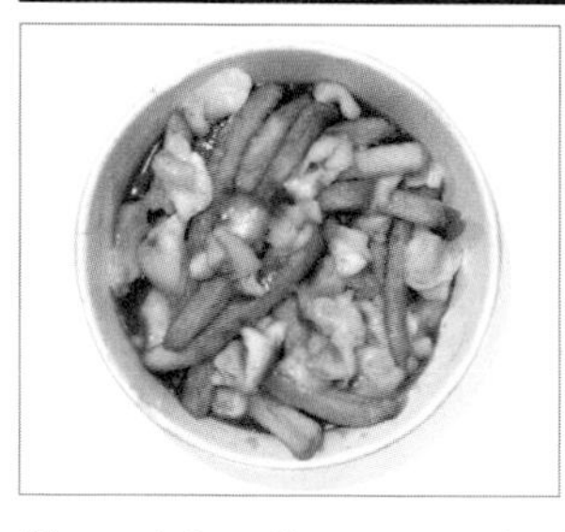

Poutine
(fries, cheese and gravy)
Calories: 840
Fat (g): 43
Saturated fat (g): 15
Sodium (mg): 2,210

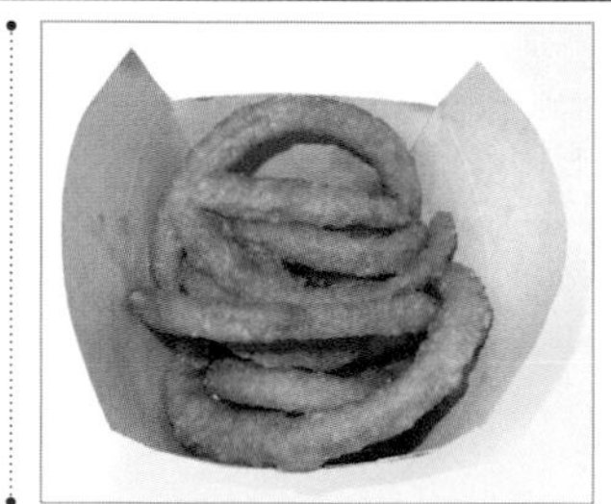

Onion Rings, Regular Size
(onion rings battered and deep-fried)
Calories: 270
Fat (g): 15
Saturated fat (g): 1.5
Sodium (mg): 790

All menu information was accurate at time of writing according to the nutritional information made available by each restaurant.

for that

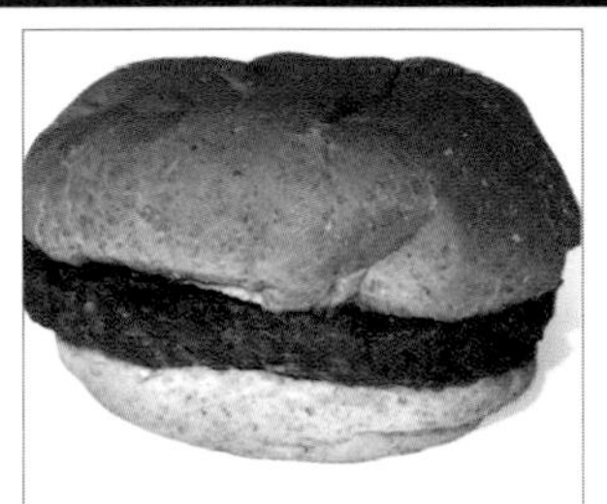

Veggie Burger

(vegetarian patty with no toppings, on whole-wheat bun)

Calories: 290
Fat (g): 10
Saturated fat (g): 1.5
Sodium (mg): 580

Switching from the first swap to the third

once a month will save you 4,800 calories in a year—more than one pound.

- Vegetarian options almost always tend to be lower in calories (unless, of course, they're slathered in cheese). It's also nice that Harvey's serves its Veggie Burger on a whole-wheat bun. Order it with low-calorie toppings like tomatoes, mustard and lettuce—skip the mayo.

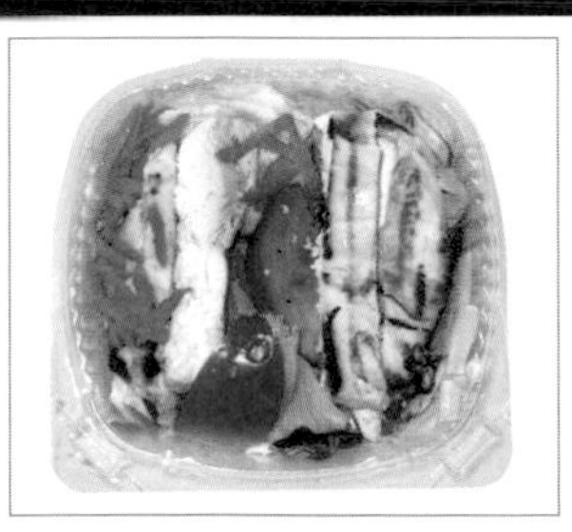

Warm Grilled Chicken Salad

(grilled chicken, lettuce, tomato, shredded cabbage and cucumbers, with half serving of Asian Sesame dressing)

Calories: 200
Fat (g): 4.25
Saturated fat (g): 1.1
Sodium (mg): 682

Switching from the first swap to the third

once a month will save you 3,240 calories in a year—almost one pound.

- Although the Grilled Chicken Sandwich is a pretty low-cal lunch choice, the salad is much healthier thanks to the vegetables in it.

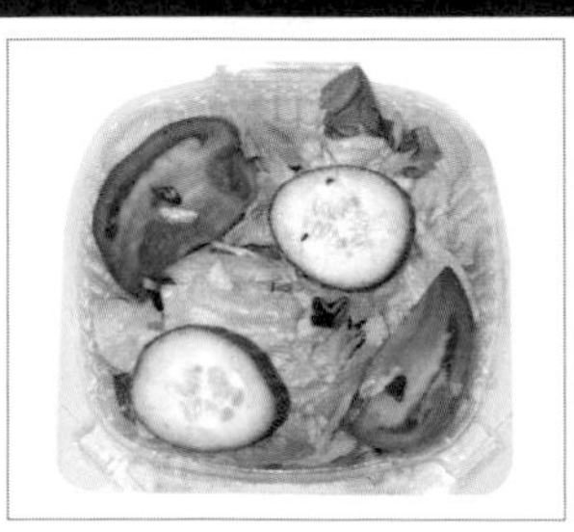

Side Garden Salad

(lettuce, tomato, cucumber and shredded cabbage, with no dressing)

Calories: 40
Fat (g): 0.2
Saturated fat (g): 0
Sodium (mg): 20

Switching from the first swap to the third

once a month will save you 9,600 calories in a year—almost three pounds.

- Harvey's 28 mL salad dressings range from 60 calories and 2.5 g of fat (Asian Sesame), up to 108 calories and 11 g of fat (Creamy Garlic Peppercorn Ranch). Ask for nutritional info before ordering if you're unsure which dressing to choose.

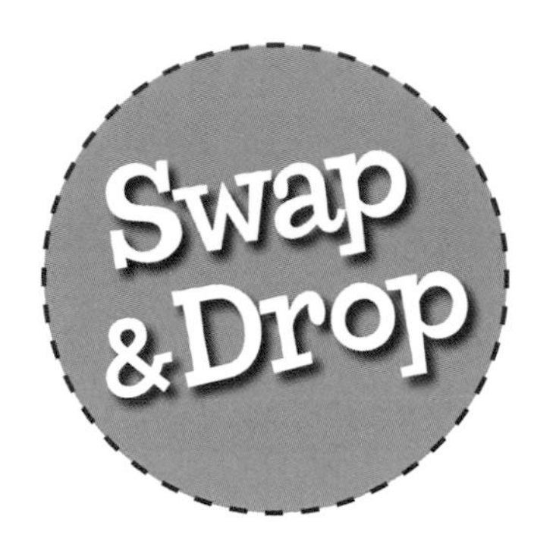

THE KEG

In the mood for steak? The Keg's got you covered. This chain also offers a variety of salads, but not all are as healthy as they seem. And beware the Bearnaise sauce!

swap this | **or this**

▼ STARTERS

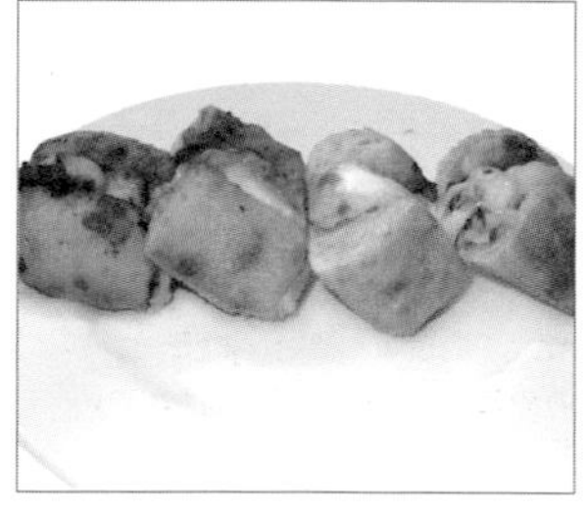

Bruschetta
(ciabatta bread topped with tomato basil salsa, bocconcini and parmesan cheese)
Calories: 1,145
Fat (g): 59
Saturated fat (g): 22
Sodium (mg): 1,384

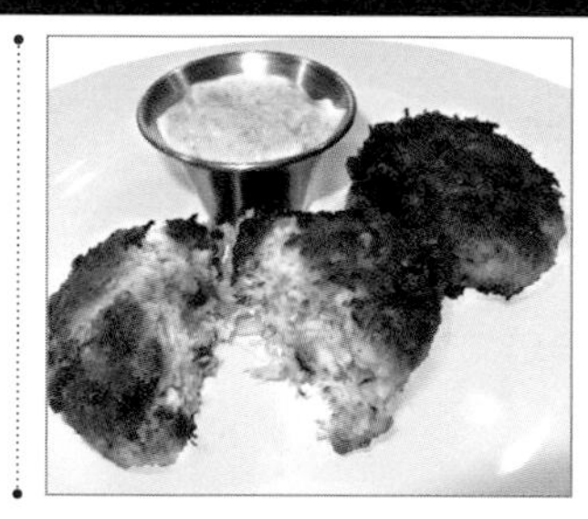

Crab Cakes
(crab meat with dill-caper mayo)
Calories: 438
Fat (g): 24
Saturated fat (g): 3
Sodium (mg): 1,356

▼ STEAKS

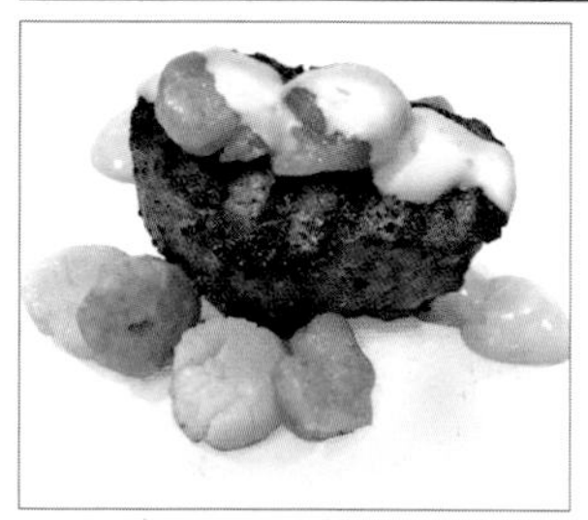

8 oz. Sirloin Oscar
(steak with shrimp, scallops, asparagus and Bearnaise sauce)
Calories: 917
Fat (g): 67
Saturated fat (g): 11
Sodium (mg): 1,110

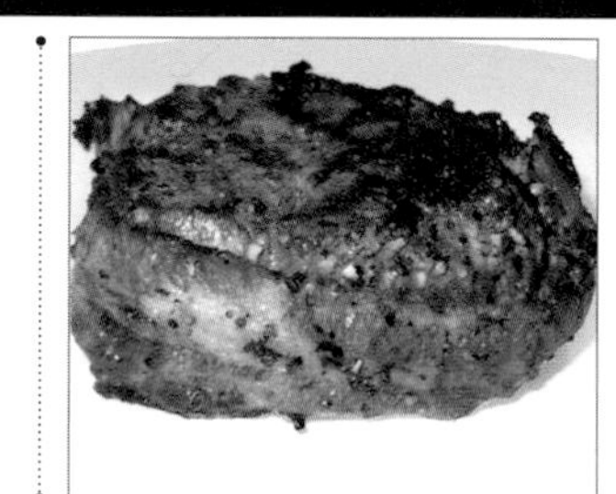

7 oz. Filet Classic
(steak wrapped in bacon—comes with salad, vegetables and mushrooms)
Calories: 783
Fat (g): 59
Saturated fat (g): 13
Sodium (mg): 1,007

▼ SALADS

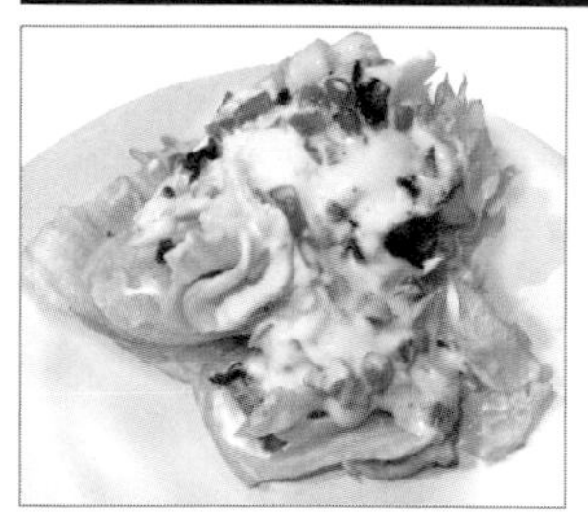

Iceberg Wedge
(lettuce wedge with tomatoes, bacon bits and your choice of ranch or Bleu cheese dressing)
Calories: 614
Fat (g): 56
Saturated fat (g): 15
Sodium (mg): 1,489

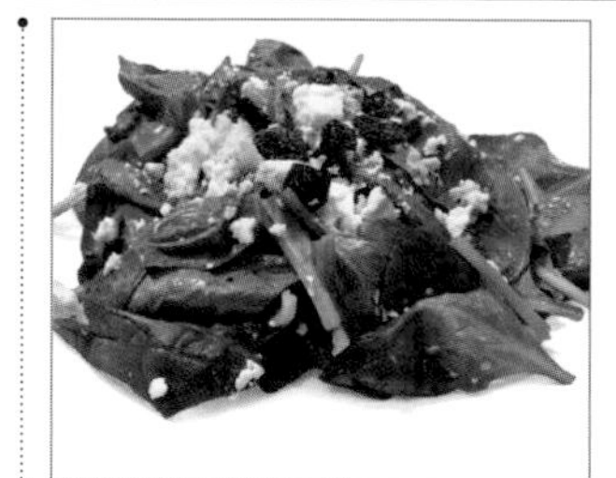

Spinach Salad
(baby spinach, mandarin oranges, dried cranberries, pecans and red onion, with your choice of goat cheese or Bleu cheese dressing)
Calories: 544
Fat (g): 29
Saturated fat (g): 10
Sodium (mg): 907

All menu information was accurate at time of writing according to the nutritional information made available by each restaurant.

for that

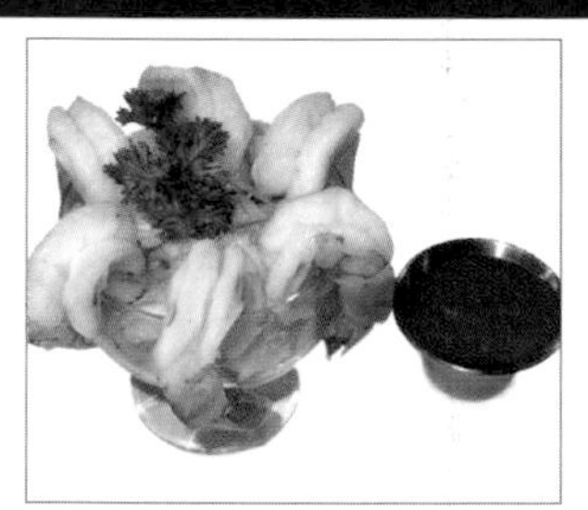

Shrimp Cocktail

(tiger shrimp with a martini cocktail sauce)

Calories: 127
Fat (g): 1
Saturated fat (g): 0
Sodium (mg): 823

Switching from the first swap to the third

once a month will save you 12,216 calories in a year—almost four pounds.

- That's one calorific bruschetta! This is a good example of why you shouldn't assume that something you recognize—something you may have prepared at home many times—will always be healthy. Don't be shy about asking exactly what's in it, or for nutritional information.

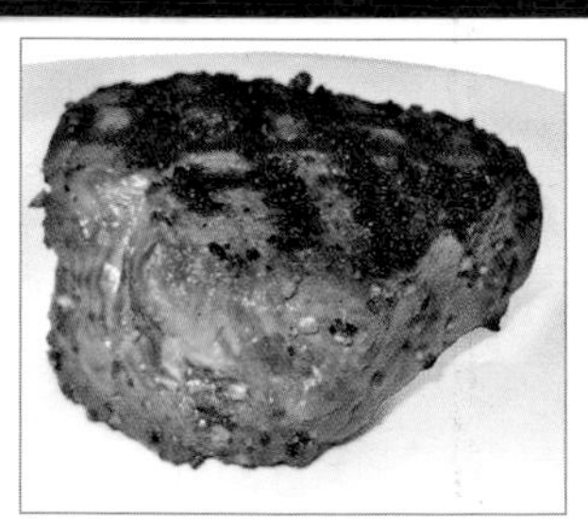

8 oz. Sirloin Classic

(steak—comes with salad, vegetables and mushrooms)

Calories: 440
Fat (g): 21
Saturated fat (g): 6
Sodium (mg): 714

Switching from the first swap to the third

once a month will save you 5,724 calories in a year—almost two pounds.

- If you want both steak and seafood in your meal, you'll get way fewer calories by ordering the Shrimp Cocktail plus the Sirloin Classic, rather than just the Sirloin Oscar on its own.

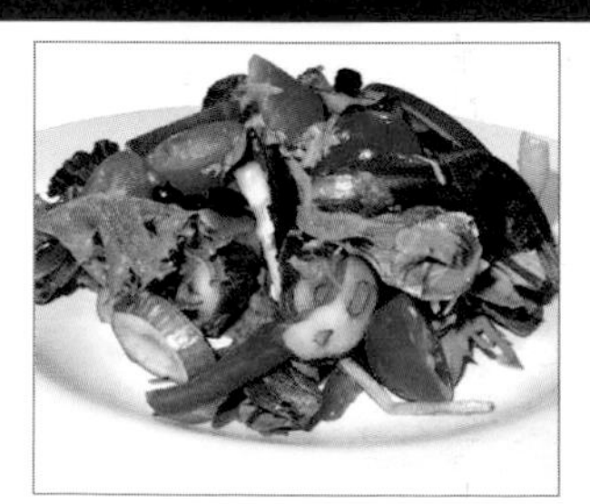

Mixed Green Salad

(field greens, tomatoes, peppers and cucumber in a vinaigrette dressing)

Calories: 232
Fat (g): 25
Saturated fat (g): 4
Sodium (mg): 585

Switching from the first swap to the third

once a month will save you 4,584 calories in a year—more than one pound.

- The Mixed Green Salad is more nutritious than the one with iceberg lettuce. But ask for the dressing on the side with this salad, since it's not exactly low-fat.

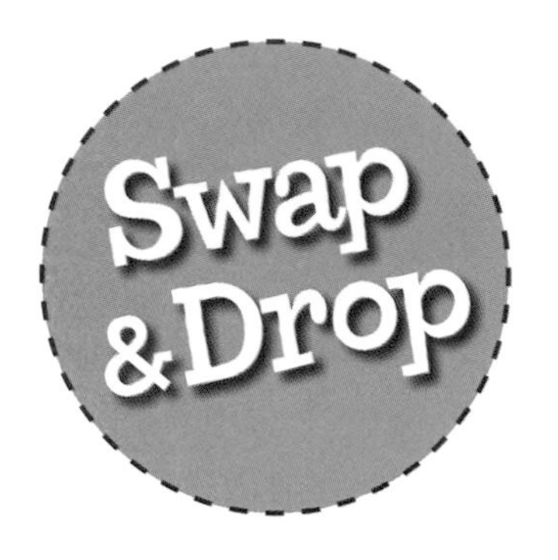

KFC

Many dishes from KFC (or PFK, as it's known in Quebec) are sodium bombs—check out the tally on the poutine, below. The key to eating here is small portions.

swap this | **or this**

▼ SANDWICHES

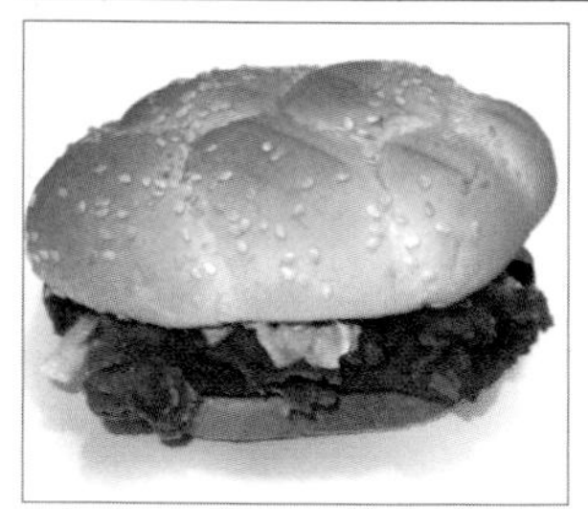

Zinger Sandwich

(breaded fried chicken, spicy seasoning, mayonnaise and lettuce on a bun)

Calories: 530
Fat (g): 26
Saturated fat (g): 4
Sodium (mg): 1,330

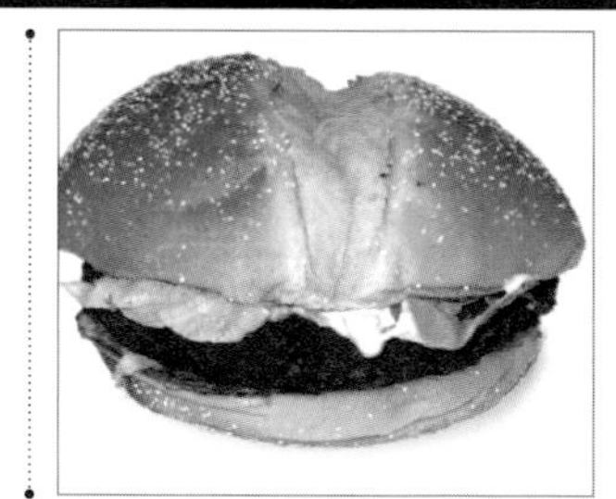

Classic Sandwich

(breaded fried chicken, lettuce and mayonnaise on a bun)

Calories: 450
Fat (g): 21
Saturated fat (g): 3
Sodium (mg): 890

▼ OTHER CHOICES

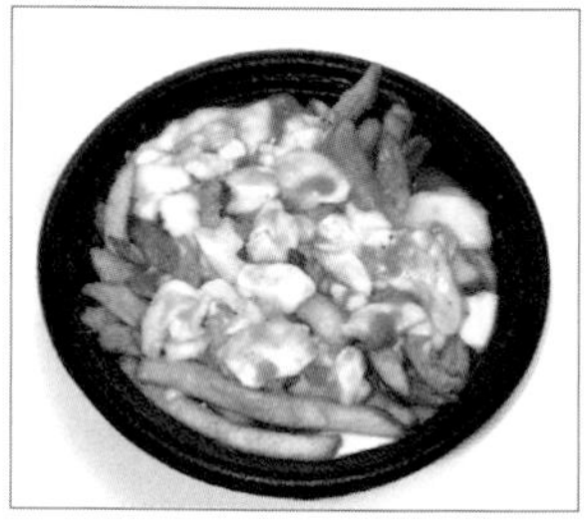

Poutine

(fries with gravy and cheese)

Calories: 860
Fat (g): 48
Saturated fat (g): 12
Sodium (mg): 2,450

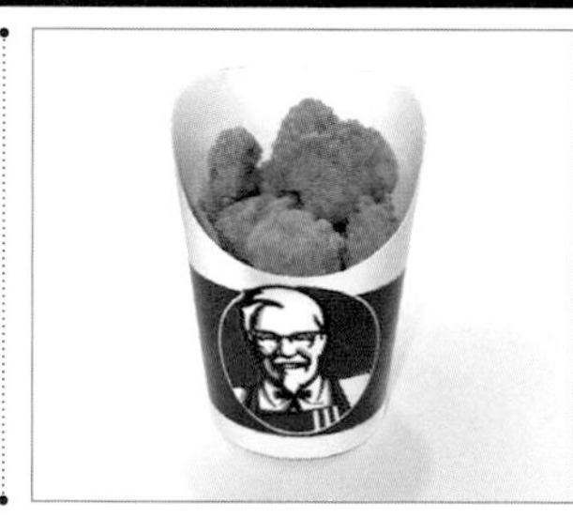

Popcorn Chicken (Small)

(bite-size pieces of fried, breaded chicken)

Calories: 525
Fat (g): 34
Saturated fat (g): 3
Sodium (mg): 1,290

▼ SIDES

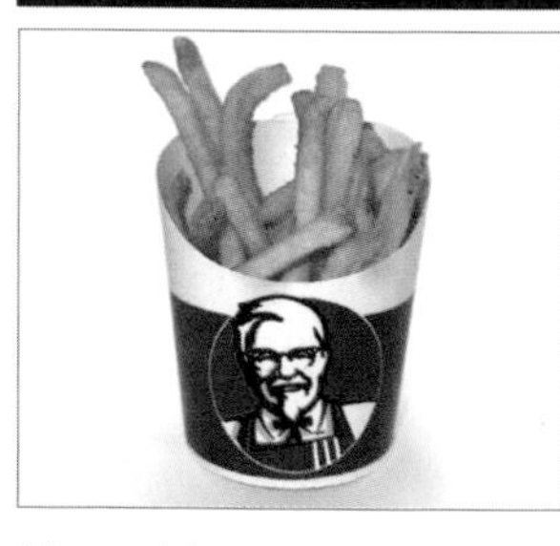

Individual-Size Fries

Calories: 340
Fat (g): 17
Saturated fat (g): 1
Sodium (mg): 770

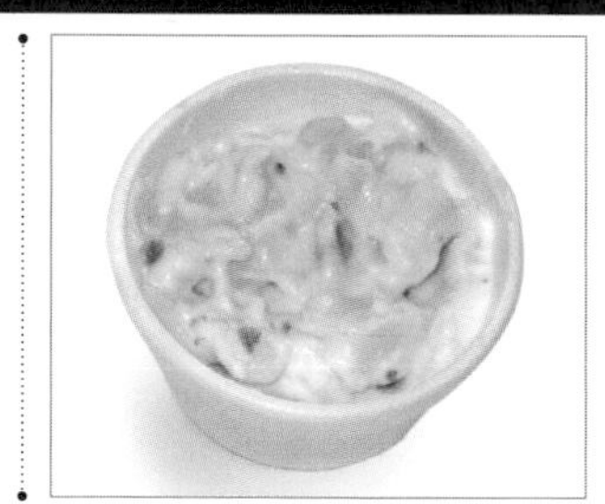

Individual-Size Potato Salad

Calories: 200
Fat (g): 9
Saturated fat (g): 2
Sodium (mg): 460

All menu information was accurate at time of writing according to the nutritional information made available by each restaurant.

for that

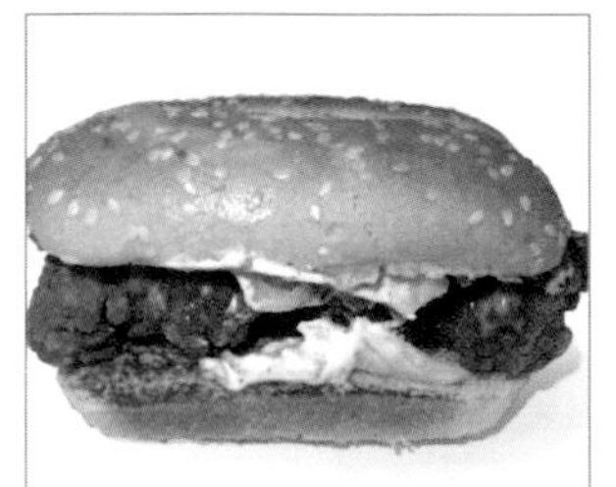

Colonel's Snacker Sandwich

(breaded fried chicken and lettuce on a bun)

Calories: 260
Fat (g): 11
Saturated fat (g): 2
Sodium (mg): 650

Switching from the first swap to the third
once a month will save you 3,240 calories in a year—almost one pound.

- Beware: Breaded, fried chicken is delicious, but it's a huge no-no if you are trying to drop a few pounds.

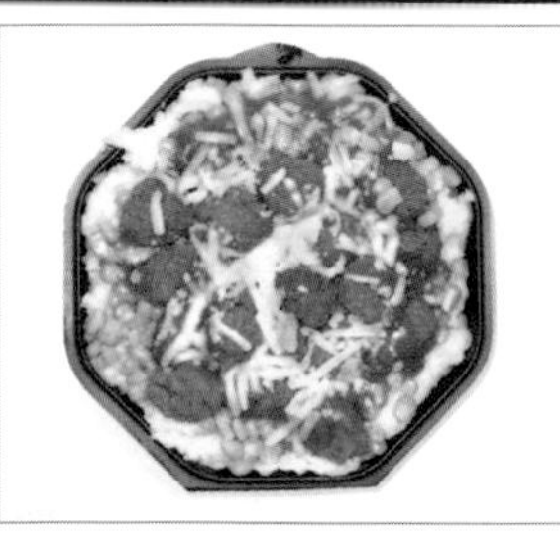

Chicken Bowl (Regular Size)

(mashed potatoes, popcorn chicken, corn, gravy and cheese)

Calories: 410
Fat (g): 17
Saturated fat (g): 4
Sodium (mg): 1,110

Switching from the first swap to the third
once a month will save you 5,400 calories in a year—almost two pounds.

- The Chicken Bowl still isn't great for you, as far as nutrition goes, but it's a whole lot lower in fat than even a small serving of Popcorn Chicken.

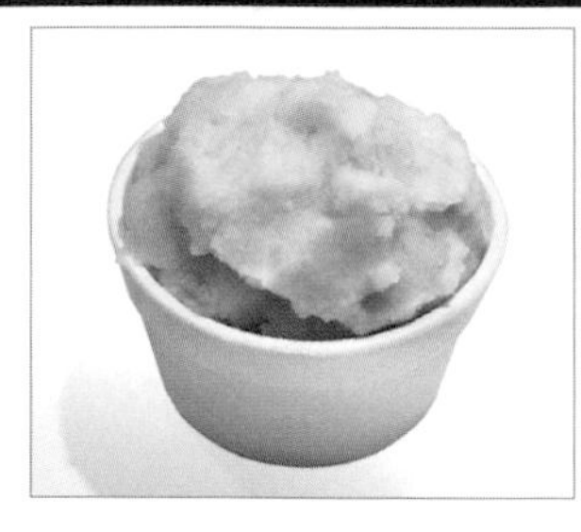

Individual-Size Mashed Potatoes

(no gravy)

Calories: 80
Fat (g): 0
Saturated fat (g): 0
Sodium (mg): 280

Switching from the first swap to the third
once a month will save you 3,120 calories in a year—almost one pound.

- Looking for something with green vegetables on the KFC menu? An order of individual-size coleslaw has 150 calories, 8 grams of fat (2 g saturated fat) and 240 mg sodium. That's about your only choice, however.

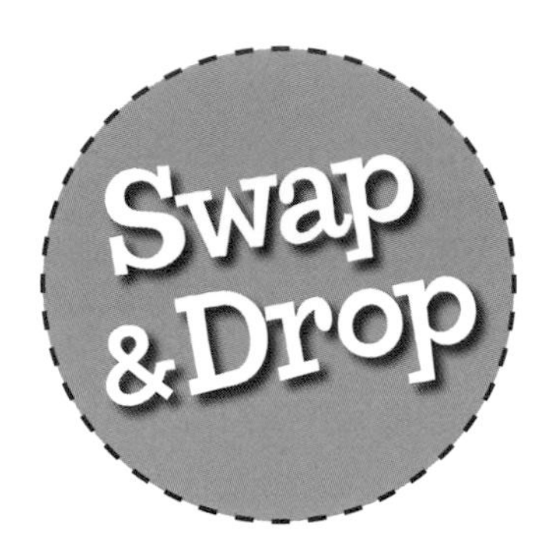

MCDONALD'S

McDonald's food has been maligned over the years, and the chain is trying to do better. But it's a good idea to keep an eye on the nutritional information of these choices.

swap this | **or this**

▼ BREAKFAST

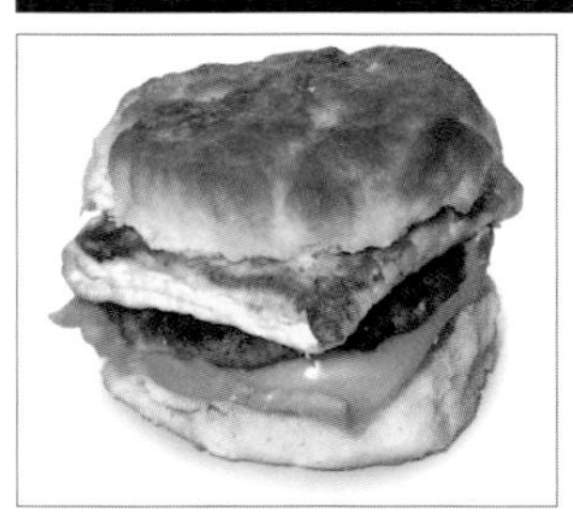

Sausage and Egg Biscuit Sandwich
(with cheese and margarine on a buttermilk biscuit)
Calories: 590
Fat (g): 37
Saturated fat (g): 19
Sodium (mg): 1,140

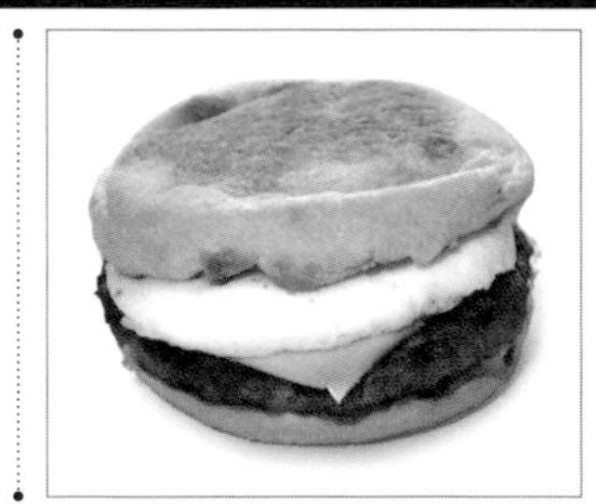

Sausage McMuffin with Egg Sandwich
(with cheese and margarine on an English muffin)
Calories: 440
Fat (g): 26
Saturated fat (g): 10
Sodium (mg): 910

▼ SANDWICHES

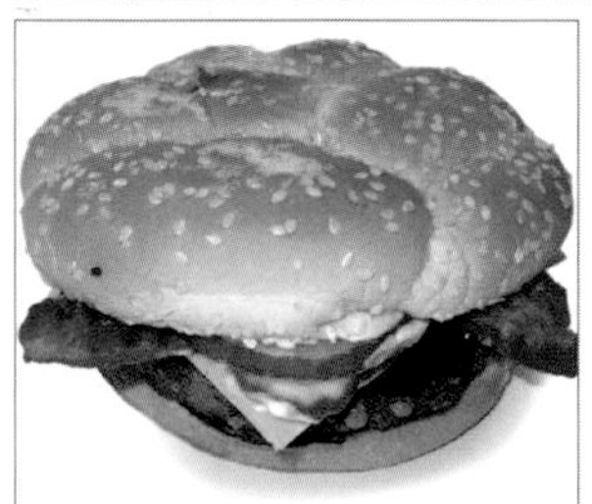

Angus Deluxe
(Angus beef patty with lettuce, mayonnaise-type sauce, mustard, pickle, cheese, red onion and tomato on a bun)
Calories: 780
Fat (g): 47
Saturated fat (g): 17
Sodium (mg): 1,660

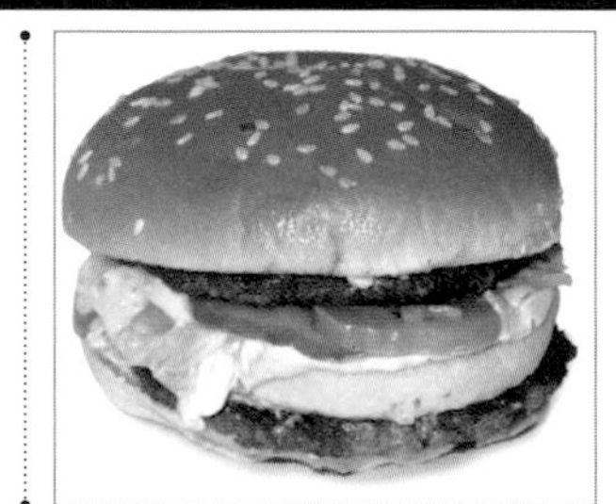

Big Mac
(two beef patties, Big Mac sauce, onions, pickles, lettuce and cheese on a three-layered bun)
Calories: 540
Fat (g): 29
Saturated fat (g): 10
Sodium (mg): 1,020

▼ ENTRÉE SALADS

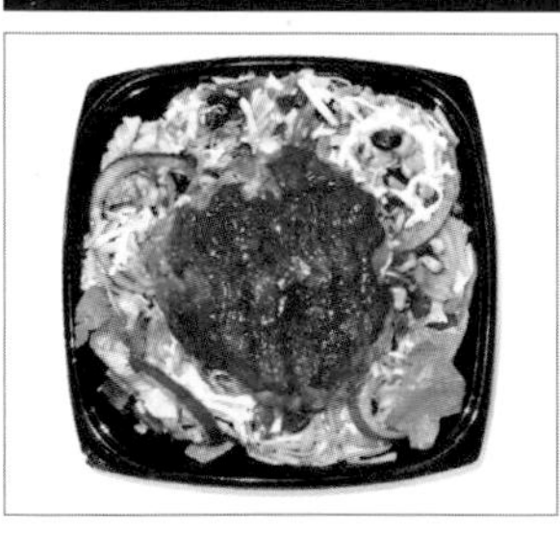

Southwest Salad with Crispy Chicken
(with Southwest Ranch dressing)
Calories: 590
Fat (g): 35
Saturated fat (g): 8
Sodium (mg): 1,610

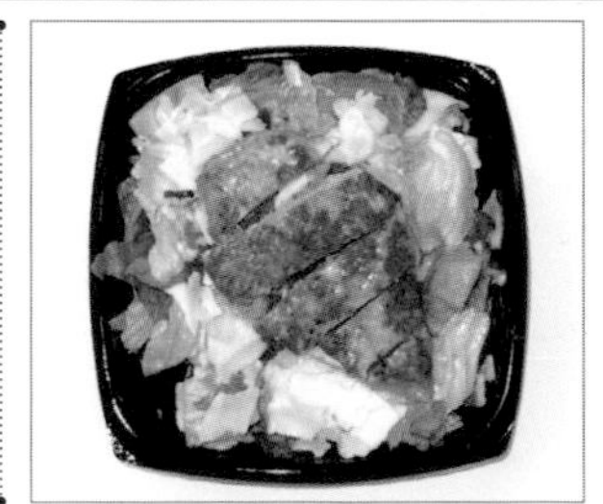

Mighty Caesar Salad with Grilled Chicken
(with Light Caesar dressing)
Calories: 490
Fat (g): 31
Saturated fat (g): 8
Sodium (mg): 1,200

All menu information was accurate at time of writing according to the nutritional information made available by each restaurant.

for that

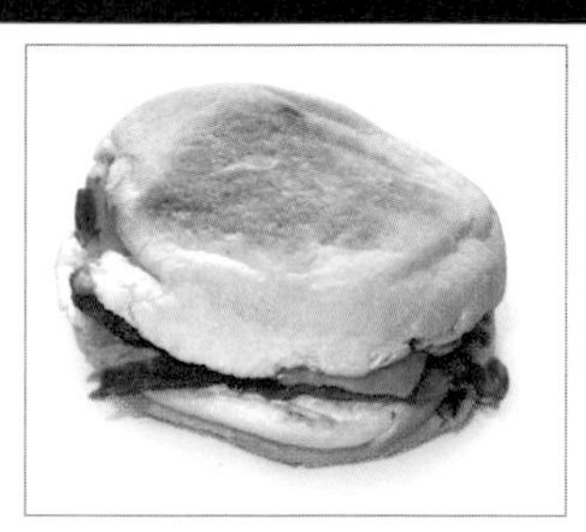

Egg McMuffin

(with Canadian bacon, cheese and margarine on an English muffin)

Calories: 290
Fat (g): 12
Saturated fat (g): 5
Sodium (mg): 760

Switching from the first swap to the third

once a month will save you 3,600 calories in a year—about one pound.

- The most well-known McDonald's breakfast sandwich is also their healthiest. The sausages in the first two options jack up the calories significantly.

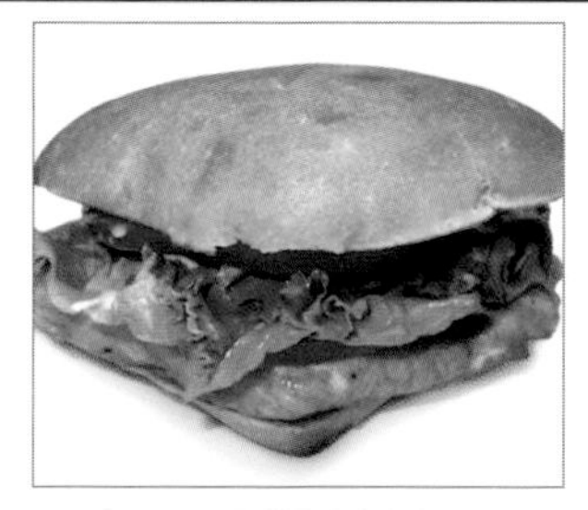

Grilled Chicken Classic

(grilled chicken with garlic sauce, lettuce and tomato on a ciabatta bun)

Calories: 390
Fat (g): 11
Saturated fat (g): 2
Sodium (mg): 810

Switching from the first swap to the third

once a month will save you 4,680 calories per year—over one pound.

- Craving a beef burger? Think smaller: A regular-size McDonald's hamburger has 250 calories, 8 grams of fat (3 grams saturated) and 510 mg sodium—much better than a Big Mac.

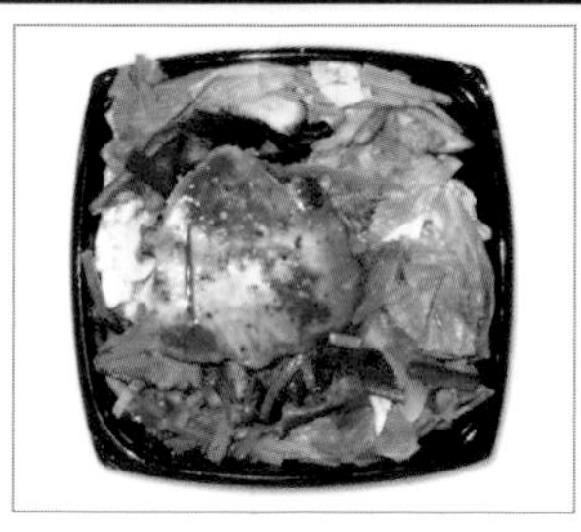

Spicy Thai Salad with Grilled Chicken

(with Asian Sesame dressing)

Calories: 360
Fat (g): 13
Saturated fat (g): 1
Sodium (mg): 910

Switching from the first swap to the third

once a month will save you 2,760 calories in a year—almost one pound.

- McDonald's salads are still high in sodium, but the chain says it's working on updating its menu selections over the next few years to make them healthier and less sodium-heavy.

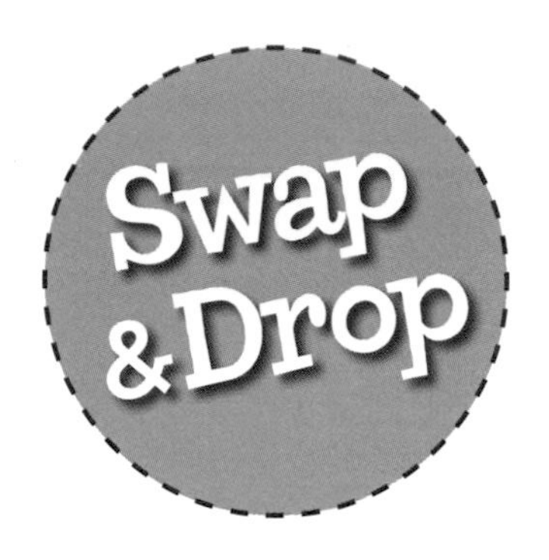

STARBUCKS

Who would've thought a coffee shop would be such a diet minefield? Not to fear: Simple coffee drinks and healthy snacks are still relatively easy to find.

swap this / **or this**

▼ ESPRESSO DRINKS (GRANDE SIZE)

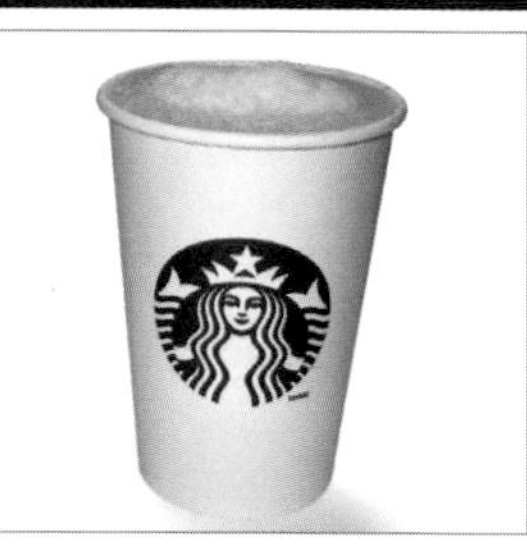

Peppermint White Chocolate Mocha

Calories: 540
Fat (g): 19
Saturated fat (g): 12
Sodium (mg): 240

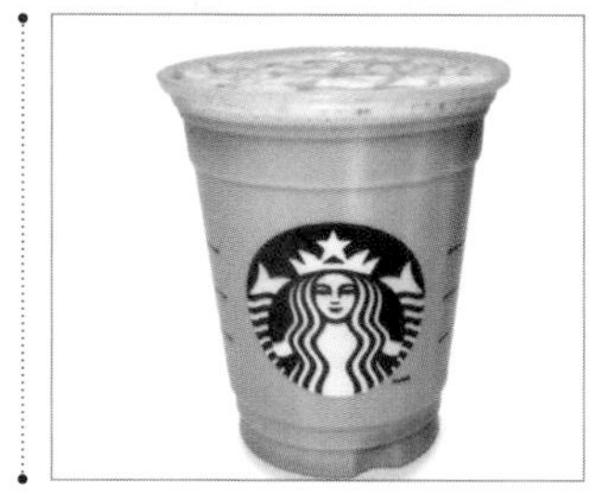

Caramel Macchiato

Calories: 240
Fat (g): 7
Saturated fat (g): 4.5
Sodium (mg) 130

▼ BAKERY ITEMS

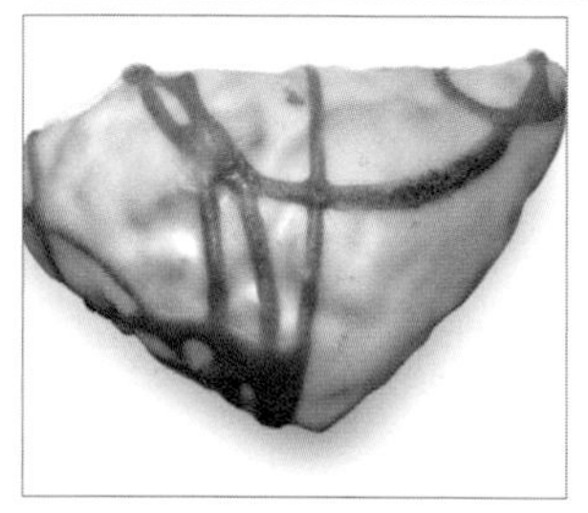

Pumpkin Scone

Calories: 480
Fat (g): 17
Saturated fat (g): 9
Sodium (mg): 280

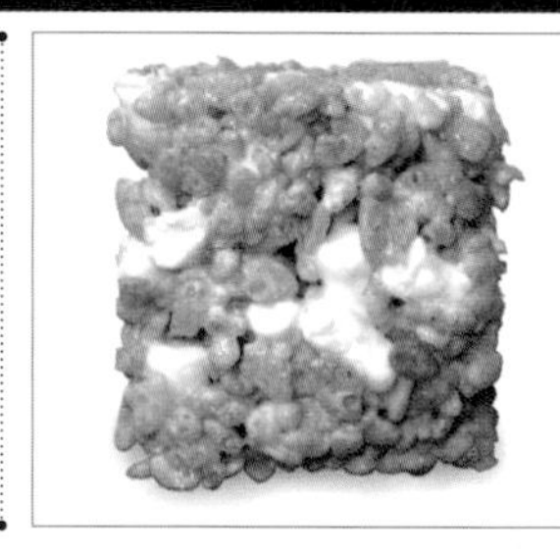

Marshmallow Dream Bar

Calories: 210
Fat (g): 4
Saturated fat (g): 2.5
Sodium (mg): 250

▼ LUNCH ITEMS

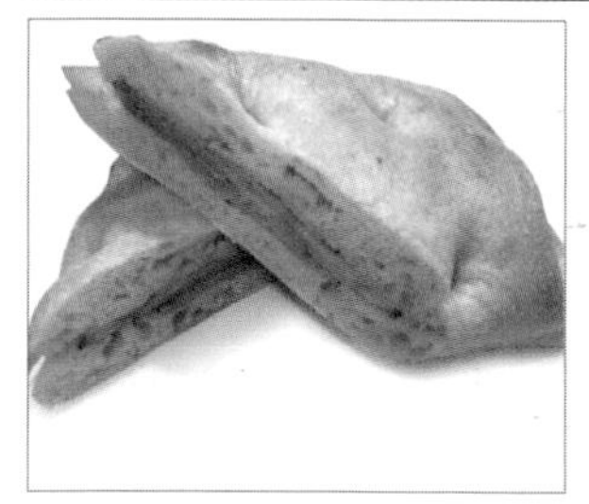

Ham & Swiss Panini
(Black Forest ham and Swiss cheese with Dijon mustard on a piccolo roll)

Calories: 430
Fat (g): 16
Saturated Fat (g): 8
Sodium (mg): 1,580

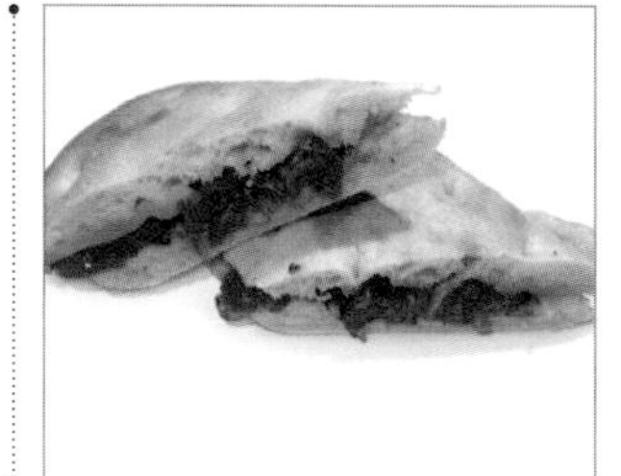

Roasted Tomato and Mozzarella Panini
(Roma tomatoes, mozzarella, spinach and basil pesto on a piccolo roll)

Calories: 380
Fat (g): 15
Saturated fat (g): 5
Sodium (mg): 780

All menu information was accurate at time of writing according to the nutritional information made available by each restaurant.

for that

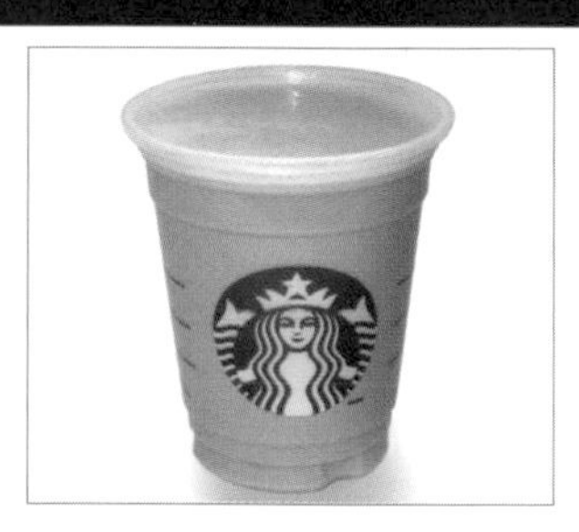

Skinny Flavoured Latte

Calories: 130
Fat (g): 0
Saturated fat (g): 0
Sodium (mg): 170

Switching from the first swap to the third

once a week will save you 21,320 calories in a year—as much as six pounds.

- Do you have a sweet tooth? Starbucks gives you the option of adding artificially sweetened syrups to any drink, so feel free to indulge in those. Just avoid the whipped cream.

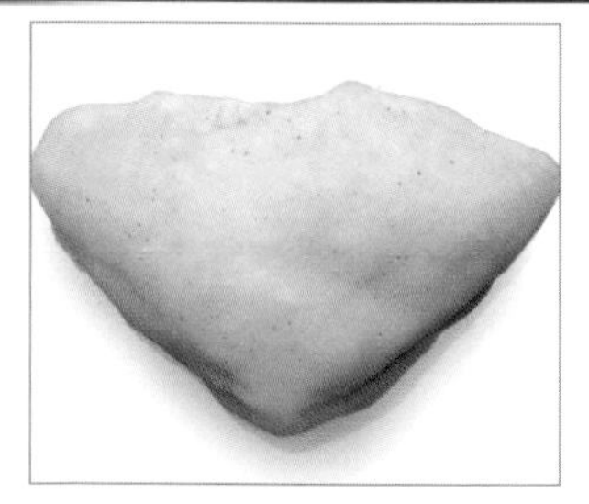

Petite Vanilla Bean Scone

Calories: 140
Fat (g): 5
Saturated fat (g): 2.5
Sodium (mg): 90

Switching from the first swap to the third

once a week will save you 17,680 calories in a year—or about five pounds.

- The word "pumpkin" conjurs up images of home-baked goods and harvest time, not calorific café treats—but this pumpkin scone won't do your diet any favours. Luckily, there are better options. Opt for a smaller choice, like the Petite Vanilla Bean Scone.

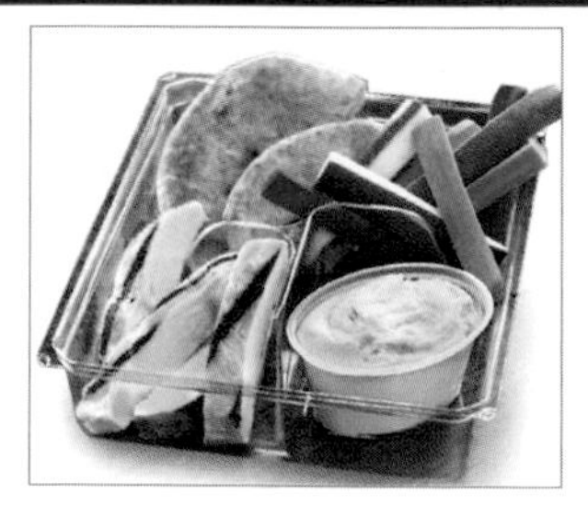

Chicken and Hummus Bistro Box

(with cucumber and carrot sticks, grape tomatoes and wheat pita)
Calories: 270
Fat (g): 10
Saturated fat (g): 1
Sodium (mg): 670

Switching from the first swap to the third

once a week will save you 8,320 calories in a year—over two pounds.

- Even the least diet-friendly sandwich at Starbucks isn't that bad, but you should still order this Bistro Box whenever possible. The variety of foods it includes will make you feel more like you're eating a complete, nutritious lunch than you would if you just ate a ham sandwich.

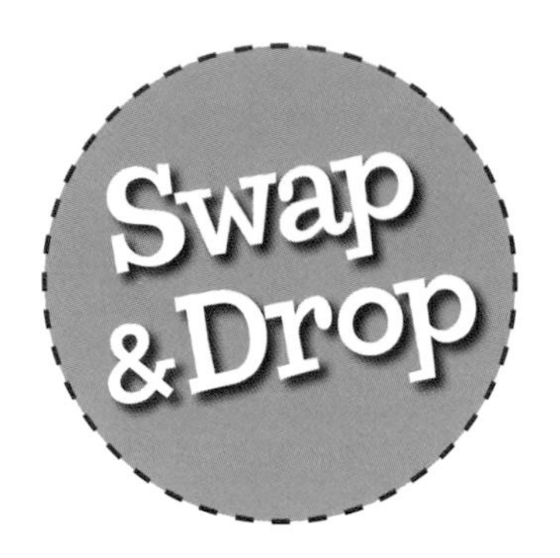

SUBWAY

We all know how well Jared did here. And yes, they do have a "6 grams of fat or less" menu. But don't let your guard down—not everything is good for you!

swap this | **or this**

▼ BREAKFAST

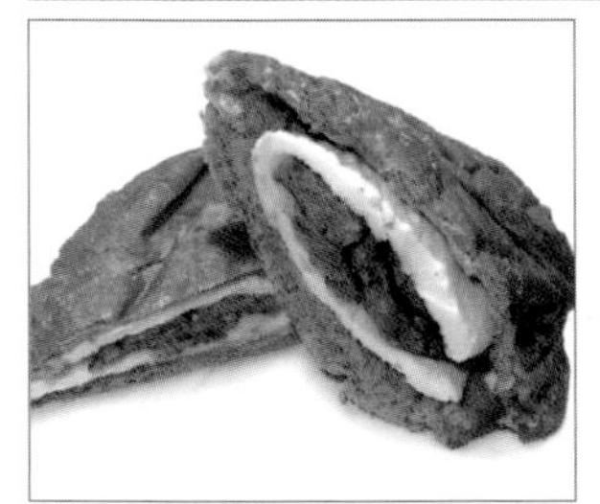

6" Sausage and Cheese Omelet Sandwich on 9-Grain Wheat Bread

Calories: 620
Fat (g): 37
Saturated fat (g): 14
Sodium (mg): 1,290

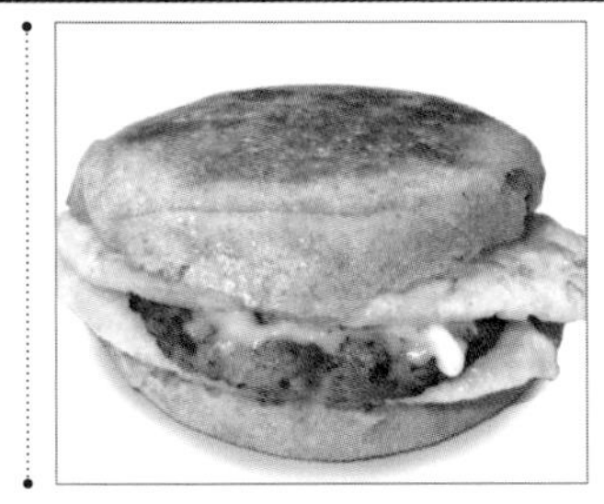

Sausage and Cheese English Muffin Sandwich

Calories: 290
Fat (g): 19
Saturated fat (g): 7
Sodium (mg): 776

▼ CHICKEN SANDWICHES

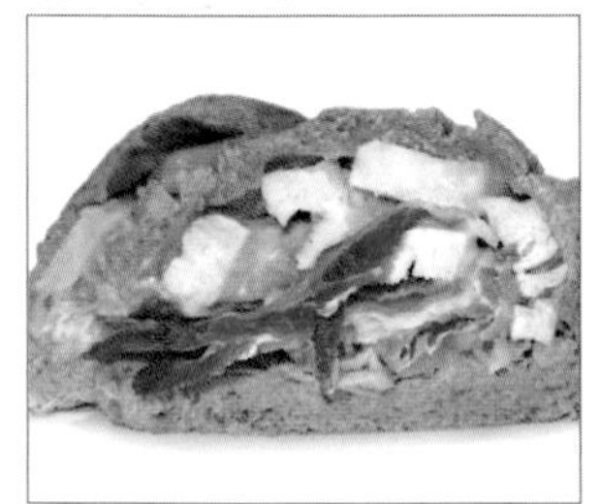

6" Chicken and Bacon Ranch
(on 9-Grain Wheat bread with lettuce, tomatoes, onions, green peppers, cucumbers and cheese)

Calories: 500
Fat (g): 23
Saturated fat (g): 7
Sodium (mg): 1,060

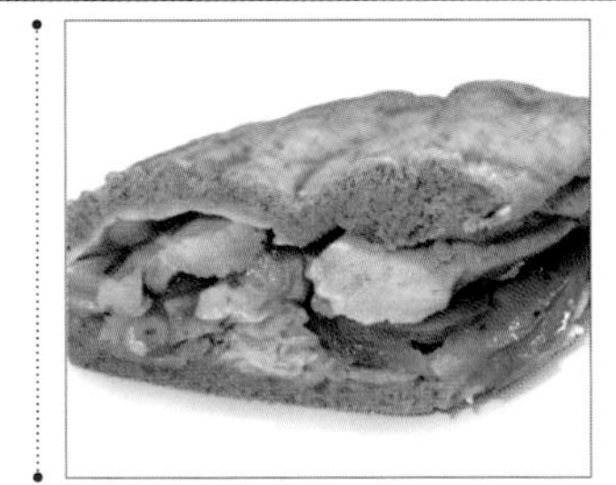

6" Sweet Onion Chicken Teriyaki Sandwich
(on 9-Grain Wheat bread with lettuce, tomatoes, onions, green peppers and cucumbers)

Calories: 380
Fat (g): 7
Saturated fat (g): 2
Sodium (mg): 1,140

▼ MEAT SANDWICHES

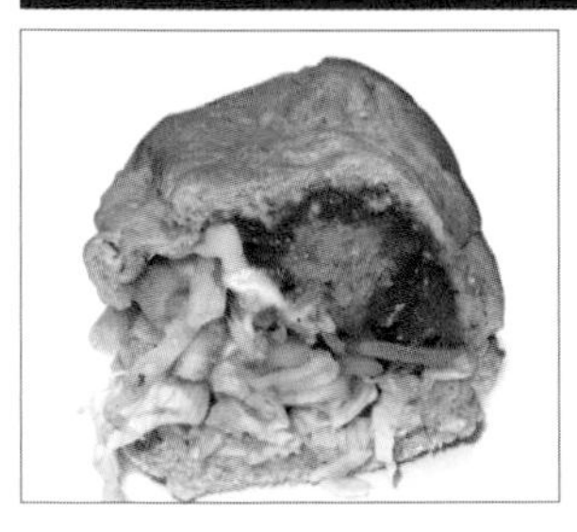

6" Meatball Marinara Sandwich
(on 9-Grain Wheat bread with lettuce, tomatoes, onions, green peppers, cucumbers and cheese)

Calories: 570
Fat (g): 22
Saturated fat (g): 9
Sodium (mg): 1,420

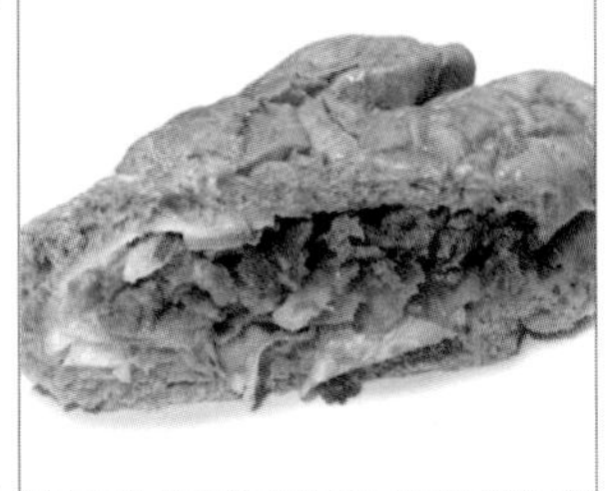

6" Steak & Cheese Sandwich
(on 9-Grain Wheat bread with lettuce, tomatoes, onions, green peppers, cucumbers and cheese)

Calories: 380
Fat (g): 10
Saturated fat (g): 4
Sodium (mg): 1,060

All menu information was accurate at time of writing according to the nutritional information made available by each restaurant.

for that

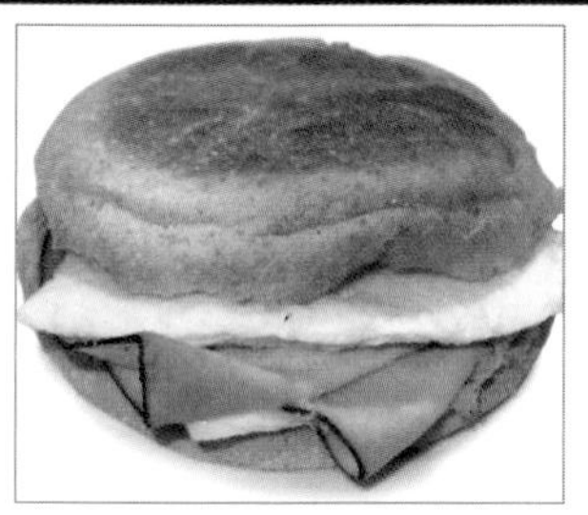

Ham and Cheese English Muffin Sandwich

(made with egg white only)

Calories: 170
Fat (g): 4
Saturated fat (g): 2
Sodium (mg): 590

Switching from the first swap to the third

once a month will save you 5,400 calories in a year—about one-and-a-half pounds.

- Once again, sausage amps up the calorie count. Opt for a much-healthier egg-white sandwich the next time you stop by Subway in the morning.

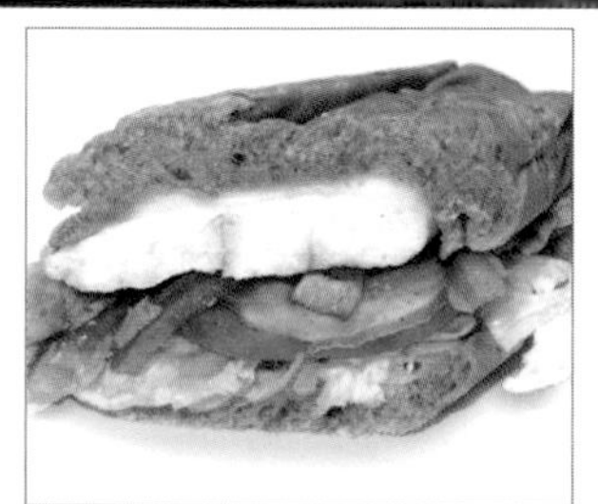

6" Oven-Roasted Chicken Sandwich

(on 9-Grain Wheat bread with lettuce, tomatoes, onions, green peppers and cucumbers)

Calories: 320
Fat (g): 7
Saturated fat (g): 2
Sodium (mg): 740

Switching from the first swap to the third

once a month will save you 1,440 calories in a year—about half a pound.

- Words like "oven-roasted" are usually good news for your calorie count. Skip the bag of chips and cookie, and you've got yourself a decently balanced lunch. And it goes without saying: Choose the 6" sandwiches, not the 12".

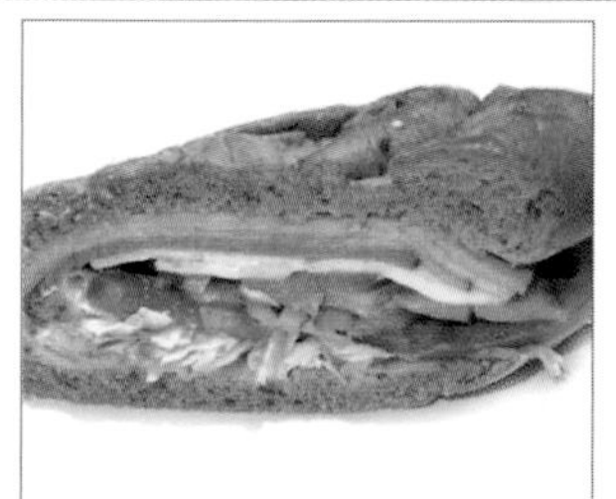

6" Club Sandwich

(ham, roast beef and turkey on 9-Grain Wheat bread with lettuce, tomatoes, onions, green peppers and cucumbers)

Calories: 300
Fat (g): 4
Saturated fat (g): 1
Sodium (mg): 720

Switching from the first swap to the third

once a month will save you 3,240 calories in a year—almost one pound.

- Sticking to the "6 grams of fat or less" menu is a pretty safe bet, while some other subs have more than 500 calories and over 20 grams of fat.

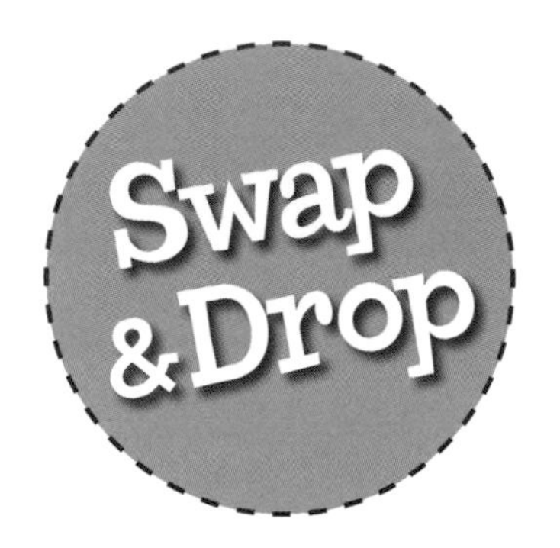

TACO BELL

Yes, taco dinners can be healthy—just be careful about what you order! Hint: Skip the cheese and the big burritos. Yo quiero my **Swap & Drop**!

swap this / or this

▼ BEEF CHOICES

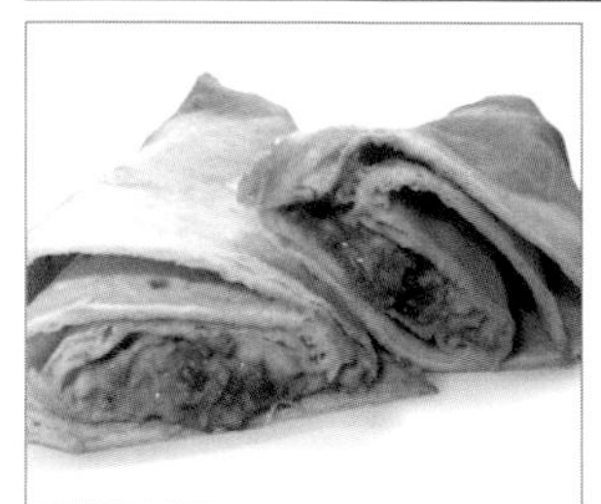

Beef Burrito
(tortilla wrapped around ground beef, topped with nacho cheese sauce)
Calories: 400
Fat (g): 18
Saturated fat (g): 7
Sodium (mg): 1,140

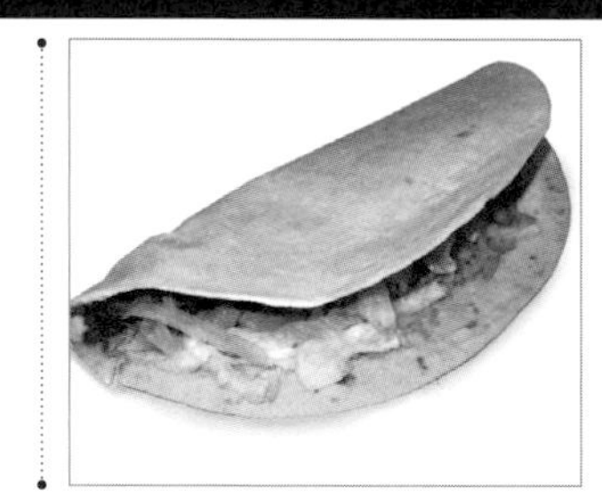

Beef Soft Taco
(tortilla filled with ground beef, lettuce and cheddar cheese)
Calories: 210
Fat (g): 10
Saturated fat (g): 4
Sodium (mg): 470

▼ CHICKEN CHOICES

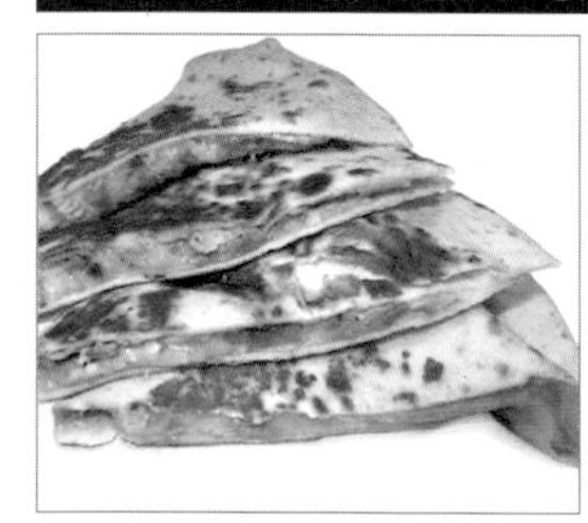

Chicken Quesadilla
(grilled chicken with Monterey Jack, cheddar and part skim mozzarella cheese plus jalapeño sauce, folded in tortilla)
Calories: 530
Fat (g): 28
Saturated fat (g): 12
Sodium (mg): 1,170

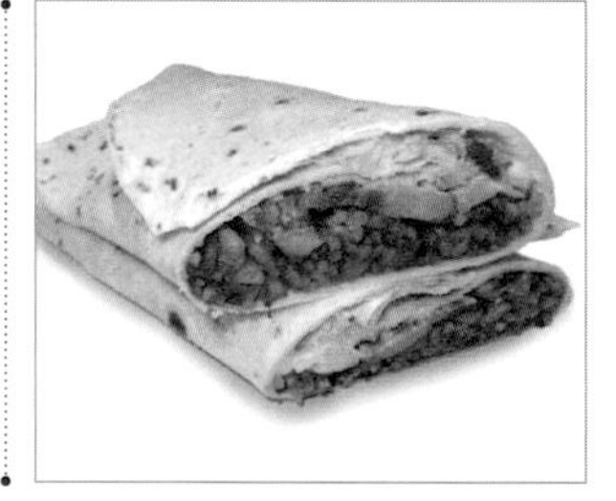

Chicken Burrito Supreme
(grilled chicken, seasoned rice, red sauce, lettuce, cheddar cheese, onions, tomatoes and sour cream in a tortilla)
Calories: 390
Fat (g): 16
Saturated fat (g): 6
Sodium (mg): 1,180

▼ SIDES

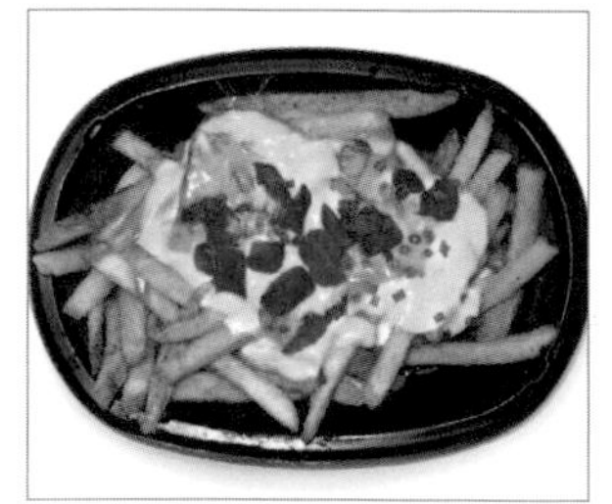

Fries Supreme
(fries with ground beef, nacho cheese sauce, tomatoes, chives and sour cream)
Calories: 540
Fat (g): 32
Saturated fat (g): 6
Sodium (mg): 1,520

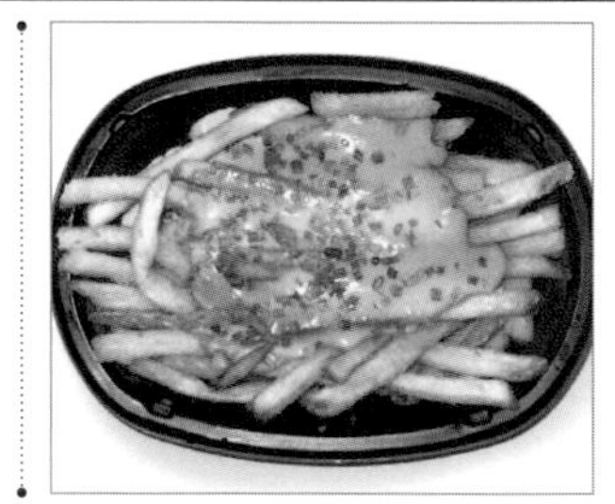

Cheesy Fries
(fries with nacho cheese sauce)
Calories: 460
Fat (g): 26
Saturated fat (g): 3
Sodium (mg): 1,380

All menu information was accurate at time of writing according to the nutritional information made available by each restaurant.

for that

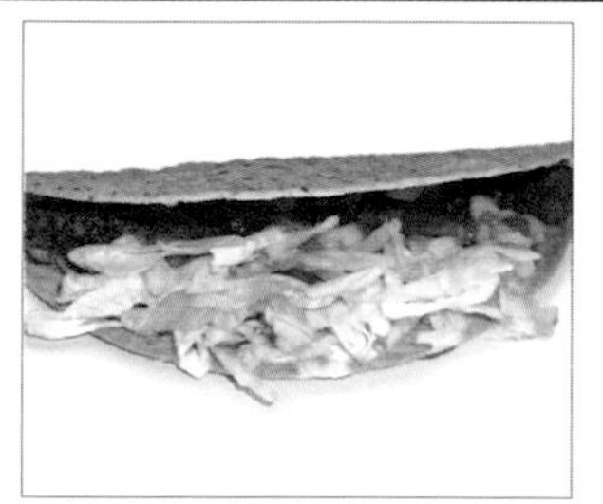

Fresco Beef Hard Taco

(taco filled with ground beef, lettuce and salsa)

Calories: 150
Fat (g): 7
Saturated fat (g): 3
Sodium (mg): 260

Switching from the first swap to the third

once a month will save you 3,000 calories in a year—almost one pound.

- It's the amount of cheddar cheese—and the portion size—that make the Beef Burrito a bad choice. One Fresco Beef Hard Taco makes a decent-sized snack, but it doesn't have a whole lot of nutritional value.

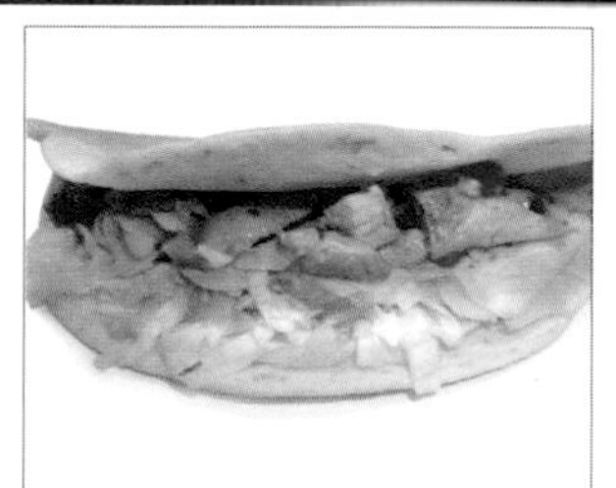

Fresco Chicken Soft Taco

(tortilla filled with grilled chicken, lettuce and salsa)

Calories: 170
Fat (g): 5
Saturated fat (g): 2
Sodium (mg): 580

Switching from the first swap to the third

once a month will save you 4,320 calories in a year—more than one pound.

- Quesadillas tend to seem like harmless snack food, but they rely entirely on melted cheese. Go for the Fresco Chicken Soft Taco instead—two would make a decent small meal.

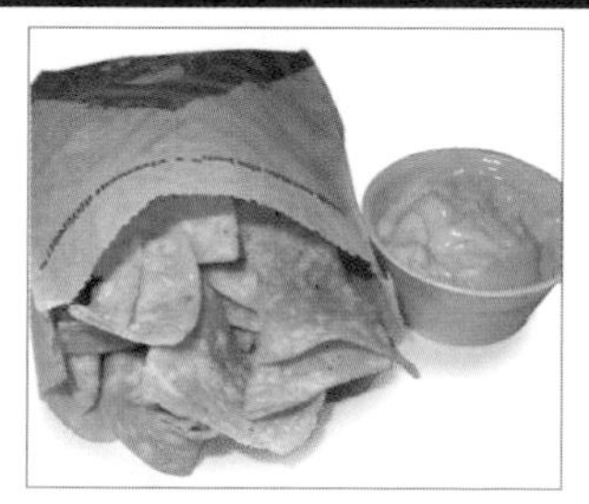

Nachos and Cheese

(tortilla chips with nacho cheese sauce on the side)

Calories: 340
Fat (g): 22
Saturated fat (g): 3
Sodium (mg): 600

Switching from the first swap to the third

once a month will save you 2,400 calories in a year—almost one pound.

- Nachos are tough to call healthy, but if you must have them, save on fat and calories by having only half the cheese and sharing with a friend.

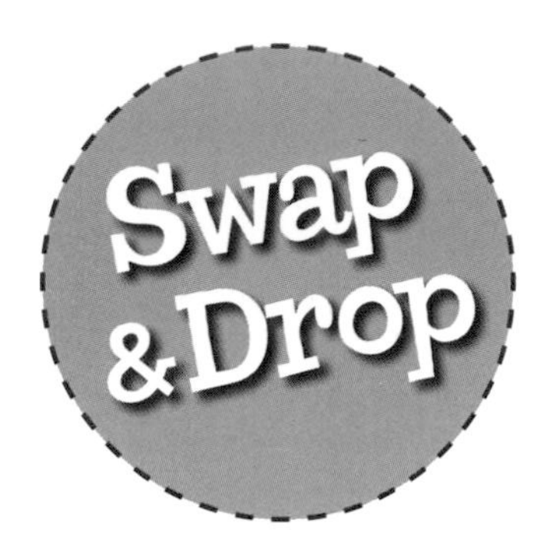

TIM HORTONS

What Canadian hasn't been to Tim's? If you're watching your weight, you already know doughnuts can't be good. But what about the other menu items? We checked it out.

swap this **or this**

▼ SNACKS

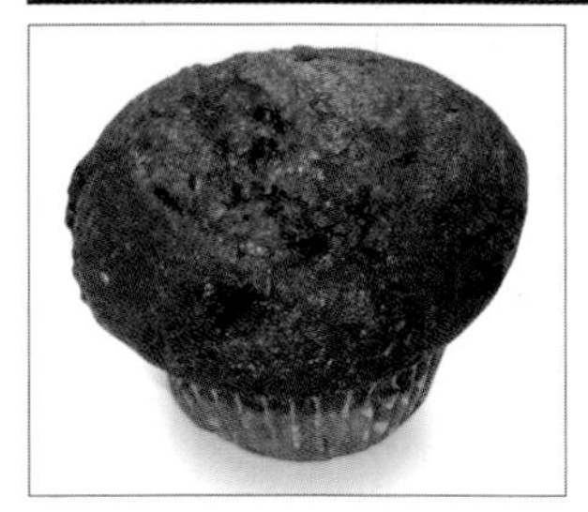

Raisin Bran Muffin
Calories: 410
Fat (g): 13
Saturated fat (g): 3
Sodium (mg): 490

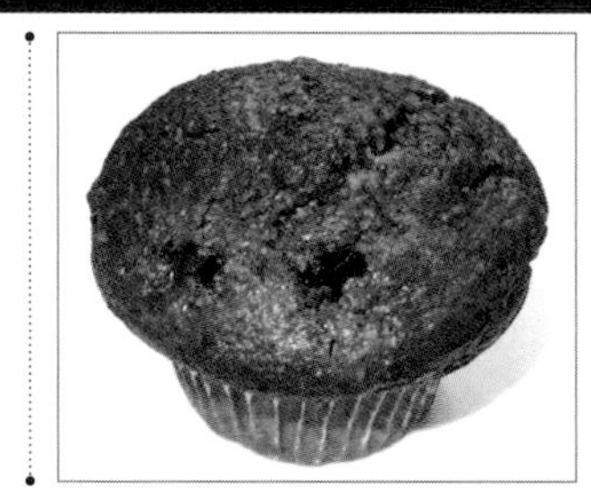

Cranberry Blueberry Bran Muffin
Calories: 340
Fat (g): 12
Saturated fat (g): 2
Sodium (mg): 460

▼ BREAKFAST

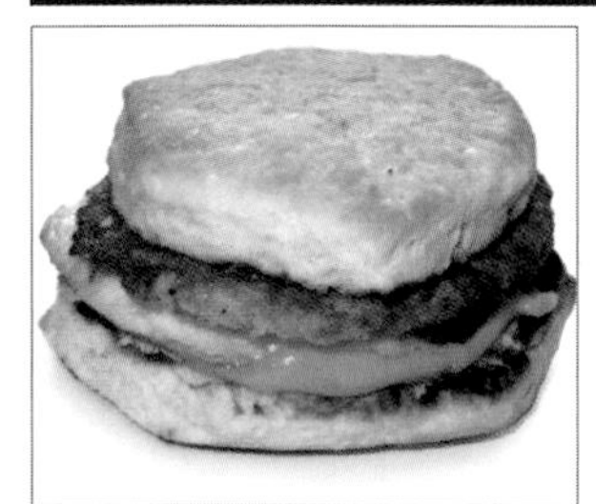

Sausage, Egg and Cheese Breakfast Sandwich on Home-style Biscuit
Calories: 530
Fat (g): 34
Saturated fat (g): 18
Sodium (mg): 1,010

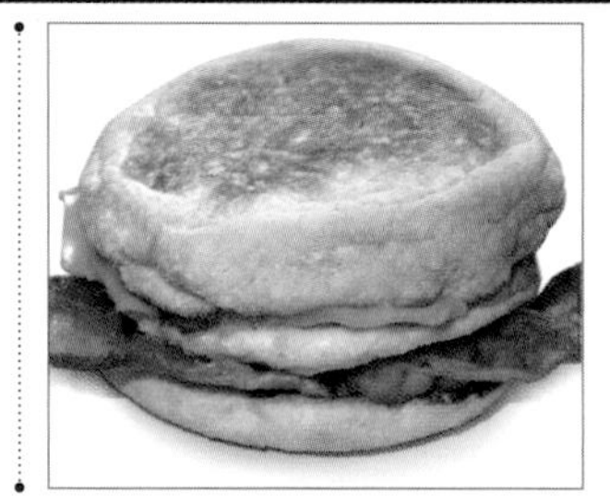

Egg, Bacon and Cheese on English Muffin
Calories: 330
Fat (g): 15
Saturated fat (g): 6
Sodium (mg): 770

▼ SIDES

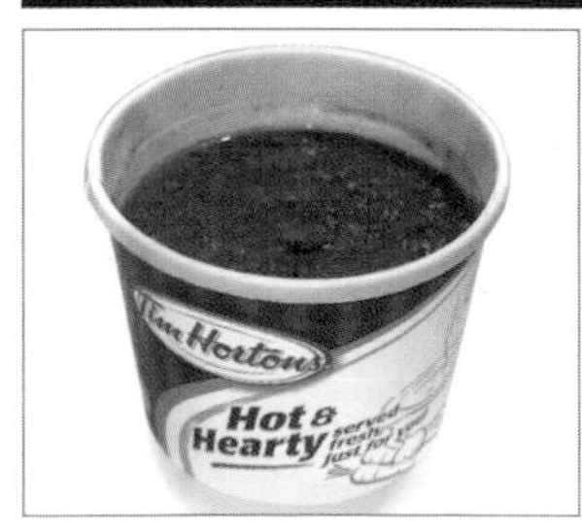

Chili
Calories: 300
Fat (g): 19
Saturated fat (g): 7
Sodium (mg): 1,320

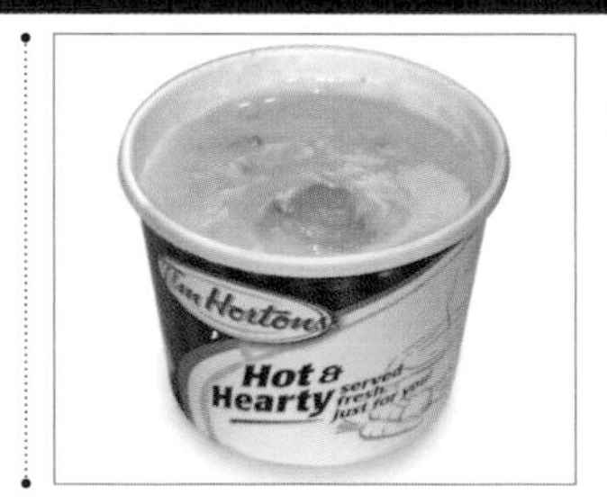

Creamy Field Mushroom Soup
Calories: 150
Fat (g): 3
Saturated fat (g): 2
Sodium (mg): 740

All menu information was accurate at time of writing according to the nutritional information made available by each restaurant.

for that

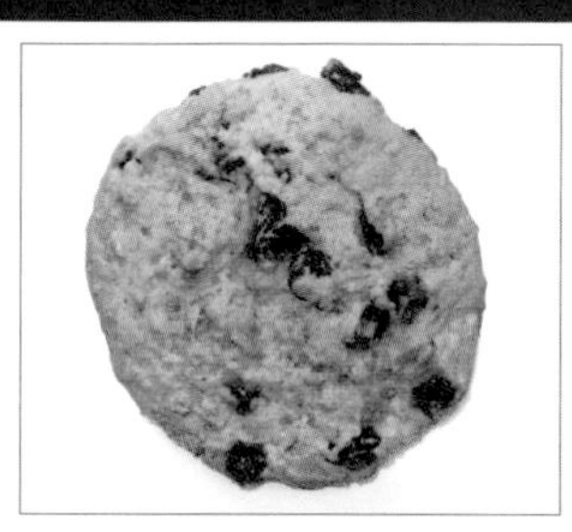

Trail Mix Cookie with Fruit and Nuts

Calories: 220
Fat (g): 8
Saturated fat (g): 3
Sodium (mg): 160

Switching from the first swap to the third

once a week will save you 9,880 calories in a year—almost three pounds.

- A bran muffin sounds healthy, but with more than 400 calories, it's not something you want to have every day.

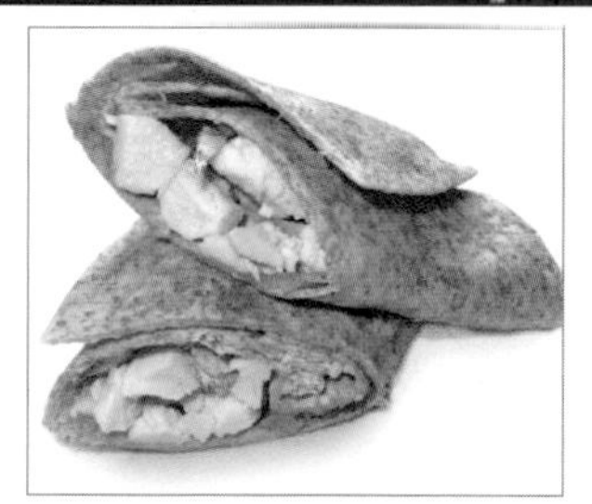

Egg and Cheese Breakfast Wrap

Calories: 270
Fat (g): 14
Saturated fat (g): 4
Sodium (mg): 690

Switching from the first swap to the third

once a week will save you 13,520 calories in a year—almost four pounds.

- When ordering breakfast at any restaurant, ham or bacon are generally lower-fat choices than sausage. If you're only given the choice between a biscuit, bagel or English muffin, choose the English muffin.

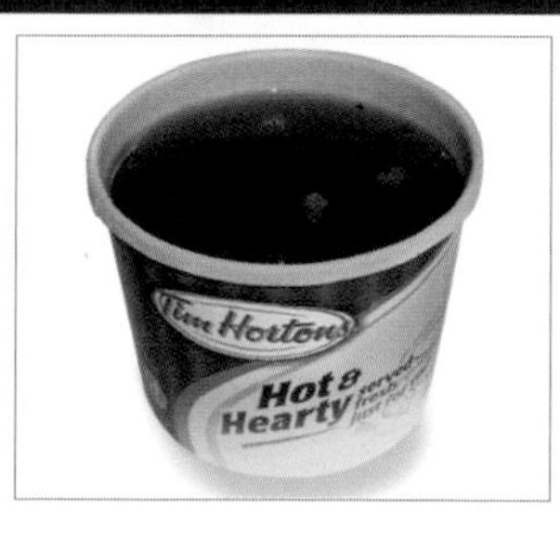

Hearty Vegetable Soup

Calories: 70
Fat (g): 0
Saturated fat (g): 0
Sodium (mg): 650

Switching from the first swap to the third

once a week will save you 11,960 calories in a year—three-and-a-half pounds.

- Many restaurant soups are high in sodium. Whenever you eat out, ask for the restaurant's nutritional information.

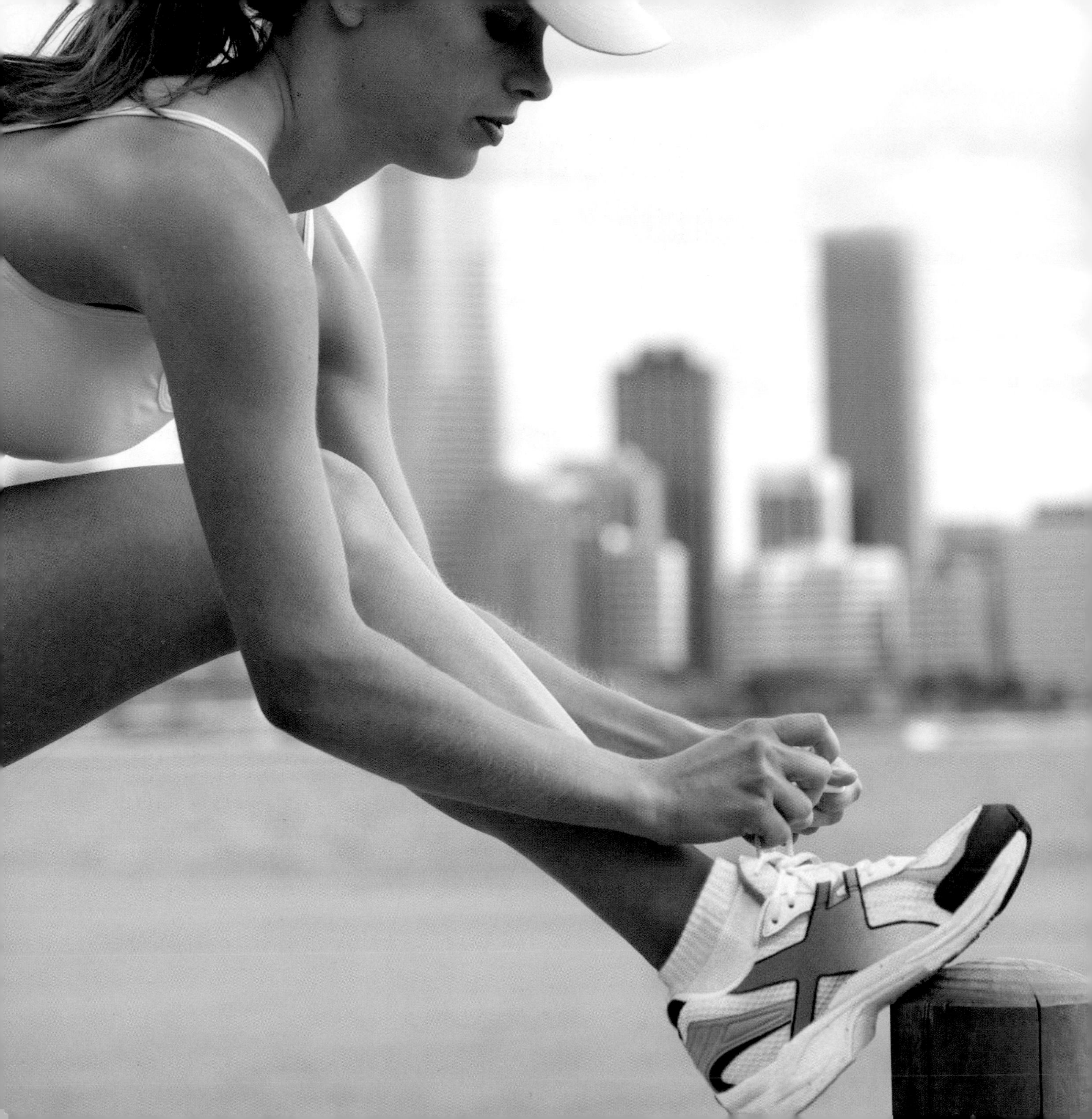

4

Walk it off in just minutes a day

I started walking when I was 15. I was going through a mildly "chubby" phase and told my mother how frustrated I felt about my weight and my body.

She told me she had discovered this magical weight-loss strategy when my sisters and I started going to a school that was a half-hour stroll from our house. "When I started walking you girls to school," she said, "I noticed that I steadily lost weight–I've walked to keep weight off ever since."

I started walking in the hills around our house that day, and quickly discovered that she was right.

I wholeheartedly applaud the idea of activity as a natural part of your life rather than an extra you have to somehow fit in. Boot camps and gym-based regimens can whip you into shape, but they won't last unless you're one of those rare people who loves the gym and lives by the words "no pain, no gain." My feeling is that, for activity to become a way of life, you have to enjoy and be able to access it easily anywhere, anytime.

I'm in pretty good shape and see the inside of a gym only once or twice a year–usually when I'm travelling and staying in a hotel. Otherwise my exercise plan is simple: I walk, dance (I'm a flamenco dancer), do low-intensity yoga stretching at home and practice strengthening exercises similar to those in this section (starting on page 238).

When I adopted a rescue dog a few years ago, I was surprised to discover how much I loved walking in any weather. Previously, I might have skipped my walk if it was pouring rain or freezing outside. Thanks to a furry friend who needs a long walk every day of the year, I learned how delicious the air smells on rainy days and how invigorating a brisk walk in the cold can be when you bundle up right.

There are few things a good, brisk walk can't cure. Go get yourself that pedometer, and welcome to the easiest exercise plan on earth.

– Dr. Susan Biali, M.D.

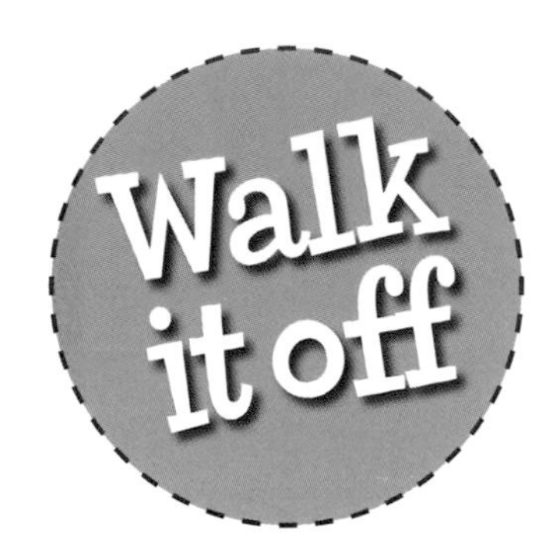

12-WEEK PROGRAM

Why walking works

The best exercise is the one you do everyday—without even realizing it. Take walking to the next level!

Imagine a "miracle vitamin" guaranteed to help you drop a clothing size or more; banish blue moods; serve up more shut-eye; slash your risk for heart disease, diabetes and cancer; and spice up life in the bedroom. Did we mention that it's also perfectly safe and costs virtually nothing?

"Physical fitness can neither be achieved by wishful thinking nor outright purchase."

—Joseph Pilates, inventor of Pilates physical fitness

WHY GYMS SHOULD MAKE YOU SWEAT

The cost of many gyms may have already discouraged you from joining. Little did you know how much you were saving yourself. The CBC reported in 2011 that the Canadian fitness industry was worth $2 billion a year, and that many gyms charged their members costly hidden fees and premiums. That's one more reason to love walking—no one will ever charge you for it!

You won't find this super supplement in any pharmacy, but you can easily pick it up on the way to the store. It's "vitamin W"–also known as walking. The perfect dose? Hit the sidewalk (or the trail, treadmill or mall) for 30 minutes, most days of the week. There's no need to buy special equipment, spring for an overpriced health-club membership or waste time (and gas) driving to the gym.

But is exercise really crucial to weight loss? Isn't it just about how much you eat? And if exercise is so important, what kind should you do and how often?

You'd think the scientific community would have solid answers to these questions. But it doesn't. Many widely held "truths" about fitness have been proved wrong in recent years, replaced by fascinating new insights which many doctors still aren't even aware of.

The good news? Recent studies show that the right type of fitness for health and weight loss is much more accessible, and less strenuous, than we've been led to believe–you already do it every day.

A brief history of weight

Scientists believe humans have been on this planet in our current form for roughly 1 million years. For 999,900 of those years, no one but athletes and warriors bothered setting aside time to exercise. They didn't need to–most of their waking hours were spent carrying, tilling, building or battling with enemies. Another plus? No fast-food restaurants. Food was scarce, given the lack of refrigeration and electricity. Needless to say, this kept them lean.

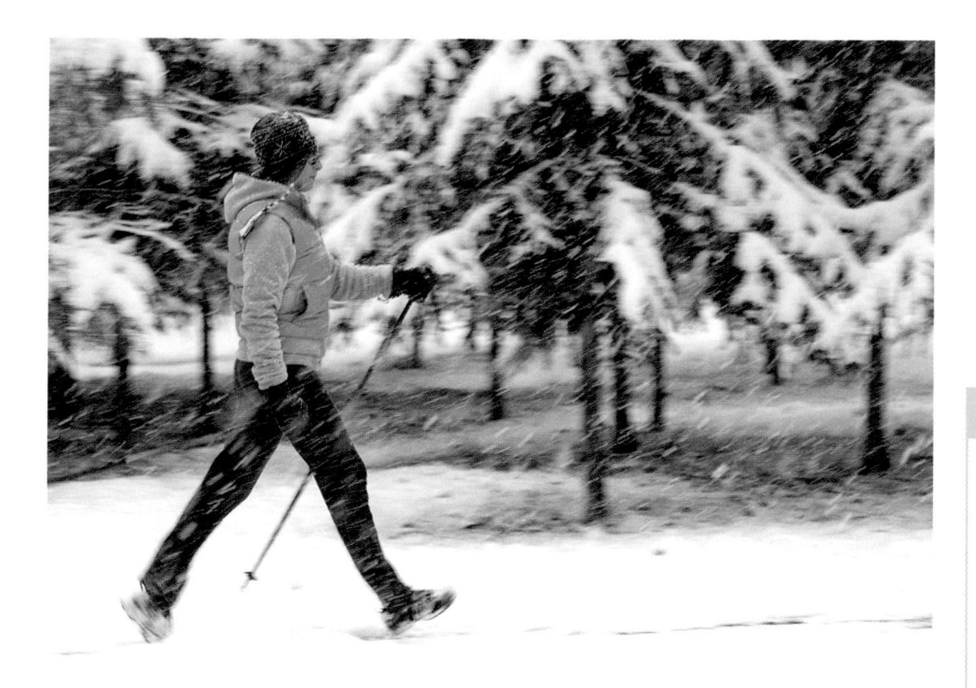

This epoch ended about a century ago. In the past 100 years, thanks mostly to technology and industry, food not only became plentiful, but food businesses discovered that the more sugar and fat they put in their products, the more people enjoyed them. Some of that is animal instinct–our bodies are naturally drawn to high-calorie foods as part of the self-preservation process.

At the same time, we became sedentary. Television, computers, desk jobs, internet shopping and socializing, long commutes by train, bus or car...it seems that life has conspired to keep our bottoms attached to our seats. Here again, animal instinct is at play: Our bodies are naturally drawn to rest as part of the energy-conservation process.

Put together much less movement with much more food, and you have the underpinnings of the modern obesity epidemic.

Yes, there are genetic causes for obesity. But for most Canadians, it's our sedentary lifestyles and our desire for convenience that result in fewer calories being burned. When was the last time you manually opened your garage door or took the stairs by choice?

Staying slim now

So how do we maintain a healthy weight in these modern, high-tech times? There is only one effective way: Move more and eat less. Not one or the other, but both. Adjusting only one rarely works. Merely eating fewer calories won't compensate for all the sitting we do. And no level of exercise can burn off all the empty calories

Get up and go, in the snow

Canadian winters aren't exactly the greatest encouragement to get up and moving. If you find yourself desperate to snuggle under the covers instead of going for a walk, try these tips:

- **Go for a walk before breakfast. Don't give yourself time to get discouraged about the weather—haul straight out of bed and out the door. Reward yourself with a steaming bowl of oatmeal.**
- **Invest in a solid pair of thermal underwear. It'll be much more bearable to walk outside if you're well-insulated.**

Obesity and exercise

If you're struggling with your weight, you're definitely not alone: The number of Canadians who are overweight or obese has skyrocketed over the last few decades. But take heart! According to a 2011 study from the Public Health Agency of Canada, eliminating physical inactivity would immediately help about 1 million obese Canadians slim down.

Active everyday movement restores the optimum daily balance between calories consumed and calories burned.

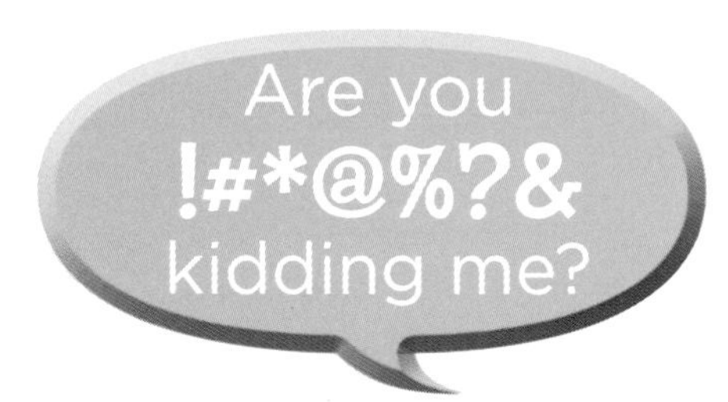

In one study, researchers examined gym records and found that people wasted an average of $700 over the course of a membership because they didn't go often enough to make the fees worth it.

in the typical diet. The remedy? A gentle, slow adjustment to both your eating and movement patterns.

By now, you know **Swap & Drop**'s rules of eating for weight loss. But how do you adjust your life for fitness? For several decades now, the government, scientists and a huge fitness industry have been telling us to put on workout clothes and get physical. They recommended at least three 30-minute sessions per week, doing some precise mix of weight lifting and aerobic exercise. There's no surprise, then, that roughly 80 percent of North Americans choose not to exercise.

And even when we try it, it doesn't work. Let's say someone–you, for example–resolves to lose weight once and for all. You know you need to exercise, so you start jogging. You've heard you have to be properly fuelled and hydrated, so you drink a flavoured electrolyte drink and hit the streets. But jogging is hard and leaves your body feeling sore and punished.

You go for it anyway, and afterward you feel you deserve a reward. So you stop by Starbucks and treat yourself to a pumpkin scone. Four weeks later (if you make it that long) you haven't shed a gram, and you despondently toss your running shoes aside.

Why didn't it work?

First, you treated exercise as a special, additional activity rather than a natural part of your day. Second, you chose an activity that was too challenging, particularly for someone who isn't used to exercising.

The result? Your workout was short and painful and left you feeling totally spent–yet you burned only the caloric equivalent of a few grams of weight. The electrolyte drink and calorific snack more than compensated for the calorie burn, effectively washing out your workout and wasting your time.

Your body is meant to move, so you should move it–but in natural, ongoing ways, as our ancestors did. Breakthrough research from recent years reveals that active daily living–including frequent short walks, taking the stairs rather than the elevator, regular stretches and movements, routinely picking up and carrying things–is healthier for you than a short, intense gym workout counterbalanced with lots of sitting.

The new fitness paradigm is to move a lot in ways that are fun and natural. No clothing changes or drives to the gym, just active daily living. Don't make it a chore, and don't think of it as just another hassle you don't have time for. Just get out of your chair and move, as often as you can, for as long as you can.

Ready to take it to the next level of fitness? Then it's time to try other great activities you'll enjoy, like walking, swimming, biking, hiking, golf or tennis–low-stress pastimes that disguise exercise as fun. You know–the things you did with friends when you were younger. Start doing these on a regular basis, and you'll return to the physically active lifestyle of our lean ancestors–even if you can't quit that desk job.

Plus, when you're starting out, you don't need energy drinks, power bars or any other special food before, during or after. Just be active and eat normally, and weight loss will follow. Let's get started! ■

THE MECHANICS OF WALKING

While there may be variables to take into account when you walk, such as speed or terrain, the only thing you really need to do when you walk is use good form. It will make walking feel easier and help prevent injuries, too. Do it like this:

HEAD
Imagine a string attached to the top of your head pulling your crown toward the sky.

SHOULDERS
Keep your shoulders relaxed, down and slightly back.

BACK
Stand up straight, not hunched forward.

ARMS
Keep your elbows bent at 90-degree angles. Pump them forward and back; they shouldn't cross in front of your body.

LEGS
Maintain a natural stride length—it shouldn't feel strained. Longer isn't better.

CHEST
Keep your breastbone lifted and facing forward.

FEET
Land first on your heel, then roll forward across the ball of your foot and push off with your toes.

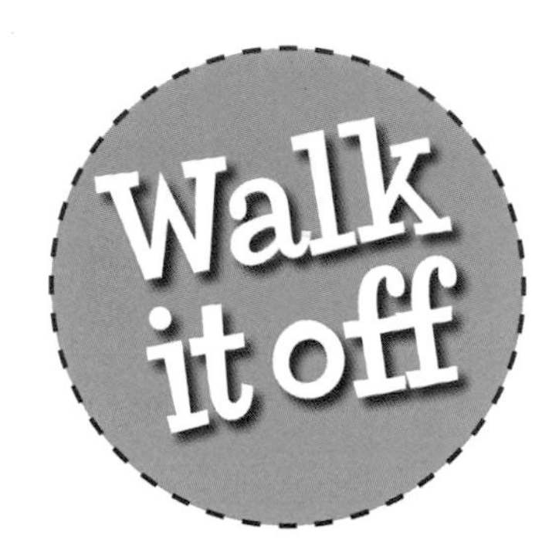

10,000 steps to a new you

The first step to getting fit? Start thinking of activity as an integral part of everyday life

"A vigorous five-mile walk will do more good for an unhappy but otherwise healthy adult than all the medicine and psychology in the world."

—Dr. Paul Dudley White, cardiologist

People who exercise know the tangible rewards. We're not talking about just health benefits, but things like this: You never miss a bus, since you can run a block to catch it. Shopping for clothes is actually enjoyable. You have more fun with your kids–bicycling, playing Wii or just roughhousing.

What Canadians need is a new way of quantifying activity. To keep from getting bigger, we need to start thinking smaller. Instead of measuring our exercise efforts in minutes and kilometres, we need to break it down to individual steps.

Canadian non-profit organization ParticipACTION recommends taking at least 10,000 steps a day. Studies have found that's the level at which you're burning enough calories to reduce the risk of obesity and chronic disease.

Despite those convincing factors, the 10,000-step rule still has yet to be widely adopted. It could be because most people don't wear pedometers, or because most of us have no clue what all those steps mean in everyday terms.

Here's a baseline to consider: People living completely sedentary lives take about 2,000 steps a day; non-exercisers, on a typical day, take closer to 4,000 steps. Anything below 5,000 daily steps should be counted as sedentary.

Spend a couple of days wearing a pedometer and your perspective on exercise will change dramatically. It will make you more conscious of being active; your concept of exercise will evolve from something you do for a specific time at a certain place (in the morning at the gym, in the afternoon on the tennis court) to something you do all day, everywhere.

Experts now believe that a shift in focus from "working out" to "being active" is the key to getting fit and staying trim for life. In fact, researchers at the University of South Carolina estimate that women who are active 75 percent of the day (run-

WALKING RULES

Runners often scoff at walking, saying it doesn't burn enough calories, but study after study shows that a regular walking program has just as beneficial an effect on your weight. And research proves that people are far more likely to stick with a walking rather than running regimen.

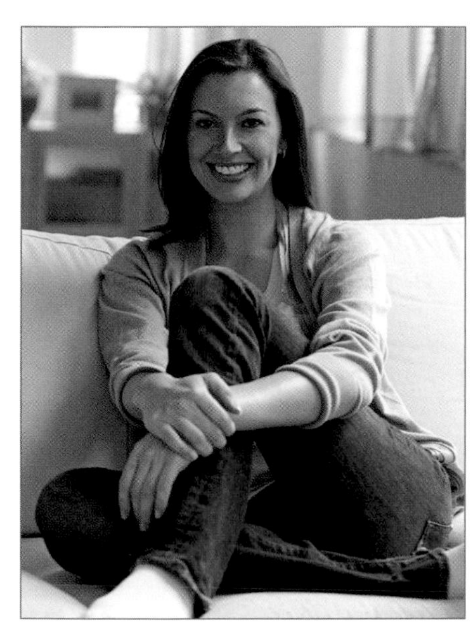

Regular activity will help you burn stress, so you feel that much more relaxed when you finally get a minute to yourself.

ning errands, gardening, cooking and so on) expend about 10 percent more energy overall than those who visit the gym for an hour but are sedentary the rest of the day (usually because they're sitting in front of a computer).

That's right: A day of housework can trump an hour on the treadmill.

Spread it around

Here's another way to look at it: Because we're so busy, most of us feel we need to put exercise in a box. Walking is something we do for a half hour before work or after lunch. It's kept separate from real life, as something that needs to be scheduled and worked around. Which means it will forever remain a chore or something easily bumped from our neverending to-do list.

To lose weight and keep it off for good, take exercise out of that box and spread it throughout your life. You can accomplish this by wiping the word "exercise" out of your vocabulary and replacing it with the word "activity." And you can do it by focusing on individual steps.

Buy a pedometer

Here's what you're going to do: Head to your local sporting-goods store and buy a pedometer (they're usually less than $20). Put it on first thing in the morning and check it before and after doing...well, anything. Before long, you'll become a pretty good judge of how many steps you take doing your normal day-to-day activities.

Now start to think about how to increase the number of steps you take in an ordinary day. One rule of thumb is to raise your activity level about 10 to 20 percent a week.

If you're emerging from a winter of hibernation, consider yourself sedentary (you might take about 3,000 daily steps), and add about 300 to 600 steps weekly. That'll not only keep you from straining yourself, but motivate you psychologically by conveying a sense of progress.

Note that it doesn't matter how long or short your strides are, or whether your daily steps are taken uphill or down, indoors or out. For simplicity's sake, a step is a step is a step. Note, too, that all the step counts in this section are estimates based on anecdotal rather than scientific evidence.

STEP-TASTIC EQUATIONS

The shopping workout

Park in the last row at the mall
+ use the far entrance
+ take the stairs, not escalators
+ shop for 3 hours
= **10,000 steps!**

The night-on-the-town workout

Don't valet park
+ mingle at a big cocktail party
+ dance the night away
= **10,000 steps!**

The stay-at-home-mom workout

Walk kids to bus stop
+ 1 hour grocery shopping
+ 2 hours of housework
+ pace while on phone with the kids' principal
+ walk kids home from bus stop
+ cook and serve dinner
= **10,000 steps!**

The spring-cleaning workout

Cut grass with push mower
+ wash and wax car
+ garden for 1 hour
= **10,000 steps!**

The desk-job workout

Park in last row of company lot
+ take the stairs
+ walk around the office every 90 minutes
+ take a 40-minute walk at lunch
= **10,000 steps!**

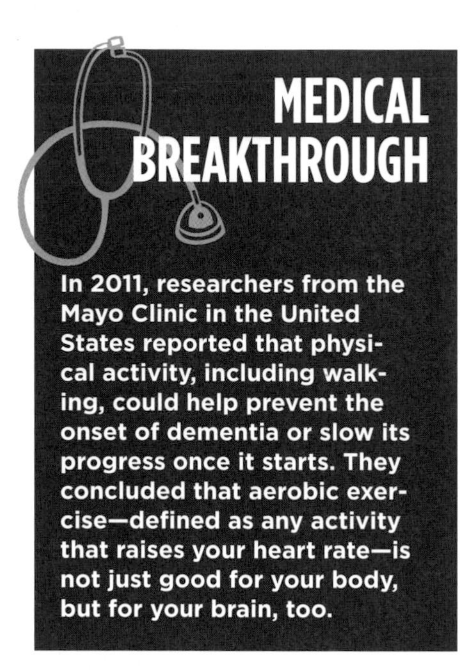

MEDICAL BREAKTHROUGH

In 2011, researchers from the Mayo Clinic in the United States reported that physical activity, including walking, could help prevent the onset of dementia or slow its progress once it starts. They concluded that aerobic exercise—defined as any activity that raises your heart rate—is not just good for your body, but for your brain, too.

Target: 10,000

To start, put on your pedometer first thing in the morning and don't take it off until bed. Note the number of steps you take every day. At the end of the week, calculate your daily average.

Once you have a good sense of how many steps you're taking (or not taking) every day, begin to look for easy ways to beef up your step numbers by 10 to 20 percent. Brainstorm how you can add more steps every day, when you're running errands, working or tidying up.

Once you've succeeded in increasing your steps by 20 percent, calculate the number it would take to increase by another 20 percent. Work your way up gradually, and never feel that you have to exhaust yourself. You'll soon find that 10,000 steps isn't such a huge number, after all! ■

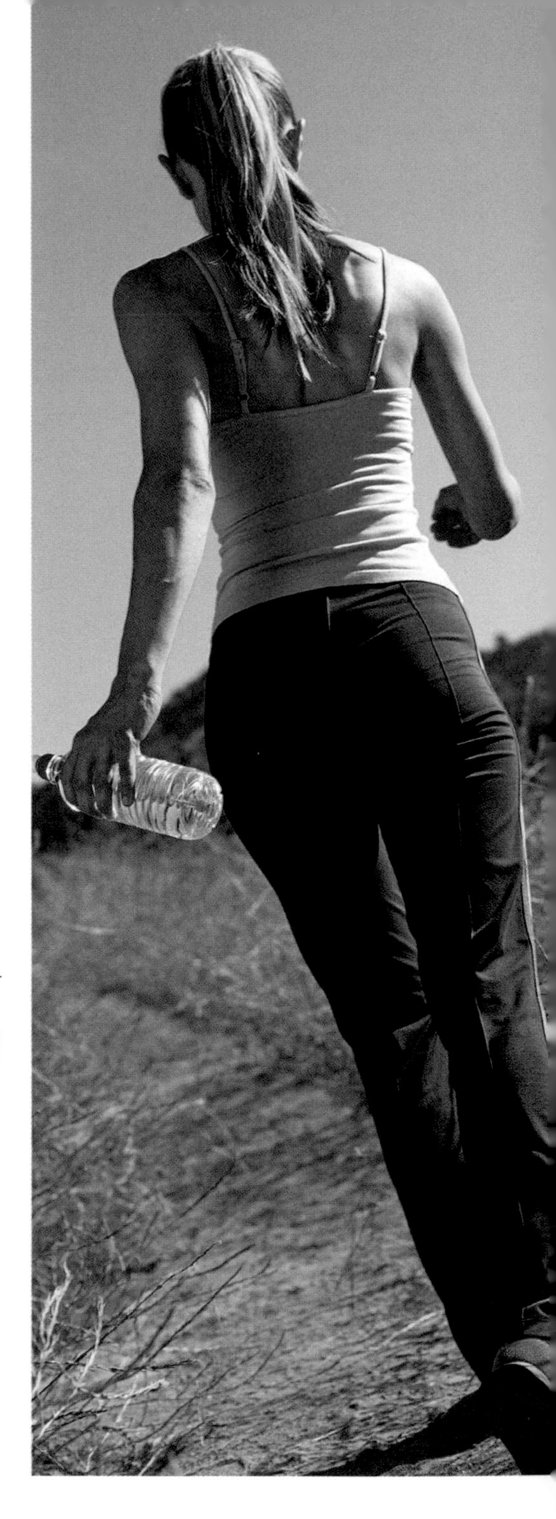

SWAP & DROP

SWAP THIS	FOR THAT
If your kids are old enough to get to the bus stop themselves, you may have been missing out on a useful early-morning stroll by letting them walk there alone.	Go along on their short walking commute at least a couple mornings a week. It'll feel good to start your day with some gentle exercise, and it's a great time to bond.
Shopping at the mall can be fun (especially when it's cold outside), but what you gain in convenience you lose in activity.	Shop downtown in the nearest city instead. You'll have to walk farther between the stores—good news if you want to lose weight.
Buying seasonal produce is the most eco-friendly and delicious way to stock up on food, but most grocery stores aren't very inspiring places to shop.	This weekend, pile the whole family in the car and head out to the closest pick-your-own apple orchard, berry farm or pumpkin patch. Nothing is more satisfying, and picking is great exercise.

Here are tons of options for reaching your own steps goal:

▼ 100-500 STEPS

- Park in the furthest row at work, the supermarket or the mall.
- After parking, take the scenic route. Use the mall or supermarket entrance farthest from your parking spot.
- Never use the drive-through at any restaurant or bank. Park and walk inside to do your business.
- Go out the back door instead of the front, and return the same way.
- Take the stairs throughout the day, rather than the escalator or elevator.
- Walk around the house for five minutes making a to-do list.
- Use the farthest bathroom from where you are sitting.

▼ 500-1,000 STEPS

- Walk the kids to a different bus stop. There's no rule that says you have to use the same one every morning.
- Pace around while you talk on the phone, making it a rule to never sit down—even during a long call.
- Cook and serve a homemade dinner to your family.
- Get up and walk down the hall so you can chat face-to-face with your coworkers, instead of emailing or phoning them.
- Spend 20 minutes tidying up around the house.
- Stroll around the house during every *Coronation Street* commercial break.
- Never use the moving walkways in airports—transport yourself.

▼ 1,000-2,500 STEPS

- Walk anywhere that takes less than five minutes to reach by car.
- Get up from your desk chair every 90 minutes during the course of an eight-hour day, and walk the full perimeter of your business or work area.
- Go for a leisurely 20-minute walk after dinner.
- Spend 15 minutes vacuuming up all the cat hair.
- Do light housework for an hour.
- Spend an hour gardening.
- Wash and wax the car.
- Do an hour of vigorous yoga.
- Stay on your feet and mingle at a cocktail party, instead of spending the whole night hovering around the cheese plate.

▼ 2,500-5,000 STEPS

- Go to the mall, forget where you parked your car and spend half an hour looking for it.
- Take a leisurely 40-minute walk during your lunch hour.
- Grocery-shop for one hour.
- Go for a leisurely one-hour bike ride in a local park (pedal strokes count as steps, too).
- Prepare food for, host and clean up after a dinner party.
- Walk 30 minutes on a treadmill set at about 6 km/h.
- Spend a few hours walking around a local museum.
- Go bowling.

▼ 5,000-7,500 STEPS

- Cut a large lawn with a push mower instead of a ride-on.
- Spend an afternoon raking up all the leaves you didn't deal with last fall.
- Walk a 5k charity event.
- Spend an afternoon walking around the downtown of a large city.
- Dance the night away.

▼ 7,500-10,000 STEPS

- Stroll back and forth to church (or temple, etc.) once a week.
- Go golfing using a pull cart.
- Volunteer at a hospital for 8 hours.
- Take the dog for a brisk 60-minute walk in the park.
- Get a part-time job as a waitress.

▼ 10,000+ STEPS

- Walk 10 km.
- Spend the day shopping in downtown Toronto or Montreal.
- Walk 90 minutes at a leisurely pace.
- Babysit a four year old for 8 hours.

> Walking lowers high blood pressure and improves cholesterol ratios.

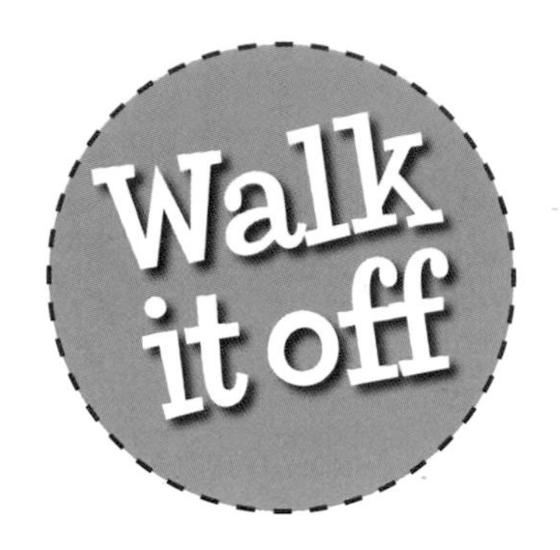

Get started on your journey

Calculate your fitness level, stretch your muscles and relearn how to walk—the right way

Starting a new activity can be intimidating. Luckily, walking is just about the most user-friendly activity there is. Follow our guide, and you'll discover that exercise is easier (and safer) than you might have thought. If you're careful not to strain yourself, you'll quickly make strides–in more ways than one!

"Small and steady victories, with minimal sacrifice and suffering, are the best way to create lasting change in your weight, your health and your life."

— *Dr. Susan Biali, MD*

STRETCH AFTER EVERY WALK

Your muscles are at their most flexible and pliable after your workout, making your stretching more effective. After any activity designed to boost your heart rate, spend about 5 to 10 minutes cooling down and bringing your heart rate back to normal. Then do the full sequence of stretches outlined on page 232.

If the last exercise you remember doing was in high-school gym class, ease into walking gradually, starting with 15 minutes at a time and working up to 20- and 30-minute walks. Pay attention to your heart rate and stop if you feel discomfort anywhere in your body. It takes almost no time for your body to adapt to walking–which, if you're able-bodied, it naturally knows how to do–and you will be comfortable handling 30-, 45- and even 60-minute walks before you know it.

At first, though, focus on shorter walks that will allow you to become familiar with how your body feels when you walk at varying paces. Pay attention, too, to the way you carry your body when you walk. It's important to walk correctly, with good posture, balanced movement and a clean gait, in order to get the most bang for your exercise buck–and, of course, to help avoid injury. (See page 215 for more tips.)

Tracking your heart rate

To track your heart rate during your walks, invest in a heart-rate monitor. Good brands start at about $60. With many models, you can input your age as well as your resting and maximum heart rates so the device automatically calculates your heart-rate status. (To calculate your resting heart rate, check your pulse when you first wake up. Count the number of heartbeats in 30 seconds, then multiply by 2.)

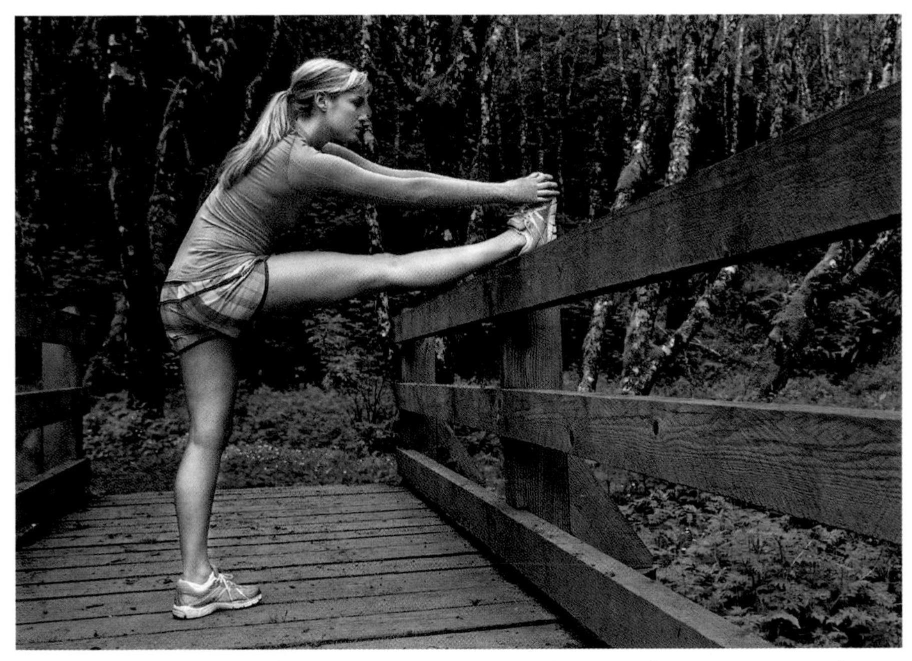

Don't have a heart-rate monitor? You can still track your heart rate. All you need is a watch with a second hand. Simply place the tips of your first two fingers on your inner wrist, or on your lower neck on either side of your windpipe. Press lightly until you feel your pulse. Count the number of pulses over 6 seconds, then multiply that number by 10 to get a rough estimate of your heart rate.

If you don't want to bother with a monitor or taking your pulse, see below for a sense of how hard you'll need to work to get your heart rate into the various target zones.

Guesstimate

- **50% to 60% of your max:** Brisk walking. You can carry a conversation, though you might breathe a little hard.
- **60% to 70% of your max:** Very fast walking. You can speak only in short sentences.
- **70% to 80% of your max:** Walking as fast as you can. You can utter only a few words because you're breathing hard.
- **80% to 85% of your max:** Walking as fast as you can up a big hill, pumping your arms aggressively. Speaking is nearly impossible.

The 5 biggest walking missteps

We know what you're thinking: How can anyone screw up walking? That's like botching breathing or sleeping. Well, it's actually more common than you might think. Many new walkers get bored, discouraged or injured, or just don't have as much fun as they should, because they're unwittingly doing some things wrong.

LEARNING TO REALLY WARM UP

A warm-up should not consist of heavy or strenuous stretching—this could actually tire out your muscles and cause injury. Save the serious stretching for your cool-down—see page 232 for stretches.

Five minutes of strolling or gentle stretching is all you need to increase the temperature and blood flow in your muscles. Try these:

Toe points. Standing, lift one foot off the floor, point your toes and hold for 5 seconds. Now flex the same foot and hold for 5 seconds. Do this 5 times for each foot.

Quad stretch. Standing, bend one leg at the knee and reach behind you to grasp your foot or ankle. Gently pull your foot to stretch the front of the thigh, holding for up to 10 seconds. Repeat same steps on the other side.

Overhead stretch. Standing with feet hip-width apart, reach your hands up over your head, palms facing forward with your arms forming a V. Gently move your hands back, as if someone is pushing against them, and hold for up to 10 seconds.

Next, bend one elbow and drop your hand to touch your back, holding for 5 seconds. Relax the first arm and repeat with the other.

WHAT'S YOUR MAX?

To calculate your maximum heart rate, simply subtract your age from 220.

220 - _____ = _____

your age in years — your maximum heart rate

If you're 40 years old, for example, your maximum heart rate is 180 beats per minute. If you want to work out at 50 percent of your maximum, multiply it by 0.5.

Walk It Off PLAYLIST

- **Crazy in Love**
  Beyoncé
- **Run To You**
  Bryan Adams
- **Forget You**
  Cee Lo Green
- **Knock You Down**
  Keri Hilson featuring Kanye West and Ne-Yo
- **Kiss (Extended Version)**
  Prince
- **Fallin'**
  Alicia Keys
- **You Oughta Know**
  Alanis Morissette
- **You Know I'm No Good**
  Amy Winehouse featuring Ghostface Killah
- **Give It To Me**
  Timbaland featuring Nelly Furtado and Justin Timberlake
- **I Feel Good**
  James Brown

Here are five frequent mistakes that could be hurting you or holding you back.

• **Wearing worn-out shoes**
The cushioning properties of even the best sports shoes break down with use. This can lead to discomfort and eventually injury, especially if you're overweight. There's no mystery to knowing when it's time for a new shoe; if you see worn areas on the soles, it's time to get yourself a new pair. To get the best fit, shop in the afternoon when your feet are biggest, wear the socks you'll be walking in, make sure there's a little space between your big toe and the end of the shoe, and walk around the store to be sure the heel doesn't slip.

• **Walking without warming up**
Most people don't think of walking as a strenuous activity, but if you spend most of your day sitting at a desk, then you're asking your body to spring out of the blocks. Before you start, you need to elevate your core body temperature, get the blood and oxygen flowing to the muscles, and lubricate your joints. Take 3 minutes to do slow ankle, hip and arm circles (not all at once!) and you'll be ready to roll.

• **Using poor technique**
Overstriding, foot-slapping, head-hanging, chicken-winging–these are just a few of the common flaws that can lead to injury. Remember to square up your posture, swing your arms bent at 90 degrees close to your body, push off evenly (heel to midfoot to toes) with every step and maintain an even stride, no matter how fast or slow you're walking.

• **Not stretching afterward**
Most new walkers forgo cool-downs. But just as muscles and tendons need to ease into an activity, they also need to ease out. Otherwise, they can get tight and cramp. The older you get, the more important it is to stretch after being active.

Take 3 minutes to do slow standing lunges. Gently bend at the waist with slightly flexed knees and stretch your bent arms overhead, as if you're scratching the top of your back.

• **Not setting specific goals**
As with everything else in life, if your goals aren't clear, realistic and measurable, it's unlikely you'll reach them. Measure your success in steps. Use a pedometer all day, every day. Find ways to add 10 to 20 percent more steps each week until you reach 10,000 steps a day. Your body will continue to reset itself to its increased capacity and you'll actually crave the benefits this amount of movement provides.

Three walks to get the ball rolling

Don't worry: No one expects you to walk out the door and make it to the top of Mt. Kilimanjaro and back on your first walk. Take it slowly if that works for you.

In fact, no matter how enthusiastic you're feeling about starting your walking program, if you haven't exercised for a long time, you will still need to ease into walking with short 15-, 20- and eventually 25-minute walks that will help your body acclimate to the activity. Luckily, it's easy to squeeze walking into a busy work schedule–just spread your activity throughout the day.

Turn the page for three simple walking programs to get you started on the walking-for-weight-loss journey. ■

SNEAK IN MORE STEPS

You can put on your gym clothes, sneakers and pedometer and put in an hour of vigorous walking–or you can just amble along on a sunny morning alive with birdsong. Do a lap around the mall before hitting the clearance sales–or hoof it to the neighbourhood mailbox, instead of dropping off letters while you run errands in the car. Opportunities to walk are endless, and by now you know that the activity math is stunningly simple: The more steps you take, the more calories you'll burn. Here are some ways to sneak more walking into your life and get the most out of every step you take.

Pick a charity and pledge to yourself to contribute $1 for every kilometre you walk

You'll take pride in the fact that you're walking for a larger cause–and who knows, maybe it will motivate you to go longer and faster. After every walk, mark the amount you owe on a chart. When you reach $100, send in a cheque. Whoever thought exercise could be tax-deductible?

Take the dog with you

Once Fido gets used to your walks, he'll look forward to them and give you a gentle nudge on the days you try to skip. Don't have a dog? Offer to walk a neighbour's, or inquire about walking dogs at a local shelter.

Walk for fun once a week

Instead of strolling around your neighbourhood, hit the zoo, an art museum or an upscale shopping mall.

Take the crew for a walk

This is a perfect way to model good fitness habits for your children. If your children walk slowly, ask them to ride their bikes or rollerblade alongside.

Once a week, do your errands on foot

If you live within a couple kilometres of town or even a convenience store, start from your house. If you live out in the middle of nowhere, drive to within a kilometre of your destination, park and walk the rest of the way there and back. You'll be surprised how many people you'll meet along the way.

Explore near and far

Rather than walking the same old tired route day in and day out, use your walks as a way to experience your surroundings. Check out the houses one neighbourhood over, walk to a town landmark that you've never been inside, or drive to a park or trailhead to take in the great outdoors.

Burn calories at the kid's soccer field

Instead of taking your folding chair and a crossword puzzle, wear comfortable shoes and take a jaunt around the field.

Walk and talk

Use your cellphone or cordless and walk around the house as you chat with friends or conduct business. This is a great way to make use of those long times spent on hold with the bank or internet-service provider. The exercise will also help you maintain your cool when you've been waiting for 45 minutes!

Walk with a friend

If someone is expecting you, you're more likely to get out of bed than you would if no one was holding you accountable. At work, look for colleagues to walk with during lunch break.

Climb up and down a flight of stairs for 2 minutes

You'll get your heart rate up in a hurry and build thigh and calf muscles that will propel you faster on your walks.

Park in Siberia

Don't fight the hordes for a space near the mall entrance. Instead, park at the perimeter of the lot. You'll save yourself stress and get more steps in, to boot.

Walk in the evening

After-dinner walks get you away from the television (and the snacks you munch in front of it), keep you from eating too much at dinner and give you a chance to bump into like-minded neighbours.

A 12-week walking plan

This program focuses on two key goals: building endurance and burning fat.

You'll build up to working out at 85 percent of your maximum heart rate for a few minutes at a time. Boosting your heart rate requires incorporating bursts of faster walking, hilly terrain and aggressive arm pumping, which in turn will help you burn more fat. Introduce variety to your routine and build endurance.

WEEK ▶ ONE

DAY 1
5 minutes at 50% maximum heart rate (HR)
20 minutes at 60% maximum HR
10 minutes at 50% maximum HR
Total: 35 min

DAY 2
5 minutes at 50% maximum HR
Repeat this sequence 5 times:
1 minute at 60% maximum HR;
1 minute at 70% maximum HR
10 minutes at 50% maximum HR
Total: 25 min

DAY 3
5 minutes at 50% maximum HR
20 minutes at 60% maximum HR
10 minutes at 50% maximum HR
Total: 35 min

DAY 4
5 minutes at 50% maximum HR
Repeat this sequence 5 times:
1 minute at 60% maximum HR;
1 minute at 70% maximum HR
10 minutes at 50% maximum HR
Total: 25 min

DAY 5
5 minutes at 50% maximum HR
30 minutes at 60% maximum HR
10 minutes at 50% maximum HR
Total: 45 min

WEEK ▶ TWO

DAY 1
5 minutes at 50% maximum heart rate (HR)
10 minutes at 60% maximum HR
5 minutes at 70% maximum HR
10 minutes at 60% maximum HR
10 minutes at 50% maximum HR
Total: 40 min

DAY 2
5 minutes at 50% maximum HR
Repeat this sequence 5 times:
1 minute at 60% maximum HR;
1 minute at 70% maximum HR;
1 minute at 80% maximum HR
10 minutes at 50% maximum HR
Total: 30 min

DAY 3
5 minutes at 50% maximum HR
10 minutes at 60% maximum HR
5 minutes at 70% maximum HR
10 minutes at 60% maximum HR
10 minutes at 50% maximum HR
Total: 40 min

DAY 4
5 minutes at 50% maximum HR
Repeat this sequence 5 times:
1 minute at 60% maximum HR;
1 minute at 70% maximum HR;
1 minute at 80% maximum HR
10 minutes at 50% maximum HR
Total: 30 min

DAY 5
5 minutes at 50% maximum HR
35 minutes at 60% maximum HR
10 minutes at 50% maximum HR
Total: 50 min

WEEK ▶ THREE

DAY 1
5 minutes at 50% maximum heart rate (HR)
5 minutes at 60% maximum HR
10 minutes at 70% maximum HR
5 minutes at 60% maximum HR
10 minutes at 50% maximum HR
Total: 35 min

DAY 2
5 minutes at 50% maximum HR
Repeat this sequence 5 times:
1 minute at 60% maximum HR;
1 minute at 80% maximum HR
10 minutes at 50% maximum HR
Total: 25 min

DAY 3
5 minutes at 50% maximum HR
5 minutes at 60% maximum HR
10 minutes at 70% maximum HR
5 minutes at 60% maximum HR
10 minutes at 50% maximum HR
Total: 35 min

DAY 4
5 minutes at 50% maximum HR
Repeat this sequence 5 times:
1 minute at 60% maximum HR;
1 minute at 80% maximum HR
10 minutes at 50% maximum HR
Total: 25 min

DAY 5
5 minutes at 50% maximum HR
30 minutes at 60% maximum HR
10 minutes at 50% maximum HR
Total: 45 min

WEEK ▶ FOUR

DAY 1
5 minutes at 50% maximum heart rate (HR)
5 minutes at 60% maximum HR
15 minutes at 70% maximum HR
5 minutes at 60% maximum HR
10 minutes at 50% maximum HR
Total: 40 min

DAY 2
5 minutes at 50% maximum HR
Repeat this sequence 5 times:
1 minute at 60% maximum HR;
2 minutes at 80% maximum HR
10 minutes at 50% maximum HR
Total: 30 min

DAY 3
5 minutes at 50% maximum HR
5 minutes at 60% maximum HR
15 minutes at 70% maximum HR
5 minutes at 60% maximum HR
10 minutes at 50% maximum HR
Total: 40 min

DAY 4
5 minutes at 50% maximum HR
Repeat this sequence 7 times:
1 minute at 60% maximum HR;
2 minutes at 80% maximum HR
9 minutes at 50% maximum HR
Total: 35 min

DAY 5
5 minutes at 50% maximum HR
45 minutes at 60% maximum HR
10 minutes at 50% maximum HR
Total: 60 min

6 Tips for walking in hot weather

- If you're planning a long walk, try to do it early in the morning or later at night. Avoid the hottest part of the day and you'll save yourself from overheating.
- Remember to wear sunscreen. You should be doing this every day anyway, but it's extra important if you're going to spend an extended period outside. That goes for people with darker skintones, too.
- Always bring water. Better yet, try this trick: Freeze a half-full water bottle overnight and bring it out on your walk. It'll melt as you go, providing you with a cool, refreshing drink even on the hottest days.
- Stroll in the shade whenever possible. That could mean walking on the less sunny side of the street, or below the trees at your local park.
- Dress for the weather. That means light-coloured, natural or sweat-wicking fabrics, thinner socks and breathable shoes—preferably runners with mesh on the sides. Ask an employee at a sporting-goods store to help you find appropriate summer workout clothes.
- Take it easy, especially right at the beginning of the season. If you start to feel faint or dehydrated, relax in the shade.

Walking in suburbia

A 2009 study from Queen's University found that 70 percent of Canadians had walked for exercise over the last few months. However, only 30 percent said they walked regularly—a number that had stayed the same for almost a decade.

This could be because of our harsh winters, but it could also be a side effect of suburban sprawl. Canadian suburbs are still growing faster than cities, and they're great for a lot of reasons, but not for walking—when the grocery store is a 30-minute walk away but only a few minutes by car, it's hard to want to hoof it.

If your neighbourhood isn't conducive to running errands on foot, schedule time to get out to a nearby park and go for a stroll. When you drive somewhere, park a little further away than necessary. Get creative, and you too will be hitting the 10,000-steps-a-day mark before you know it—no matter where you live.

WEEK ▶ FIVE

DAY 1

5 minutes at 50% maximum heart rate (HR)
5 minutes at 60% maximum HR
20 minutes at 70% maximum HR
5 minutes at 60% maximum HR
5 minutes at 50% maximum HR
Total: 40 min

DAY 2

5 minutes at 50% maximum HR
Repeat this sequence 6 times:
 1 minute at 60% maximum HR;
 2 minutes at 80% maximum HR;
 1 minute at 85% maximum HR
11 minutes at 50% maximum HR
Total: 40 min

DAY 3

5 minutes at 50% maximum HR
5 minutes at 60% maximum HR
20 minutes at 70% maximum HR
5 minutes at 60% maximum HR
10 minutes at 50% maximum HR
Total: 45 min

DAY 4

5 minutes at 50% maximum HR
Repeat this sequence 6 times:
 1 minute at 60% maximum HR;
 2 minutes at 80% maximum HR;
 1 minute at 85% maximum HR
11 minutes at 50% maximum HR
Total: 40 min

DAY 5

5 minutes at 50% maximum HR
40 minutes at 65% maximum HR
10 minutes at 50% maximum HR
Total: 55 min

WEEK ▶ SIX

DAY 1

5 minutes at 50% maximum heart rate (HR)
5 minutes at 60% maximum HR
25 minutes at 70% maximum HR
5 minutes at 60% maximum HR
5 minutes at 50% maximum HR
Total: 45 min

DAY 2

5 minutes at 50% maximum HR
Repeat this sequence 7 times:
 1 minute at 65% maximum HR;
 2 minutes at 80% maximum HR
9 minutes at 50% maximum HR
Total: 35 min

DAY 3

5 minutes at 50% maximum HR
5 minutes at 60% maximum HR
25 minutes at 70% maximum HR
10 minutes at 50% maximum HR
Total: 45 min

DAY 4

5 minutes at 50% maximum HR
Repeat this sequence 7 times:
 1 minute at 65% maximum HR;
 2 minutes at 80% maximum HR
9 minutes at 50% maximum HR
Total: 35 min

DAY 5

5 minutes at 50% maximum HR
45 minutes at 65% maximum HR
10 minutes at 50% maximum HR
Total: 60 min

WEEK ▶ SEVEN

DAY 1

5 minutes at 50% maximum heart rate (HR)
5 minutes at 60% maximum HR
30 minutes at 70% maximum HR
5 minutes at 60% maximum HR
5 minutes at 50% maximum HR
Total: 50 min

DAY 2

5 minutes at 50% maximum HR
Repeat this sequence 6 times:
1 minute at 65% maximum HR;
2 minutes at 80% maximum HR;
1 minute at 85% maximum HR
11 minutes at 50% maximum HR
Total: 40 min

DAY 3

5 minutes at 50% maximum HR
5 minutes at 60% maximum HR
30 minutes at 70% maximum HR
5 minutes at 60% maximum HR
5 minutes at 50% maximum HR
Total: 50 min

DAY 4

5 minutes at 50% maximum HR
Repeat this sequence 6 times:
1 minute at 65% maximum HR;
2 minutes at 80% maximum HR;
1 minute at 85% maximum HR
11 minutes at 50% maximum HR
Total: 40 min

DAY 5

5 minutes at 50% maximum HR
50 minutes at 65% maximum HR
10 minutes at 50% maximum HR
Total: 65 min

WEEK ▶ EIGHT

DAY 1

5 minutes at 50% maximum heart rate (HR)
5 minutes at 60% maximum HR
15 minutes at 70% maximum HR
5 minutes at 80% maximum HR
15 minutes at 70% maximum HR
5 minutes at 60% maximum HR
5 minutes at 50% maximum HR
Total: 55 min

DAY 2

5 minutes at 50% maximum HR
Repeat this sequence 7 times:
1 minute at 65% maximum HR;
3 minutes at 80% maximum HR
12 minutes at 50% maximum HR
Total: 45 min

DAY 3

5 minutes at 50% maximum HR
5 minutes at 60% maximum HR
15 minutes at 70% maximum HR
5 minutes at 80% maximum HR
15 minutes at 70% maximum HR
5 minutes at 60% maximum HR
5 minutes at 50% maximum HR
Total: 55 min

DAY 4

5 minutes at 50% maximum HR
Repeat this sequence 7 times:
1 minute at 65% maximum HR;
3 minutes at 80% maximum HR
12 minutes at 50% maximum HR
Total: 45 min

DAY 5

5 minutes at 50% maximum HR
55 minutes at 65% maximum HR
10 minutes at 50% maximum HR
Total: 70 min

WEEK ▶ NINE-TWELVE

Repeat routine for week 8

To make your walks more challenging, try the three interval workouts on page 231.

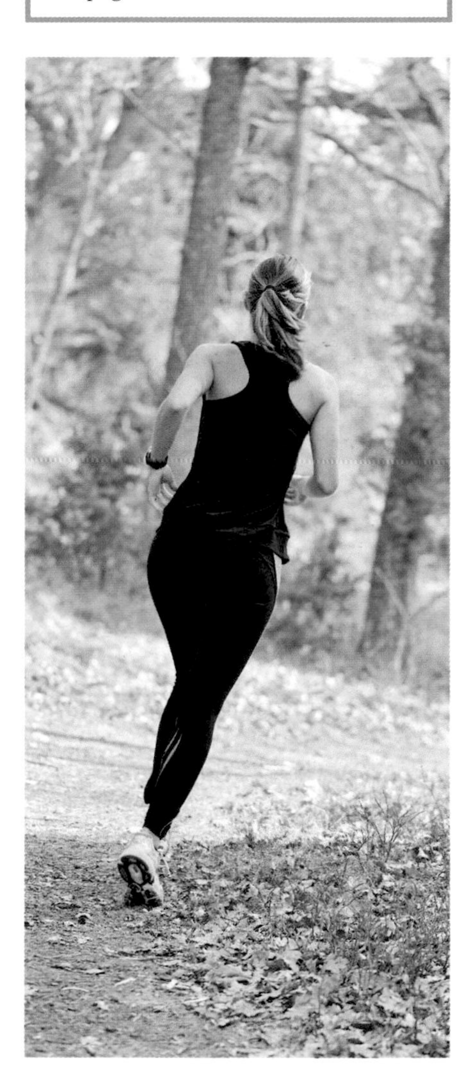

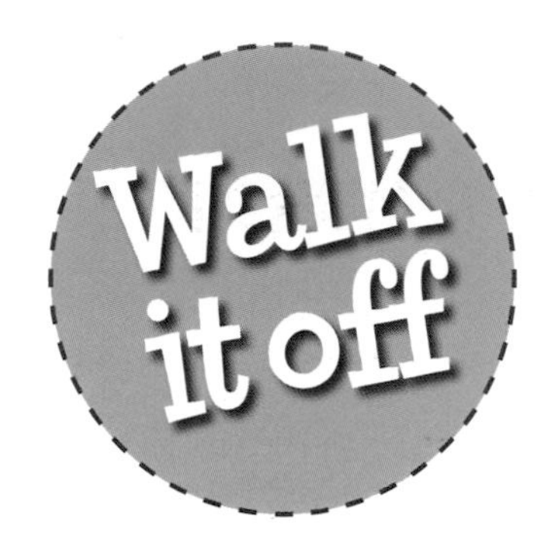

Step it up

You've started walking regularly, and you're feeling great. Now it's time to take things to the next level

"Strength does not come from physical capacity. It comes from an indomitable will."
— *Mahatma Gandhi*

It doesn't take long to fall in love with the benefits of walking: the energy it gives you, the way it buoys your mood and the feeling you get from becoming fitter with every step. But if you're walking to lose weight, chances are you'd like to see those pounds come off faster.

Most people quickly drop some weight when they start a new walking program. But after a few months, weight loss tends to slow down, and it's not unusual to hit a sticking point. Often this weight-loss plateau is a symptom of success: As you get fit, your body becomes more efficient at walking, allowing you to walk farther with less effort. All it means is that you need to step up your routine.

Cutting calories from your diet and hitting the weight room to build metabolism-boosting muscle are two surefire ways to speed your progress. But nothing will help more than interval training: incorporating short bursts of harder effort into your regular workout.

The concept is simple: The harder you walk, the more calories you burn. Now, you certainly don't want to go all-out over your entire walk. But you can still reap the weight-loss benefits of high-intensity workouts by throwing in brief bouts of faster walking. You'll speed your weight loss without adding a single extra minute to your time on the pavement.

To shed the most fat, you should walk at an intensity of at least 3 METs–meaning you're moving quickly enough to meaningfully raise your heart rate, increase your body's need for oxygen and combust calories. 1 MET, or Metabolic Equivalent of Task, equals burning 1 calorie per kilogram of body weight per hour (if you weigh 180 pounds, that's 81 kilograms, or 81 calories per hour).

Just how fast do you need to walk to reach 3 METS? Researchers at San Diego State University set out to answer that. They asked 97 men and women to walk on treadmills as they measured their METs and counted their steps. In the end, they found that the magic number is 100 steps per minute (spm). That's the minimum you need for calorie-burning aerobic benefit. To lose fat faster, you will need to step quicker.

Taking quicker steps isn't usually what people try to do when they want to get more from their walking workouts. Without thinking about it, many people try taking longer strides instead, which actually slows them down. Aim for more, faster steps, not longer ones.

If you really want to see your walking program pay off, you'll need to eat smart, too. So while the occasional "reward treat" is fine, stick to the **Swap & Drop** diet. Now let's get down to some walking.

Quick-step weight loss

To get the most benefit from your roadwork, use the 100 spm mark as a baseline, then add bursts of faster stepping to rev up your results. Research shows that interval training regularly yields significantly faster weight loss than one-speed workouts do.

Most remarkably, a study from the University of South Wales found that women who exercised for 20 minutes three days per week, alternating fast- and moderate-paced intervals, lost five times more weight (up to 18 pounds in 15 weeks, without changing their diet) than those who exercised at a steady, brisk speed for twice that amount of time. As if that isn't exciting enough, the interval exercisers sliced most of their fat from stubborn spots such as the legs and belly.

To get yourself moving more quickly, steal some tips from racewalkers–athletes who speedwalk competitively. If you watch a racewalker, you'll notice she keeps her body angles sharp: The elbows are bent at 90 degrees, as is the knee of the front leg until it makes contact with the ground. These angles are aerodynamic, helping to propel the racewalker forward. As she walks, her bent elbows shorten the pendulum action of her swinging arms, enabling her arms to swing more quickly and drive her body forward. At the same time, she's pushing purposefully off her rear toes, which helps to drive her knee forward.

These two simple actions–bending the elbows and explosively pushing off with the back foot–combine to push your body forward faster. Before you begin to integrate interval programs into your walks, practice this technique for short distances–no more than 30 seconds or so,

COUNTING OUT YOUR SPM

Calculating your steps-per-minute (spm) is easy—just count 'em out! For the best results, warm up for a few minutes. Then, using your watch, count how many steps you take in one minute. (You can also count your steps for 20 seconds and multiply by 3.)

Repeat three times and take the average. If your number is below 100, pick up the pace and repeat the test until you're in the 100–115 spm range. Every time you begin walking, count your steps again until that faster pace becomes second nature.

Repeat this process with faster step counts in order to feel what it's like to walk 115–130 spm and 130–145 spm.

SWAP & DROP

SWAP THIS	FOR THAT
Having coffee with a friend is fun, but it also involves a lot of, well, sitting. And why tempt yourself with those sweet café desserts when you could be out and about?	Make a plan to go for a walk in a nearby park instead. The fresh air and natural setting will clear your head, making for great conversation.
Buying all your food at the supermarket is convenient, but by shopping at only one place, you also miss out on a useful walking activity.	Do your shopping at a farmers' market, where you have to go to different stalls for vegetables, meat and cheese. It'll repay you in both food quality and added steps.
Relaxing with a movie in the evening can feel like a treat after a long day. But how does it help you in the long run?	Propose to your partner that you take a leisurely after-dinner walk instead. It's a romantic, active way to end the day.

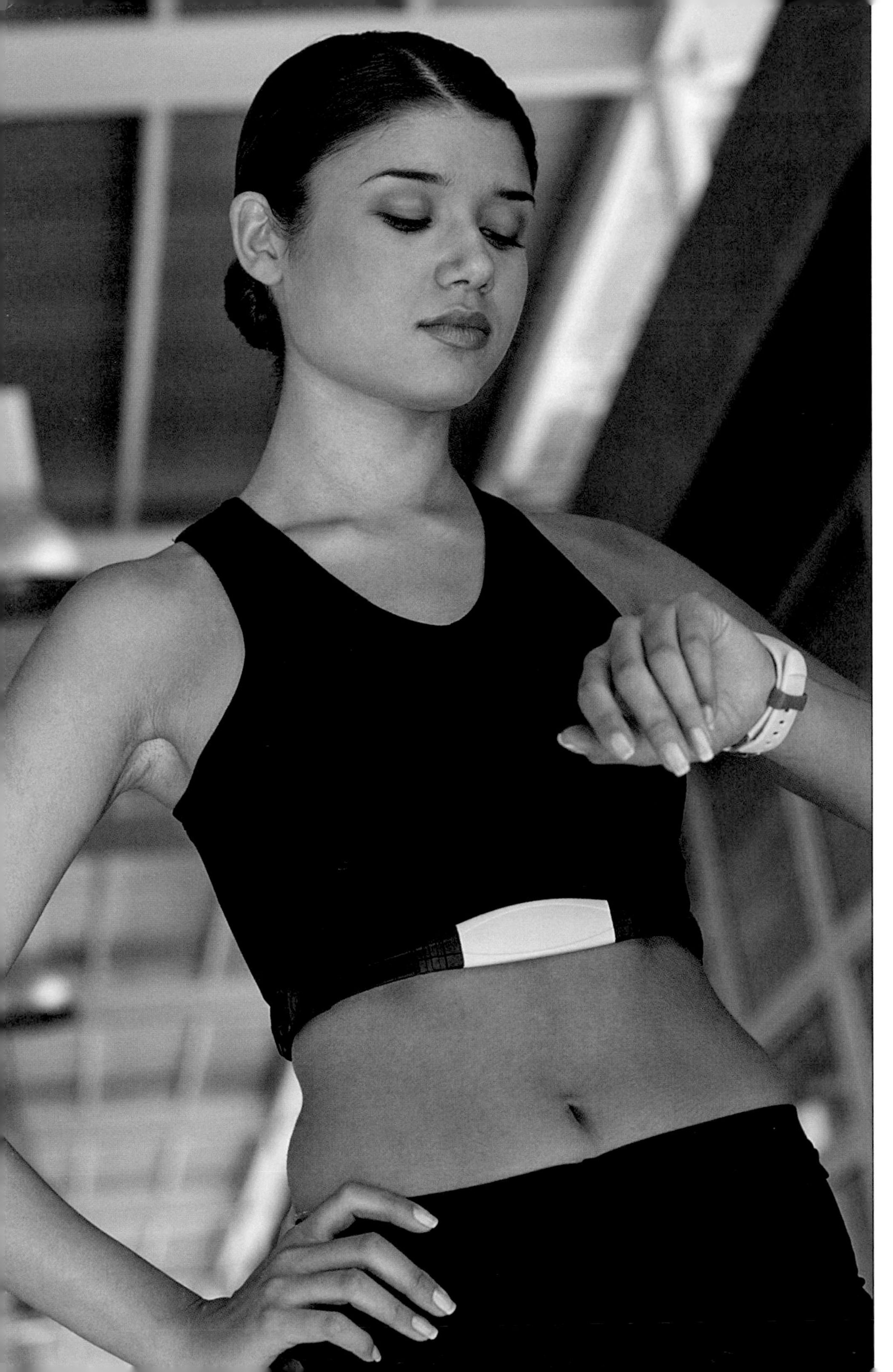

with a minimum of two minutes of regular walking in between.

Keep your neck, shoulders and hands relaxed, not tense or clenched. Swing your arms loosely but vigorously, and keep your hands and elbows close to your body. Lead with your heel, then roll right through to push off with your toes.

Notice the difference between your ordinary pace and what happens when you make like a racewalker. It may feel awkward at first, but practice it until the movement feels smooth and natural. And now you're ready to start the interval workout plan.

The plan

These three interval workouts are based on three different paces:

- *Base Pace:* 100-115 spm (about 4.5-5 km/h)
- *Burn Pace:* 115-130 spm (about 5-6 km/h)
- *Power Pace:* 130-145 spm (about 6-7 km/h)

Do the interval workouts three days a week (a different workout each day), preferably on non-consecutive days so your body can rest and recover in between. On alternate days, walk at Base to Burn Pace for 30 to 60 minutes.

Take one day off a week to relax. If you're walking on a treadmill, feel free to measure yourself using km/h instead of spm. Now get out there and work it! ■

INTERVAL WORKOUT ▸ ONE

DOUBLE DOWNS

These high-energy intervals are hard (but not exhausting), so you fry lots of fat, strengthen your heart and boost overall fitness while still reserving energy for all your other daily duties. You'll do 4 minutes at Burn Pace (aiming for the high end of the range), followed by 2 minutes at Base Pace. After 5 weeks, increase the amount of time at Burn Pace to 6 minutes and recover for 3 minutes at Base Pace. Use a stopwatch–the times below indicate when you should start each stage. Here is a sample 40-minute workout:

Start	Warm up, working to Base Pace
0:00	Burn Pace
4:00	Base Pace
6:00	Cycle through Burn to Base Pace four more times
30:00	Cool down, from the top to the low range of Base Pace
40:00	Finish

INTERVAL WORKOUT ▸ TWO

30-SECOND SURGES

During these bursts, you'll be walking as fast as your feet will carry you–that's pushing for Power Pace, 130 spm or higher if you can–for 30 seconds, followed by 1 minute of recovery at Base Pace. These intervals burn tons of calories while improving your capacity for hard exercise. That means you'll soon be walking faster and burning more calories even on your easy days, which will help put your weight loss on fast-forward. The times below indicate when you should start each stage. Here is a sample 43-minute workout:

Start	Warm up, working to Base Pace
0:00	Burn Pace
4:00	Power Pace
4:30	Base Pace
5:30	Repeat minutes 4:00 through 5:30 nine times
19:00	Burn pace
25:00	Repeat minutes 4:00 through 5:30 ten times
40:00	Cool down, from the top to the low range of Base Pace
43:00	Finish

INTERVAL WORKOUT ▸ THREE

HOT & COOL

Because you have plenty of recovery time in between, you can really push hard on these intervals to help boost your lactate threshold–science-speak for how long you can last before you need to slow down. Start by pushing for 1 minute at Power Pace followed by one minute at Base Pace. After 3 weeks increase the time at Power Pace to 2 minutes, with equal time for recovery at Base Pace. Three weeks later go for 3-minute Hot & Cool intervals. The times below indicate when you should start each stage. Here is a sample 40-minute workout:

Start	Warm up, working to Base Pace
5:00	Burn Pace
10:00	Power Pace
11:00	Base Pace
12:00	Repeat minutes 10 through 12 eleven times
34:00	Burn Pace
35:00	Cool down, from the top to the low range of Base Pace
40:00	Finish

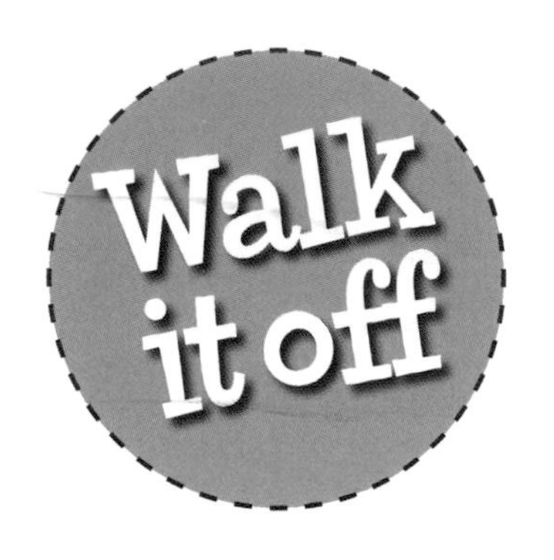

Aim to be flexible

Do this stretching routine after your workout, and you'll still feel loose tomorrow

"It's human nature to want a quick fix with no effort, but it will never get you where you really want to go."

— Dr. Susan Biali, MD

Smart stretching is great for walkers: It leaves you feeling loose, relaxed and stress-free. This routine is best done after walking to keep your body from tightening up again. Hold each stretch for 30 to 60 seconds unless otherwise indicated.

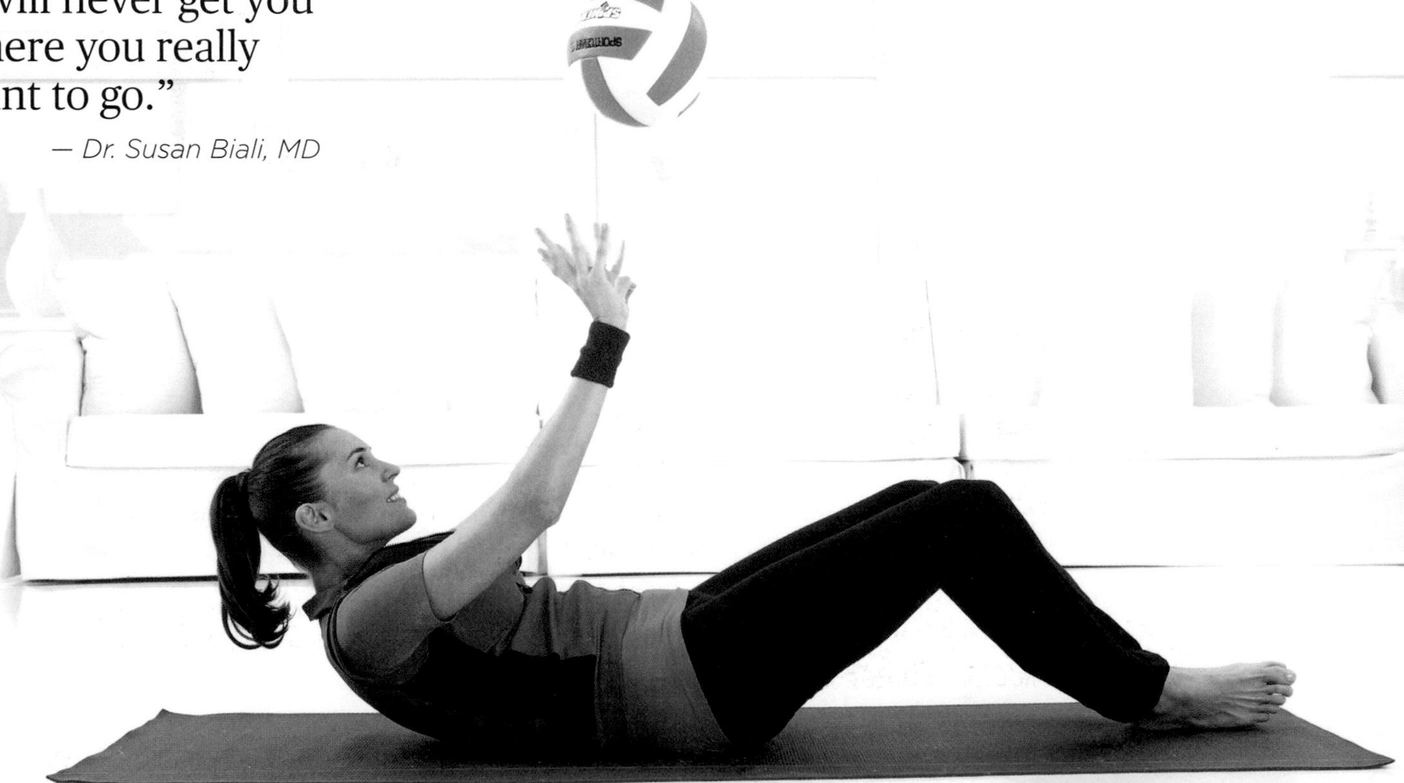

EXTENDED TRIANGLE

Stretches your upper legs, abs, back and sides

1. Start with your feet wide apart in a straddle stance. Raise your arms out to the sides, parallel to the floor, palms facing down. Turn your left foot out 90 degrees.

2. Keeping your arms extended, bend from the hip and extend your torso to the left directly over your left leg. Rest your left hand on top of your left foot (or on your ankle or shin if you can't reach) while reaching toward the ceiling with your right hand, palm forward. Turn your head to gaze up toward your right hand (right). Hold for 30 seconds. Switch sides.

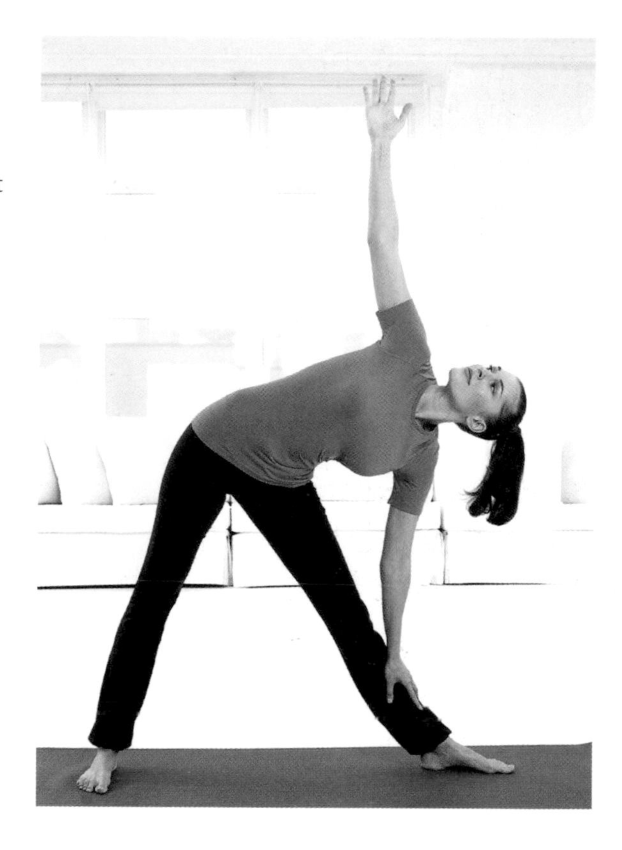

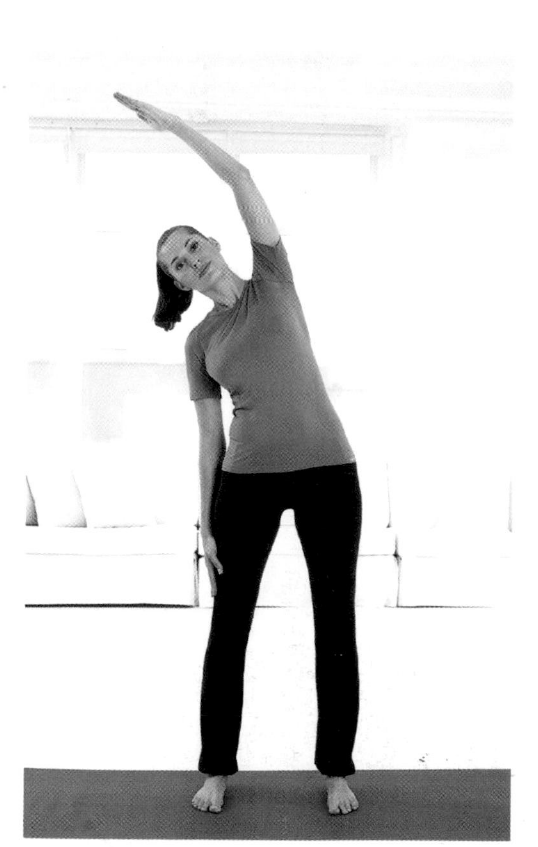

SKY REACH & BEND

Stretches sides, shoulders, arms, back and hips

1. Stand with your feet hip-width apart, arms at your sides, palms facing in.

2. Extend your left arm straight up from your side, reaching over your head to the opposite side as far as comfortably possible, keeping your shoulders down and relaxed (left). Hold for 30 seconds. Repeat on the other side.

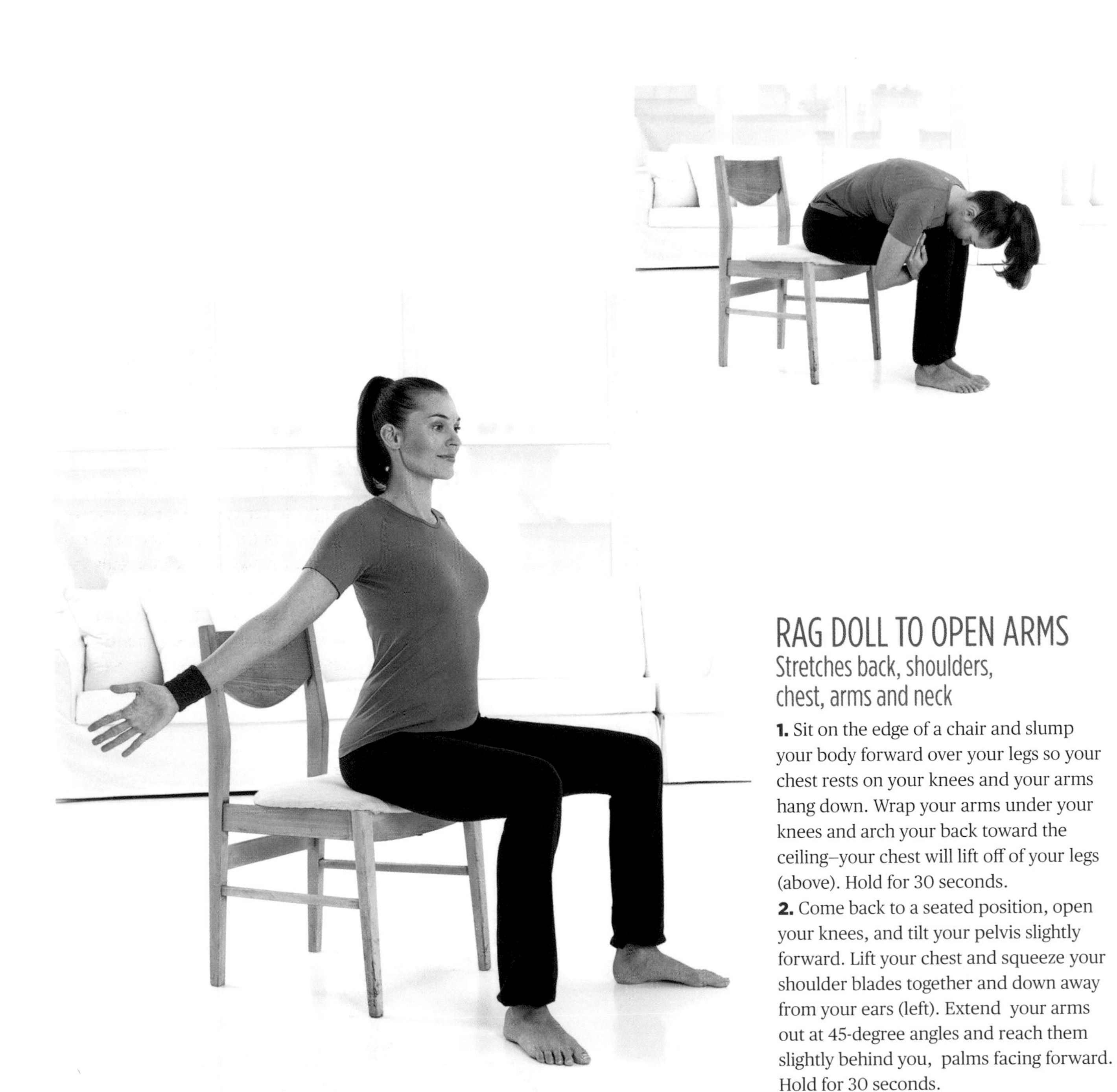

RAG DOLL TO OPEN ARMS

Stretches back, shoulders, chest, arms and neck

1. Sit on the edge of a chair and slump your body forward over your legs so your chest rests on your knees and your arms hang down. Wrap your arms under your knees and arch your back toward the ceiling–your chest will lift off of your legs (above). Hold for 30 seconds.

2. Come back to a seated position, open your knees, and tilt your pelvis slightly forward. Lift your chest and squeeze your shoulder blades together and down away from your ears (left). Extend your arms out at 45-degree angles and reach them slightly behind you, palms facing forward. Hold for 30 seconds.

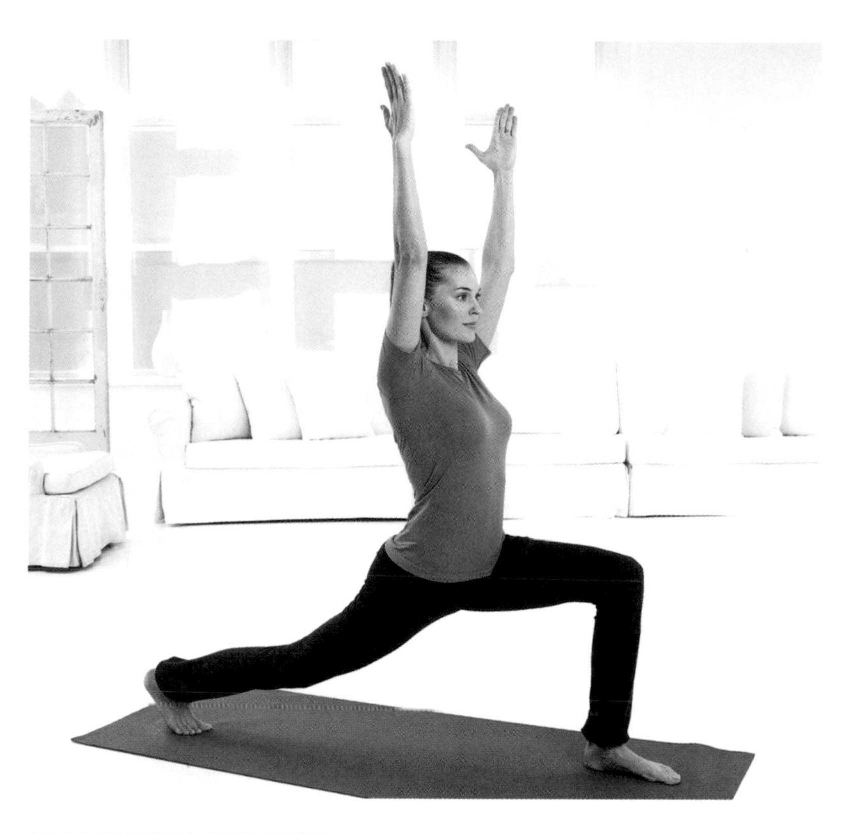

SIT BACK

Stretches back, sides and hips

1. Stand tall with your feet close together, shoulders back. Raise your arms straight out in front of you, palms down.
2. Bend your knees and sit back, trying to lower your thighs as close to parallel with the ground as possible, allowing your torso to lean slightly forward over your thighs (below). Keep your back long and straight as you hold the stretch. Then straighten your knees and lower your arms to return to a standing position.

GIANT STEP STRETCH

Stretches hips and lower legs

1. Stand tall with your feet hip-width apart. Take a giant step forward with your left foot. Bend your left knee until your thigh is as close to parallel to the ground as comfortably possible, keeping the knee directly in line with your ankle.
2. Raise your arms overhead, palms facing each other, keeping your shoulders down. Press up and forward with your rib cage as you hold the stretch (above). Hold for 30 seconds, then switch sides.

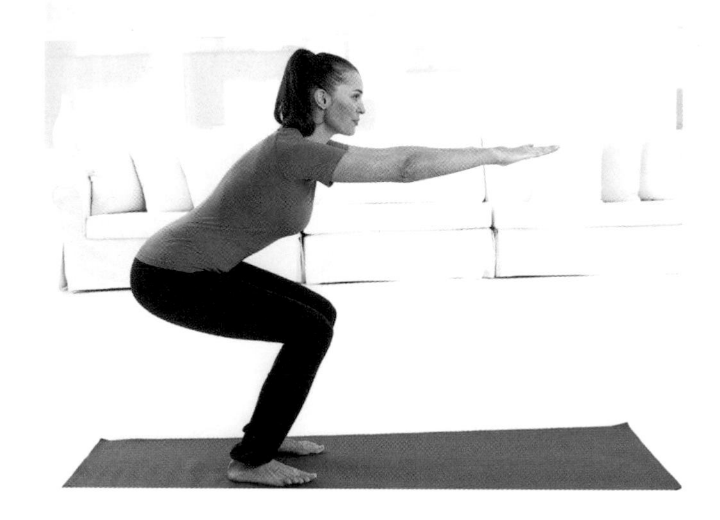

DOWNWARD DOG WITH KNEE DROP

Stretches legs, shoulders, back and hips

1. Begin on your hands and knees with your feet hip-width apart, hands directly beneath your shoulders. Press into your palms and straighten your legs, lifting your tailbone toward the ceiling while pulling your navel toward your spine so your body forms an inverted V. Gently press your torso toward your arms and your heels toward the floor. Hold for 30 seconds.

2. Begin "pedaling" your legs: Bend the left knee slightly while extending your right leg, pressing the right heel into the floor (below). Then switch legs, bending the right knee and extending the left leg. Continue alternating for another 30 seconds.

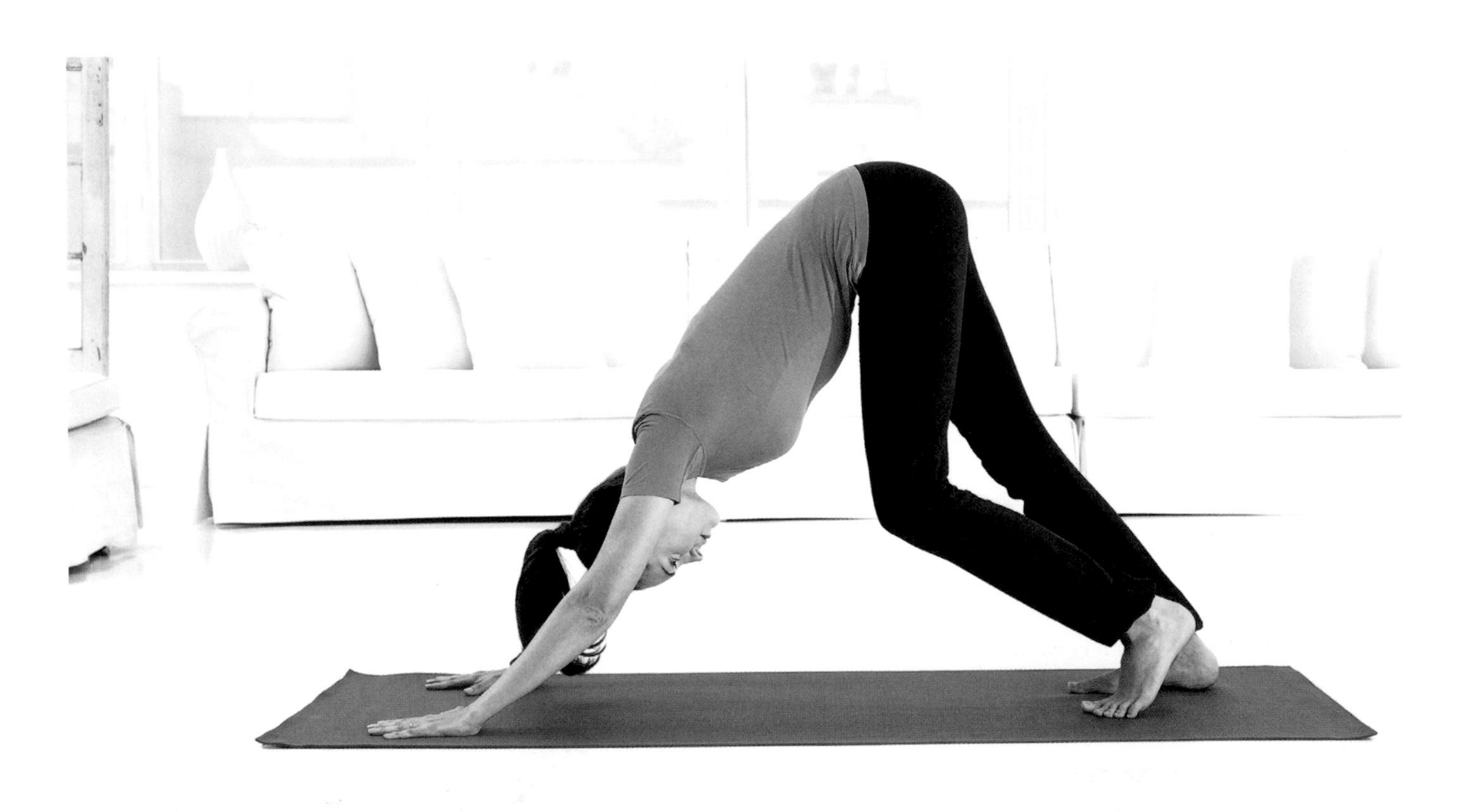

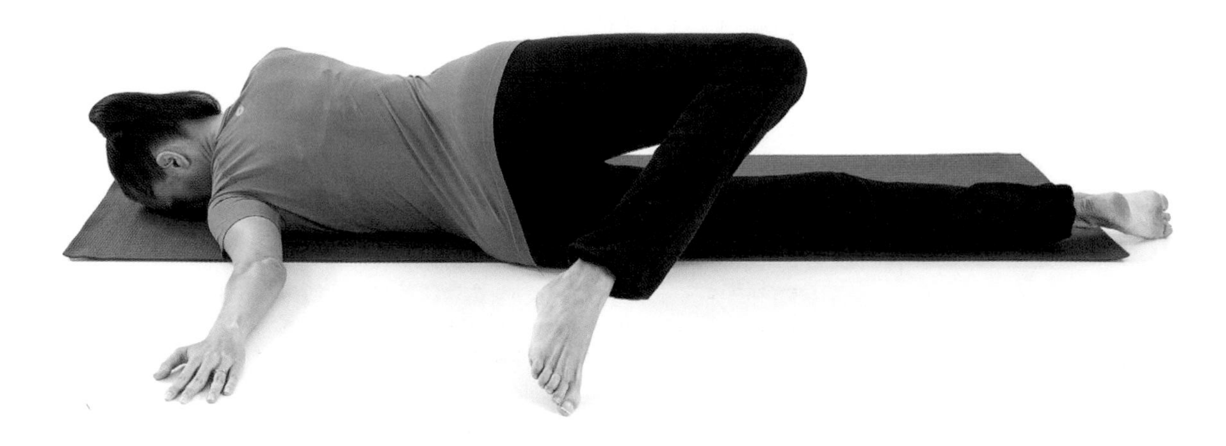

SCORPION

Stretches back, hips and core

1. Lie facedown with your arms out to the sides, shoulders flat on the floor.
2. Lift your right leg off the floor and, twisting your torso, reach it across the back of your body as far as possible toward your left hand (above). Return to start, then repeat to the other side. Repeat this motion for 30 to 60 seconds.

PRAYER POSE

Stretches back and shoulders

1. Kneel with the tops of your feet on the floor, toes pointed behind you. Sit back onto your heels and lower your chest to your thighs.
2. Stretch your arms out overhead and rest your palms and forehead on the floor, or as close as possible (right).

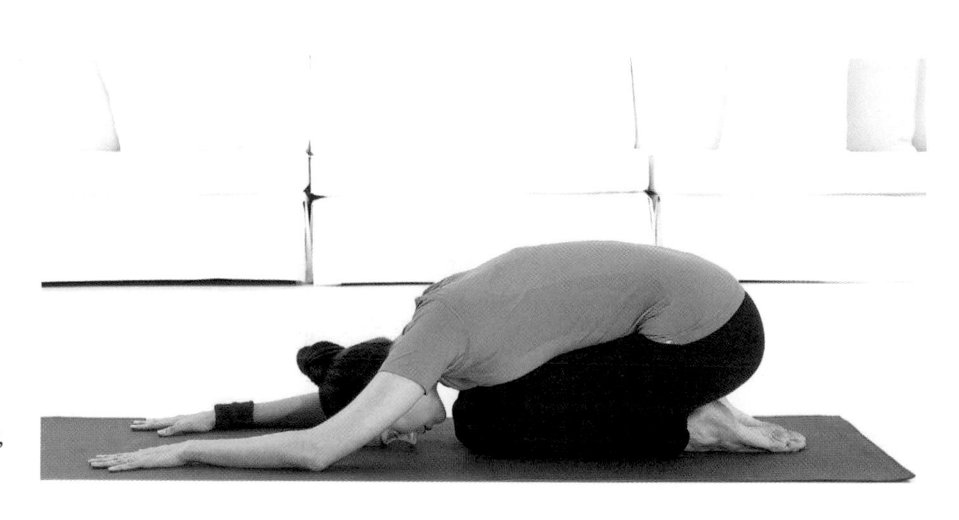

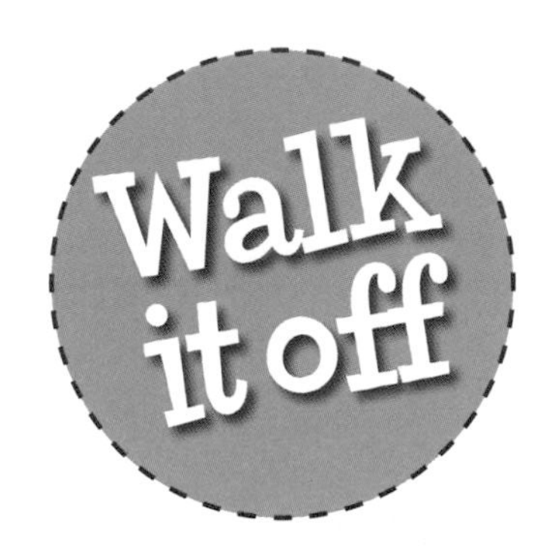

Easy moves for belly, hips and butt

Supplement your walks and show off the new, slimmer you with these easy strengthening exercises

> "Take care of your body. It's the only place you have to live."
>
> — *Jim Rohn, motivational speaker*

Forget sit-ups! Contrary to what you might have been taught, they aren't the be-all-end-all ab exercise. In fact, they work only one set of ab muscles, leaving others weak. Instead, use these six moves which work your abs from all angles. Remember: A stronger core means better posture, which automatically makes you look thinner.
Because these are the muscles that hold you upright, you'll also find that all your daily chores, such as carrying groceries or lugging your laptop, feel easier on your back and the rest of your body. Choose at least three moves to do on a given day, and plan to work your abs three times per week. Do the exercises carefully–faster isn't better.

PELVIC TILT

Tones your chest, triceps, shoulders and core

1. Lie flat on your back with your knees bent, your hands behind your head and your elbows extended to the sides (right).
2. Rotate your pelvis toward your rib cage, gently pressing your lower back into the floor. Hold for 2 seconds, then relax. Repeat the exercise in a slow, controlled manner.

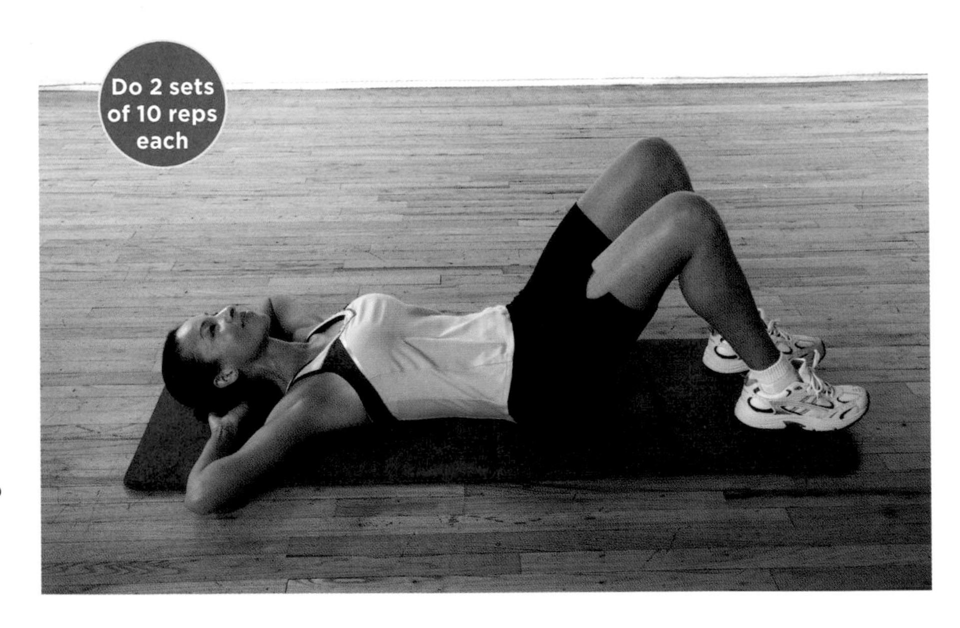

SEATED TOE LIFT

Tones your chest, triceps, shoulders and core

1. Sit straight all the way back in a chair, and place your hands on the sides of the seat in front of your hips or on the chair arms.

2. Contract your abdominal muscles, and slowly lift your feet off the floor as far as comfortably possible (right). Pause, then lower your feet back to the floor.

Do 2 sets of 10 reps each

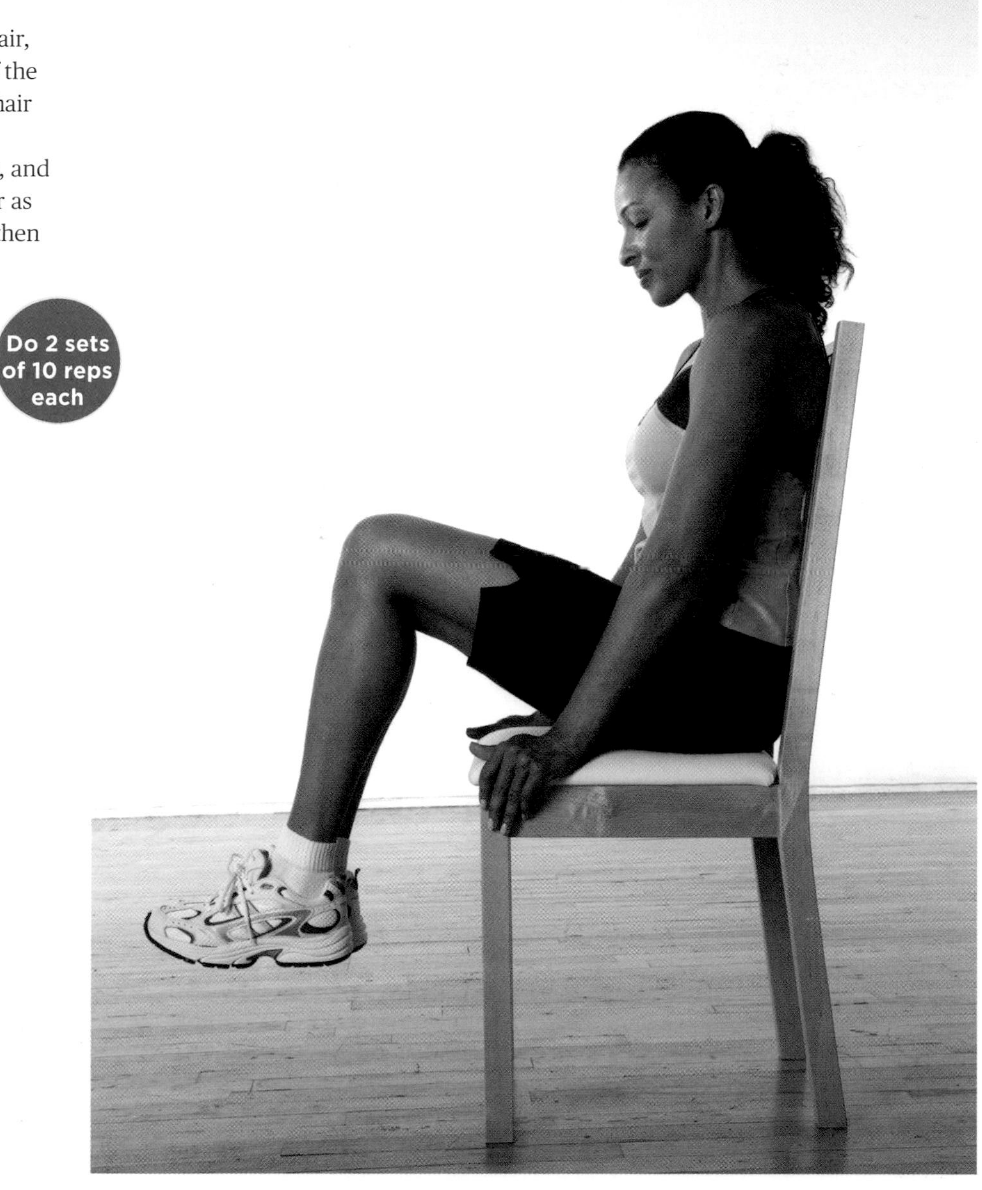

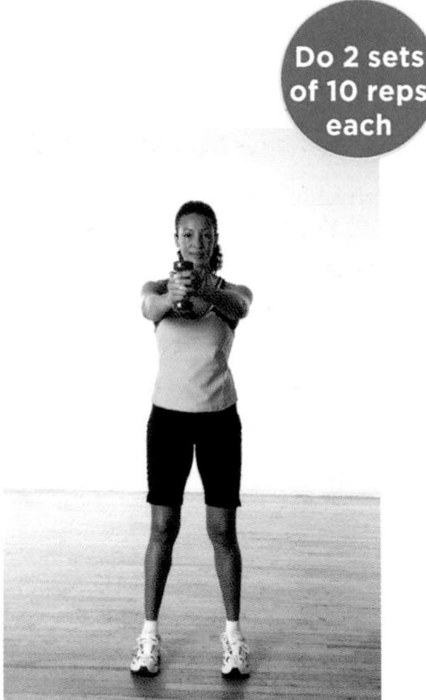

Do 2 sets of 10 reps each

STANDING TWIST

Tones your chest, triceps, shoulders and core

1. Stand straight with your legs shoulder-width apart. Hold a light dumbbell (optional) with two hands, and extend your arms straight in front of you, keeping your elbows soft (above).

2. Contract your abdominal muscles, and turn your torso to the right as far as comfortably possible (right). Pause, then return to start. Repeat on the opposite side. Continue alternating for a full set of reps on each side.

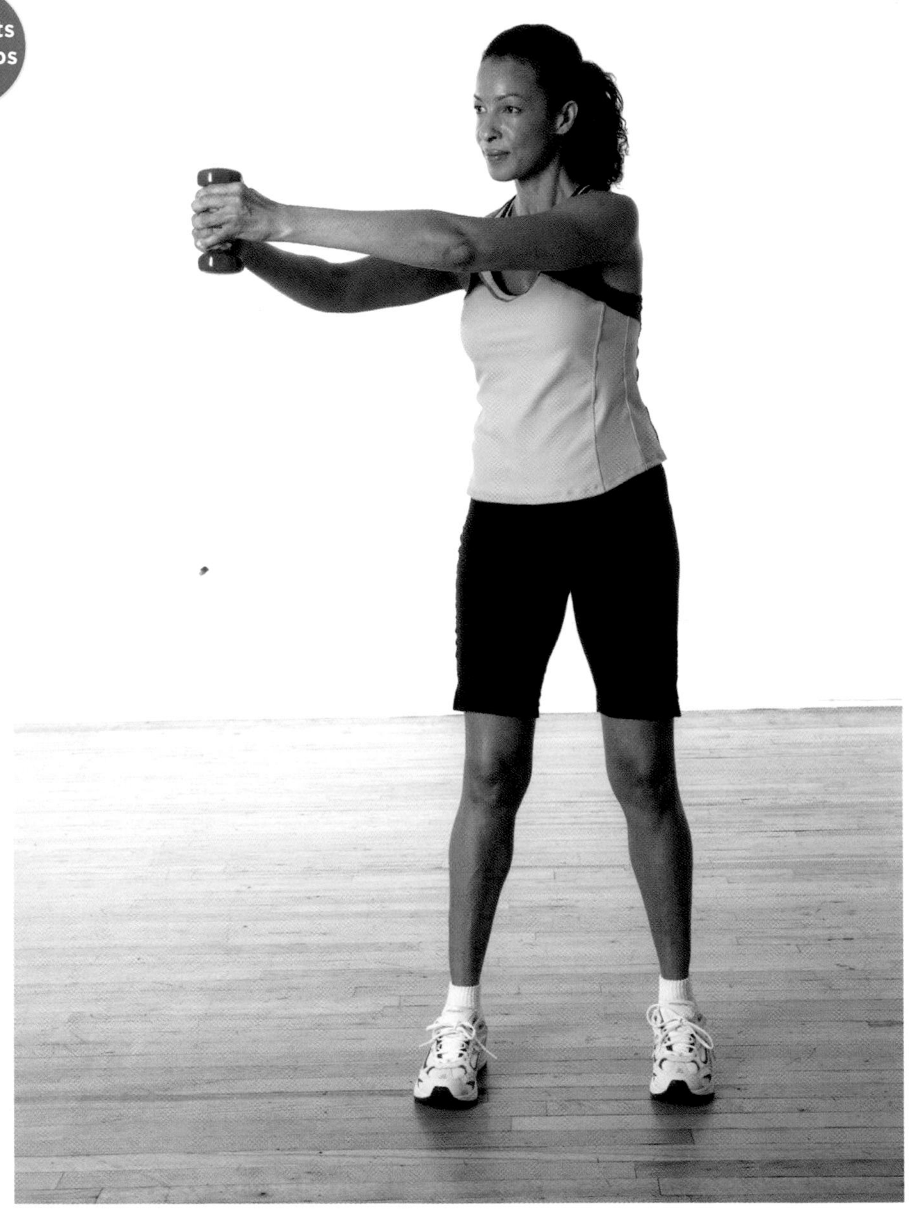

BOAT

Tones your chest, triceps, shoulders and core

1. Sit on the floor with your back straight, your knees bent and your feet flat on the floor (left).

2. Keeping your back straight, contract your abdominal muscles, lean back and extend your legs so your body forms a right angle. Extend your arms straight out on either side of your knees (below). Hold for 3 to 5 seconds, then return to start.

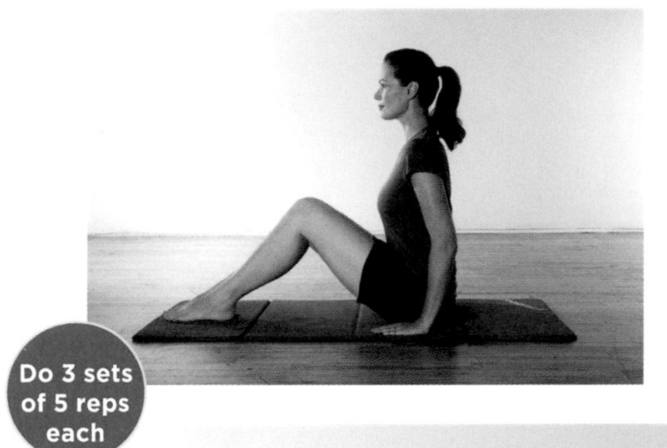

Do 3 sets of 5 reps each

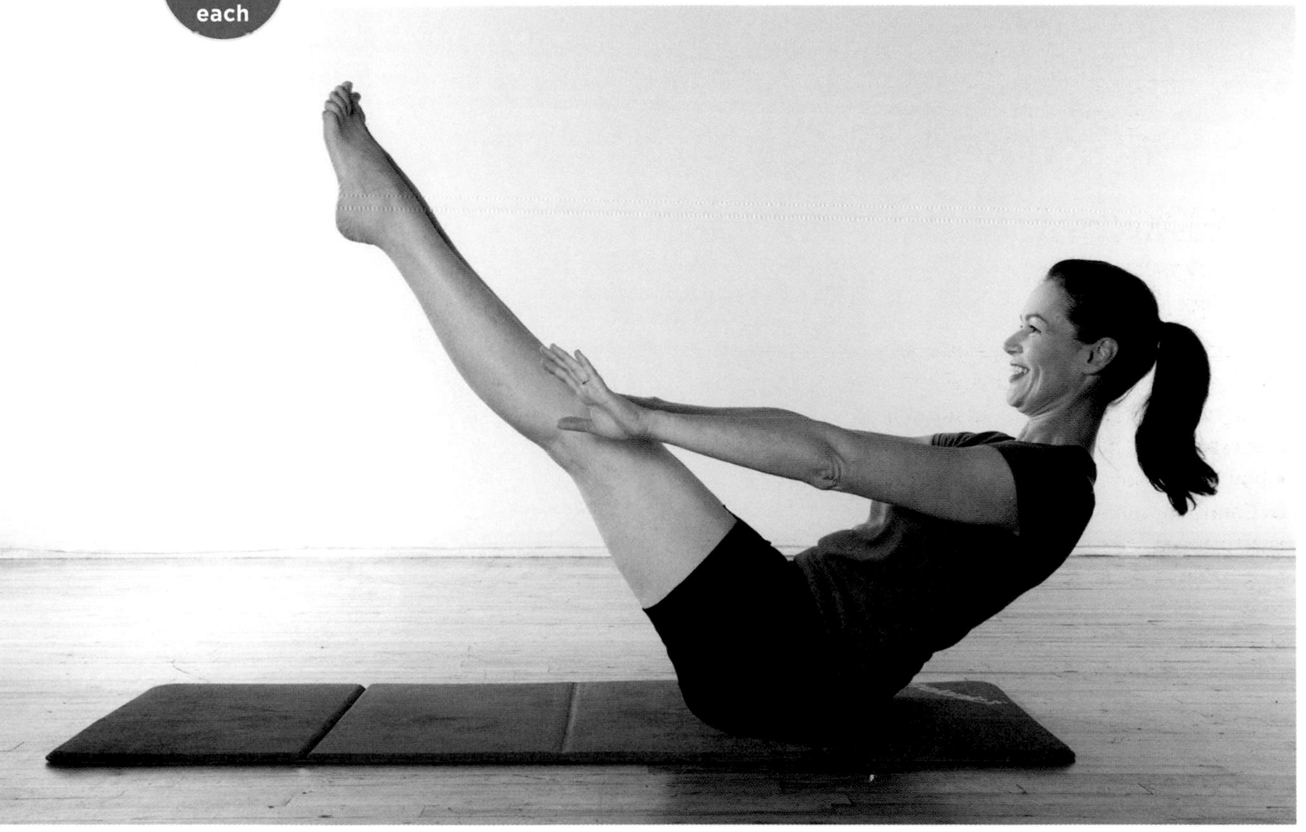

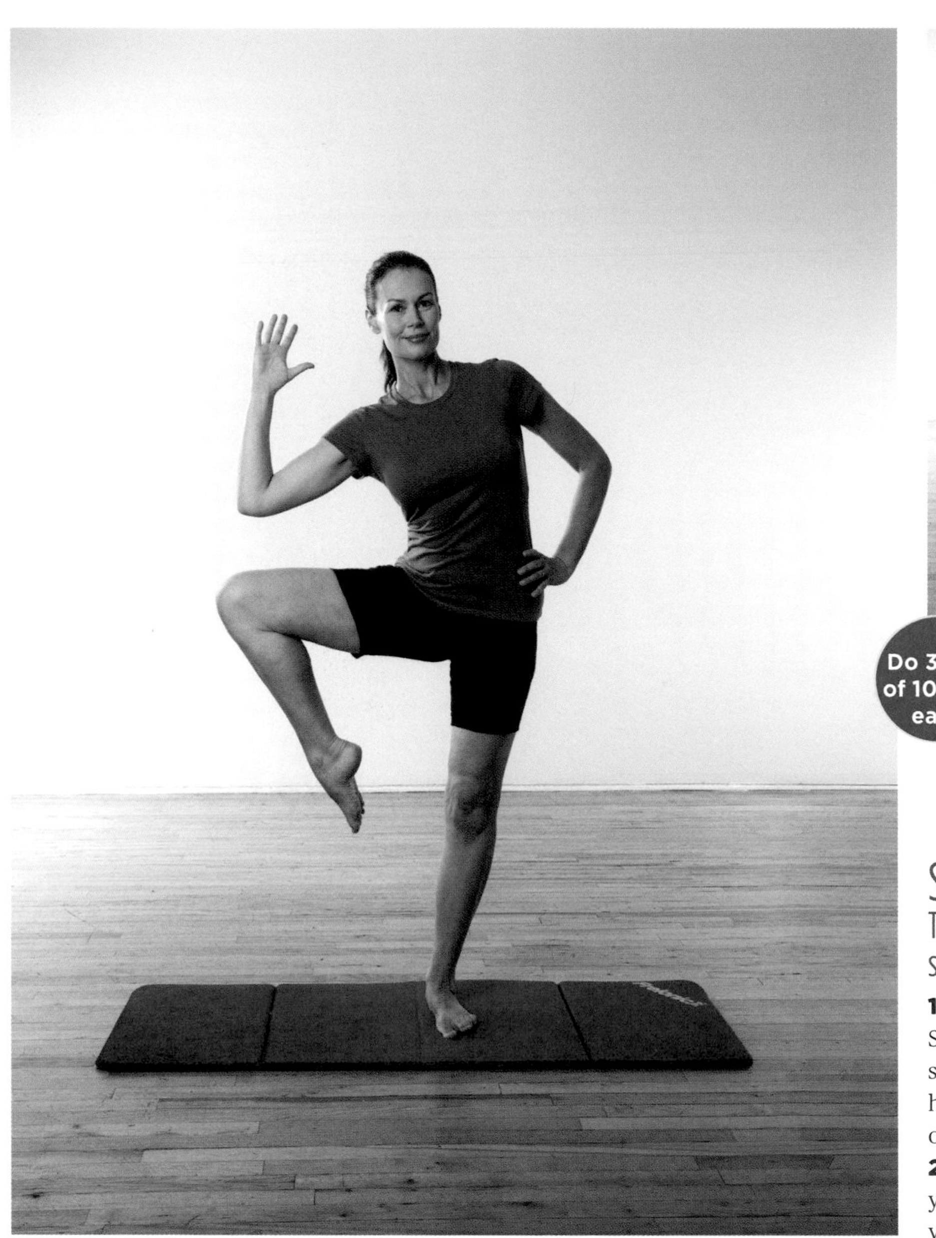

Do 3 sets of 10 reps each

STANDING SIDE-CRUNCH

Tones your chest, triceps, shoulders and core

1. Stand with your feet hip-width apart. Slightly point your right toes out to the side (above). Place your left hand on your hip, and extend your right arm straight overhead.

2. Raise your right knee to waist height as you bring your right elbow down to meet your knee (left). Complete a full set with one side before switching to the other.

STEP-UP

Tones your chest, triceps, shoulders and core

1. Stand facing a step and hold dumbbells at your sides, palms facing in.
2. Place your left foot on the step (below), then press up so your right foot is also on the step (right). Next, step down with your left foot, followed by the right. Repeat, starting with your right leg. Alternate 10 times for one set.

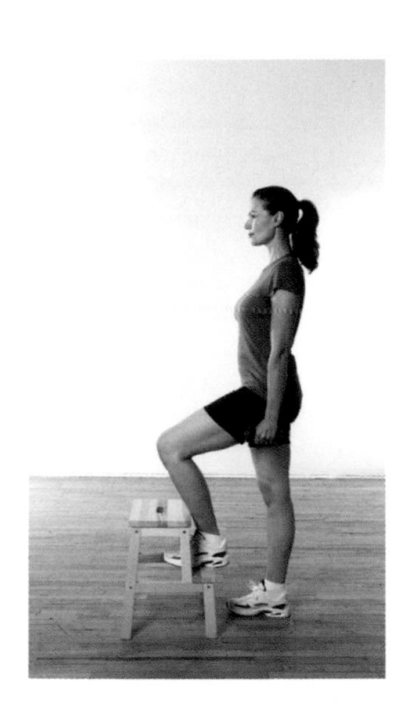

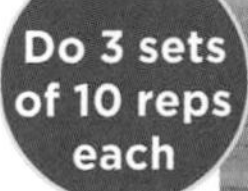

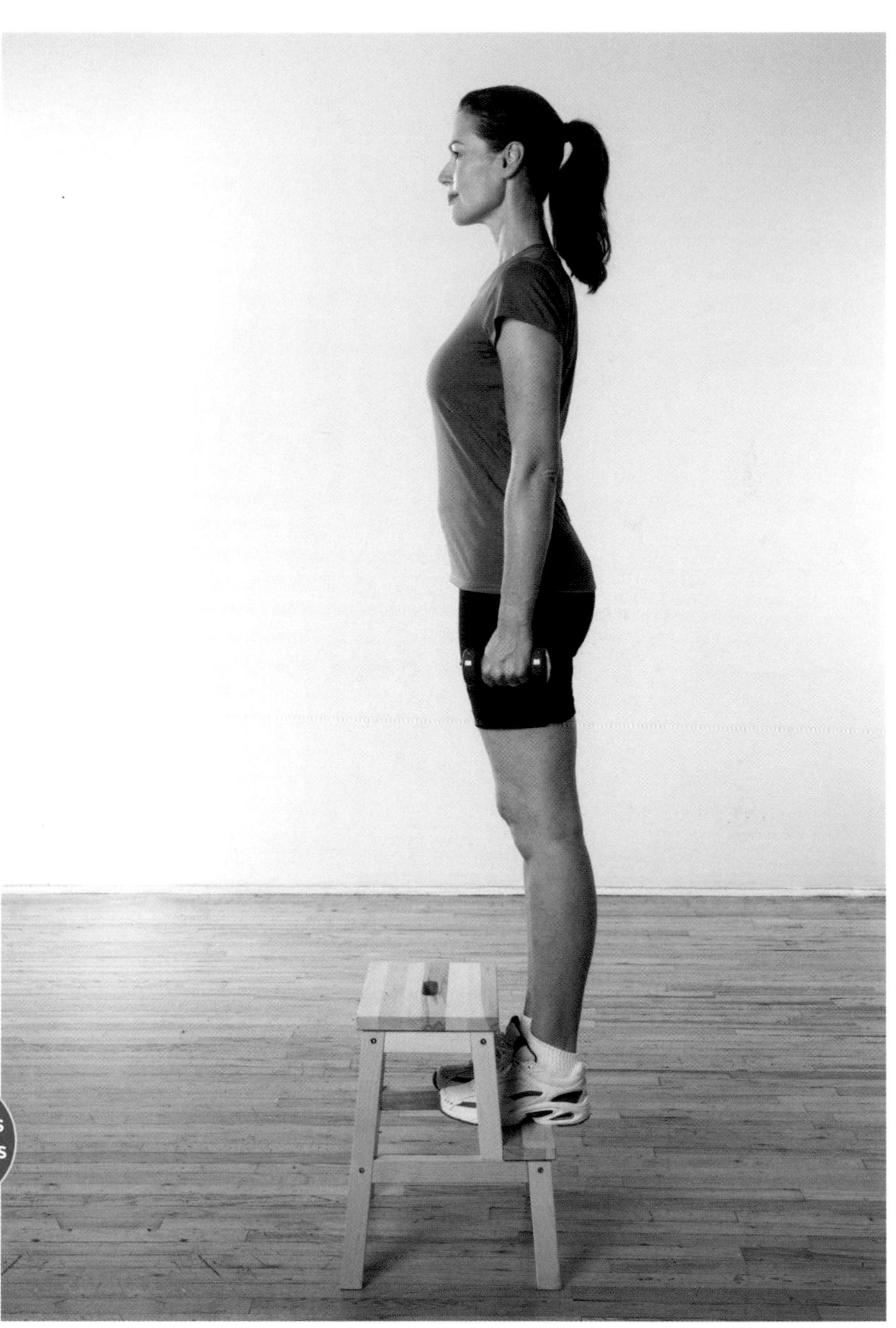

Do 3 sets of 10 reps each

MARCH & SWING

Tones your chest, triceps, shoulders and core

1. Stand with your left hand on your hip and the other on a chair back or tabletop for support. Raise your left knee until the thigh is parallel to the floor, with the foot flexed (near right).

2. Straighten your left leg, pressing the heel forward and toward the floor as you lean your torso slightly backward (far right).

3. Return to the knee-lifted position, then straighten your left leg behind you, leaning forward with your torso (below). Complete a full set with one leg before switching to the other.

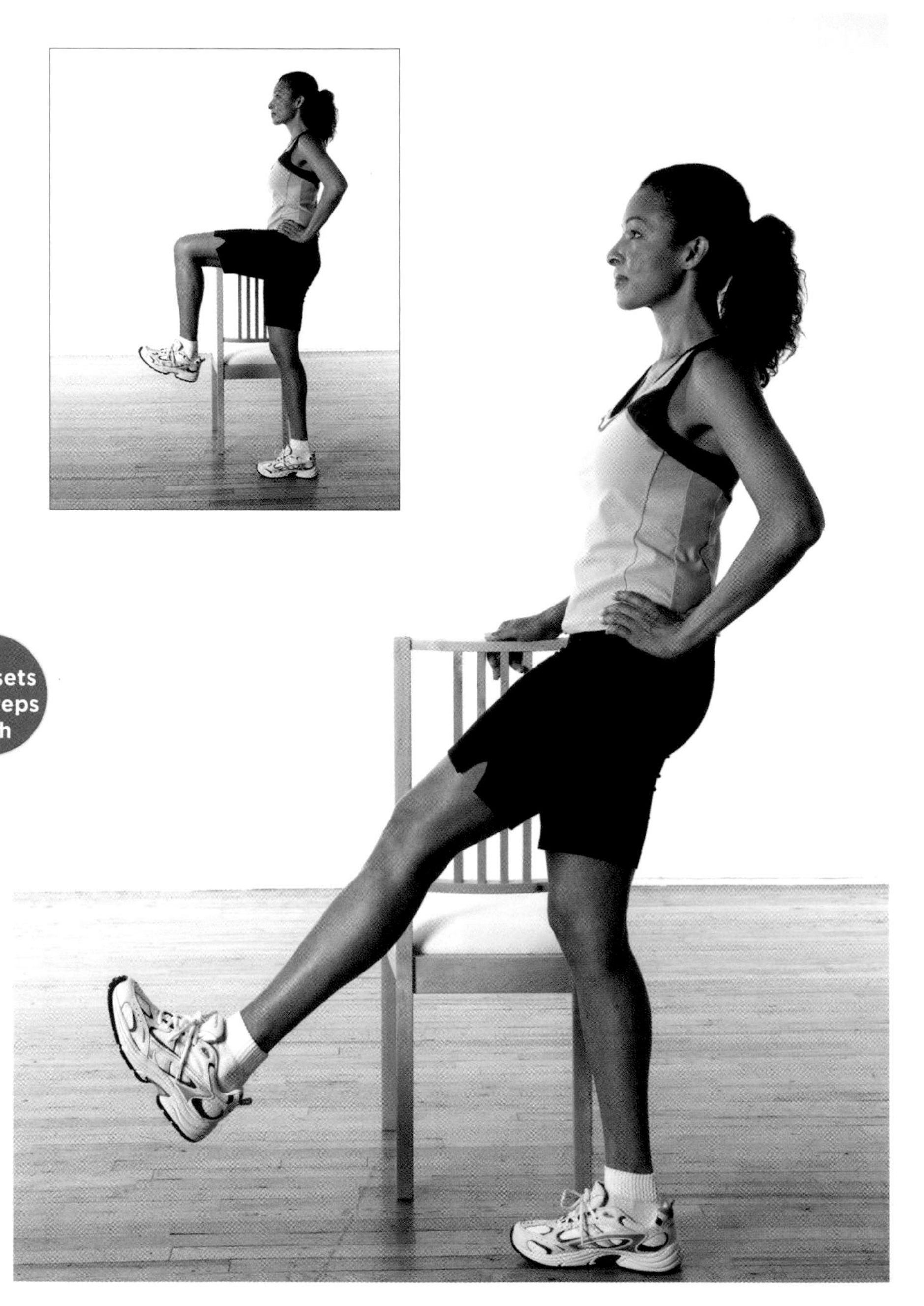

Do 2 sets of 10 reps each

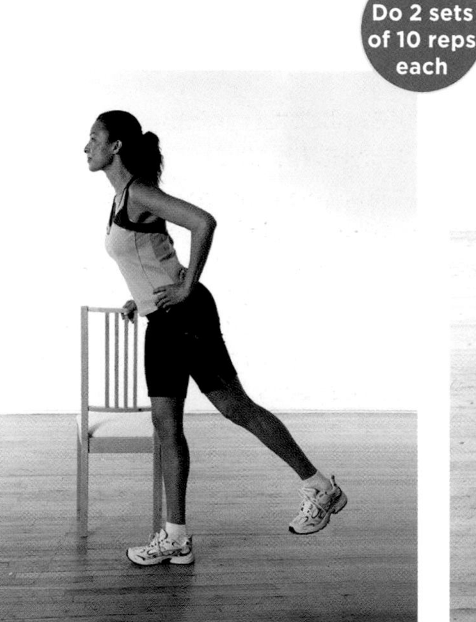

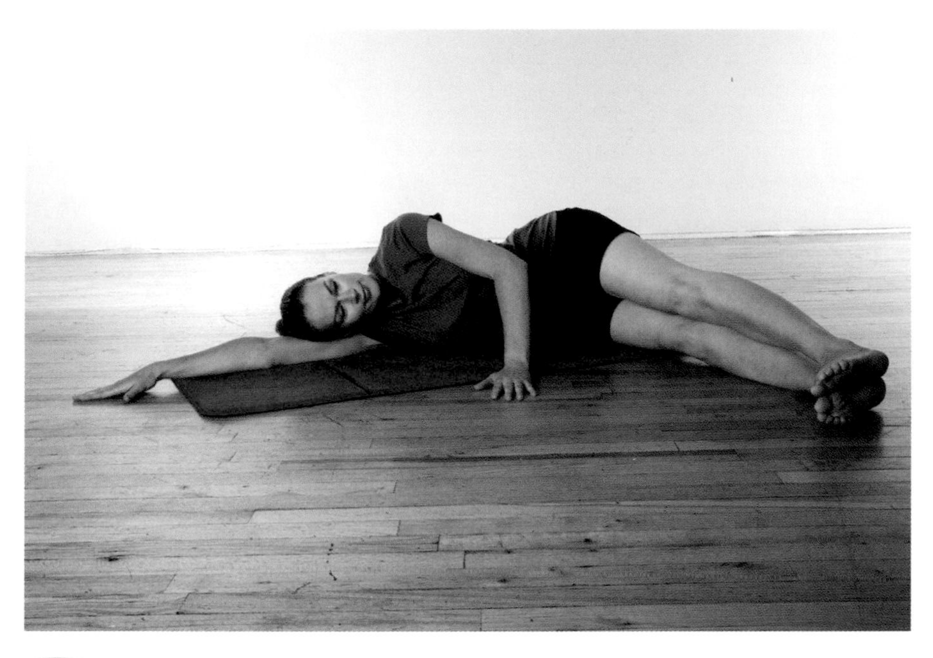

Do 2 sets of 10 reps each

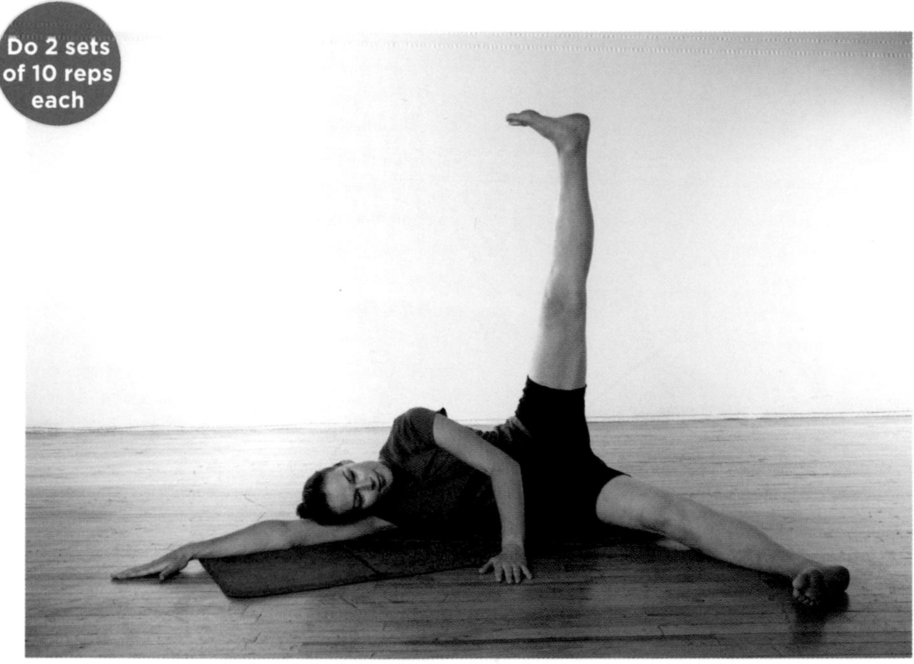

L-LIFT

Tones your chest, triceps, shoulders and core

1. Lie on your right side with both legs extended straight in front of you so your body forms an L shape. (If your back or hamstrings are tight, angle your legs at 45 degrees). Extend your right arm overhead, resting your head on your upper arm, and place your left hand on the floor in front of you for support (above left).
2. Keeping your feet flexed and your abdominal muscles tensed for back support, lift your left leg toward the ceiling as high as comfortably possible (left). Pause, then return to start. Complete a full set with one leg before switching to the other.

SINGLE BRIDGE

Tones your chest, triceps, shoulders and core

1. Lie on your back with your knees bent and your feet flat on the floor about hip-width apart (above right). Contract your buttocks, and lift your rear up so your body forms a straight line from your knees to your shoulders. (If this is as far as you get in this exercise, that's fine. Return to starting position and repeat.) Support your hips with your hands, keeping your elbows and upper arms planted on the floor.

2. If you can, straighten your left leg toward the ceiling, pointing the toe, then flex your foot (below).

3. Lower your leg until your knees line up (right), then raise the leg again. Repeat 3 times, then switch sides.

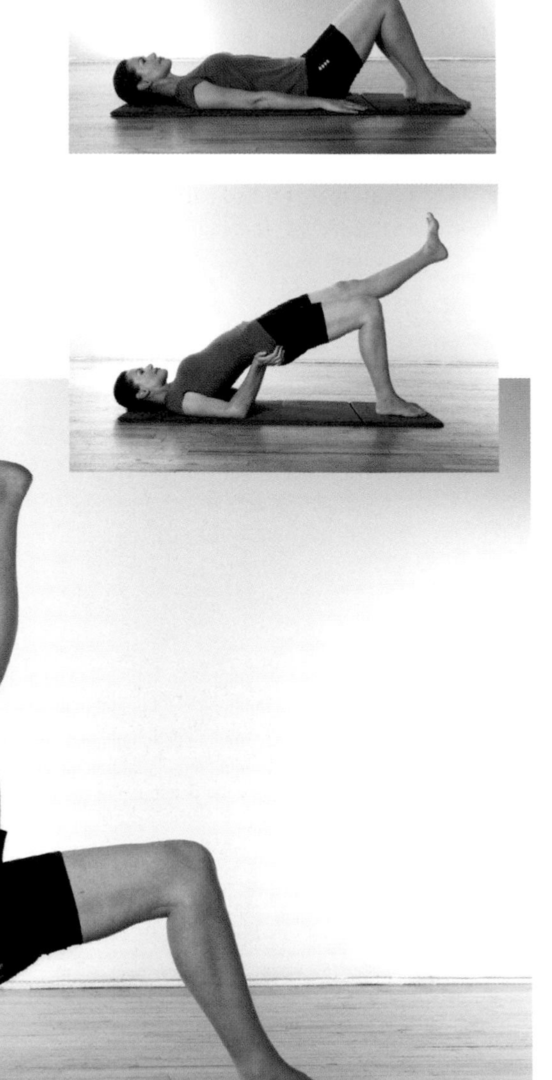

Do 2 sets of 3 reps each

WATER PITCHER RAISE

Tones your chest, triceps, shoulders and core

1. Stand with your feet shoulder-width apart and hold a dumbbell in each hand. Bend your elbows, keeping them close to your body so your forearms are straight out in front of you, palms facing each other (below).

2. Raise your upper arms and elbows to the side. The weights (pretend they are water pitchers) should rotate toward each other as if you were pouring water in front of you (below right). Pause, then return to start.

Do 2 sets of 10 reps each

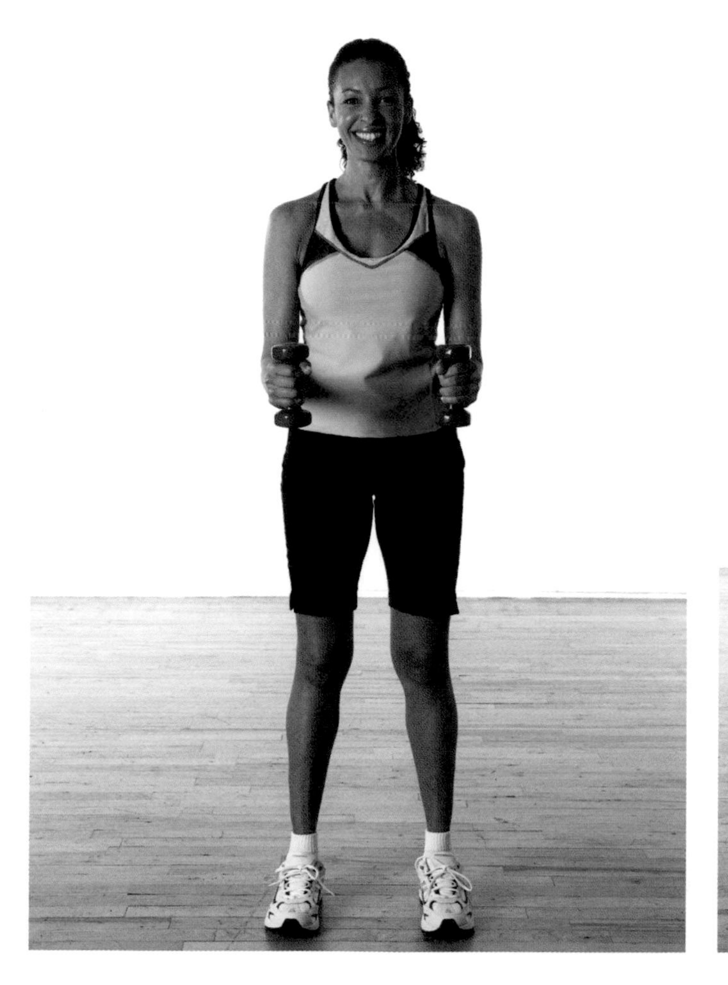

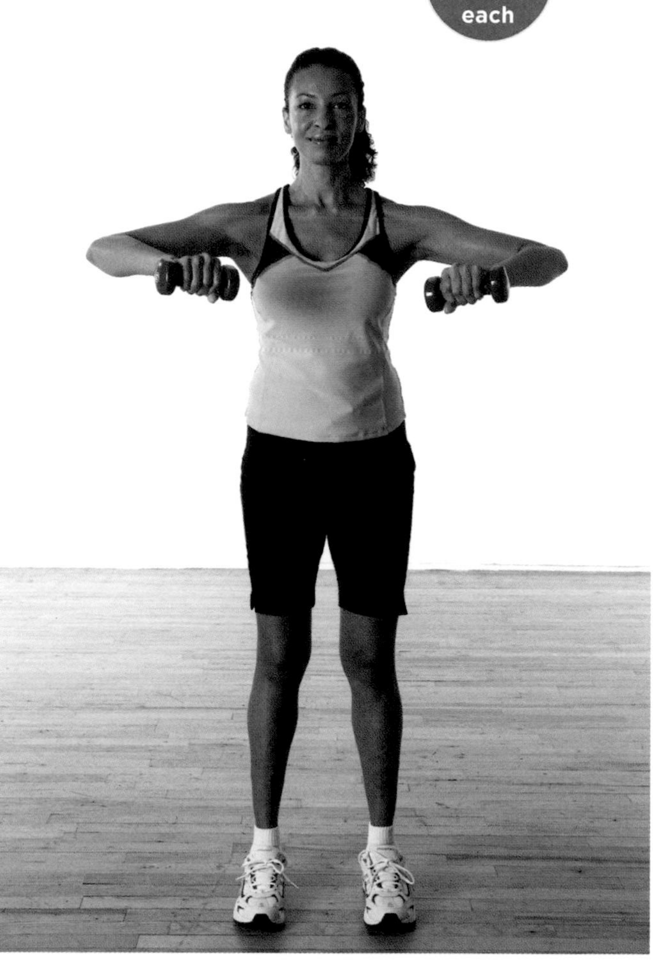

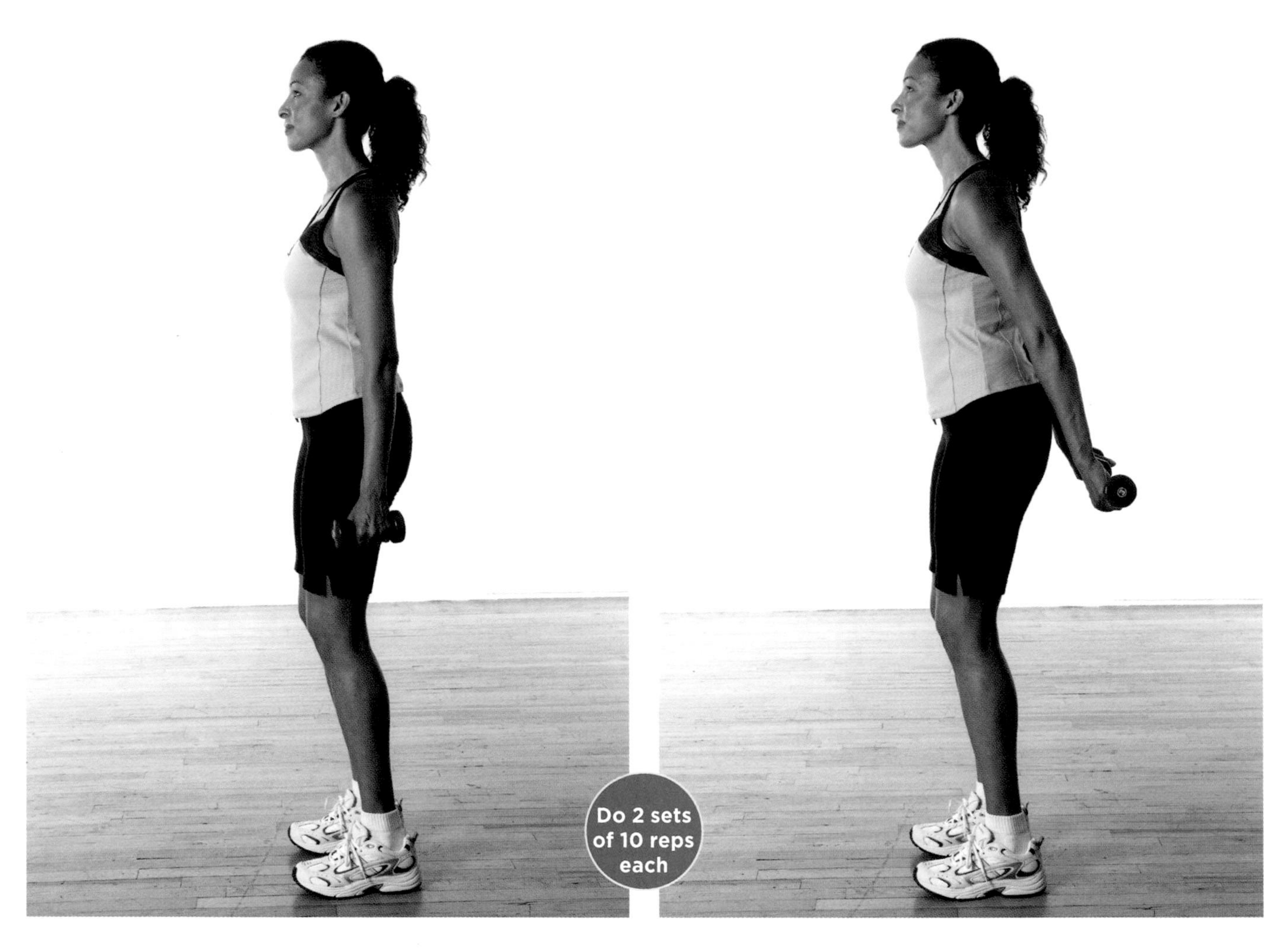

REVERSE RAISE

Tones your chest, triceps, shoulders and core

1. Stand with your feet about hip-width apart with your knees slightly bent, a dumbbell in each hand, palms facing in (above left).

2. Keeping your arms straight, slowly raise them behind you as high as comfortably possible, rotating your palms so they face the ceiling (above right). Pause, then slowly lower back to start.

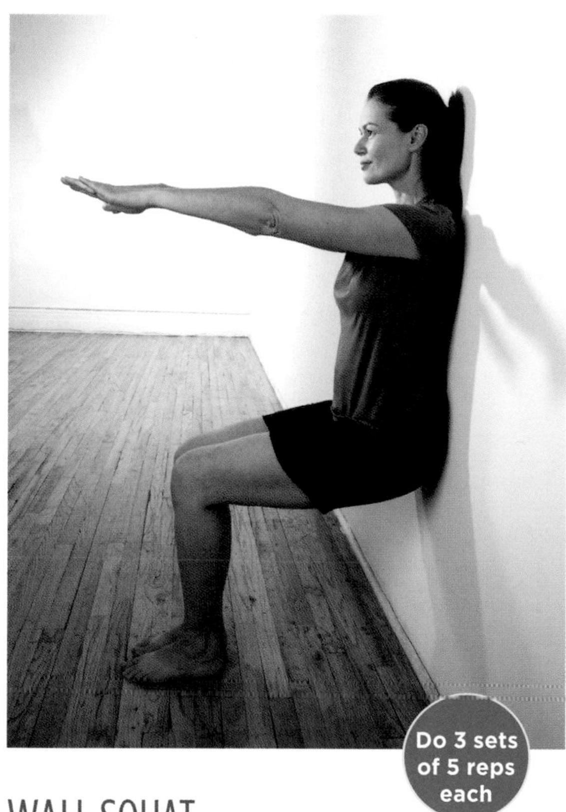

Do 3 sets of 5 reps each

WALL SQUAT

Tones your chest, triceps, shoulders and core

1. Stand against a wall with your legs straight and your feet about two feet from the wall and slightly apart.
2. Raise your arms straight in front of you and slide down the wall until your thighs are nearly parallel to the floor (above). Hold for 3 to 5 counts, then slide back up to the starting position, lowering your arms as you stand.

CHAIR DIP

Tones your chest, triceps, shoulders and core

1. Sit on the edge of a chair with your hands grasping the chair seat on either side of your rear. Slide your rear off the chair and walk your feet forward slightly.
2. Keeping your shoulders down, slowly bend your elbows, lowering your hips toward the floor (below). Pause, then push up to starting position.

Do 2 sets of 10 reps each

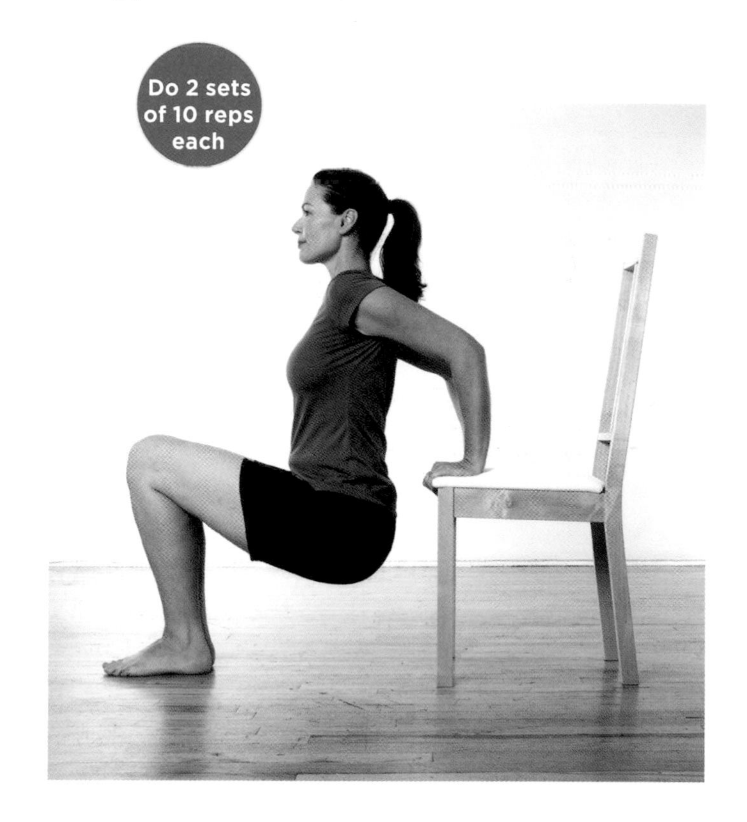

INDEX

A

Alcohol, 59, 62, 63, 65
Antioxidants, 47, 125
Apples
- Baked Apple, 98, 124
- Maple-Walnut Roasted Apples, 178
- Oatmeal with Apple and Flaxseeds, 128

Apricot-Pecan Muffins, 131
Arizona State University study, 52
Asparagus
- Pesto-Stuffed Chicken Breasts with Asparagus Ragout, 164–165

Avocado
- about, 147
- Spinach, Grapefruit and Avocado Salad, 147
- Turkey and Bean Chili with Avocado Salsa, 154

B

Basal metabolic rate (BMR), 67, 68
Basil
- Pesto-Stuffed Chicken Breasts with Asparagus Ragout, 164–165

Beans and legumes
- about lentils, 145
- Bean and Barley Soup, 142
- Bean and Halloumi Soup, 142
- Black Bean and Sweet Potato Burritos, 162
- Black-Bean Salad, 101, 109
- Curried Red Lentil Soup, 145
- Dahl with Spinach, 160
- Hearty Split-Pea Soup, 98, 102, 111
- Meatless Chili Pots with Cheddar, 102, 111
- Quick Black Beans and Rice, 103, 117
- refried beans, 93, 127
- Smoked Haddock and Cannellini Bean Soup, 142
- Turkey and Bean Chili with Avocado Salsa, 154

Beef
- Barbecue Beef on a Bun, 101, 118
- Beef Stew, 98, 115
- Orange Beef Stir-Fry with Broccoli and Red Pepper, 163
- Pot Roast with Braised Vegetables, 100, 114
- Speedy Steak Stroganoff, 158–159
- Summer Beef Salad, 144
- switching from beef to fish, 52

Benson, Herbert, 82–83
Beverages
- caffeine and stress, 80
- green tea, 31, 32
- soft drinks, 86
- Tropical Smoothie, 100, 105, 107
- water, 23, 50, 57–58, 95
- *See also* Alcohol

Biali, Susan, 5–8, 17, 97, 183, 211
Blueberries
- about, 125
- antioxidants in, 125
- Blueberry Bonanza, 98, 101, 125
- Blueberry Muffins with Lemon Glaze, 101, 102, 106
- Cantaloupe and Blueberry Compote with Green Tea and Lime, 181
- Lemony Blueberry Cheesecake Bars, 172

Boston Pizza, 99, 190–191
Breads
- calories in dinner rolls, 59
- Cinnamon-Raisin Bread, 130
- Cranberry Scones with Orange Glaze, 99, 107
- Peach Quick Bread, 102, 106
- serving size, 24
- whole-wheat bread, benefits of, 37
- *See also* Flatbreads; Muffins; Sandwiches

Breakfast
- cereal options, 35
- fruit with, 26–27, 33
- importance of, 30–32
- as lunch, 34
- meal planner, 32, 98–103
- Swap & Drop ideas, 32, 184
- time-saving tips, 31
- *See also* Breakfast dishes

Breakfast dishes
- Apricot-Pecan Muffins, 131
- Blueberry Muffins with Lemon Glaze, 101, 102, 106
- Cinnamon-Raisin Bread, 130
- Cottage Cheese Melba, 99, 105
- Cranberry Scones with Orange Glaze, 99, 107
- Eggs Benedict, 136
- Fresh Fruit Muesli, 132–133
- Herbed French Toast with Mushrooms, 128
- Huevos Rancheros, 127
- Mint and Berry-Scented Melon Cup, 129
- Multi-Grain Waffles, 135, 184
- Oatmeal with Apple and Flaxseeds, 128
- Peach Quick Bread, 102, 106
- Silver Dollar Pancakes, 99, 101, 103, 105
- Spinach and Goat Cheese Omelette, 134
- Tropical Smoothie, 100, 105, 107
- Upside-Down Nectarine Muffins, 137
- Vegetable-Cheddar Omelette, 99, 104
- Vegetable Frittata, 103, 107
- Yogourt Parfait, 98, 101, 102, 104

Brigham and Women's Hospital study, 7
Broccoli
- Chicken and Broccoli Stir-Fry, Italian Style, 102, 112
- Orange Beef Stir-Fry with Broccoli and Red Pepper, 163
- Whole-Wheat Pizza with Broccoli and Olives, 157

Brownie Bites, 99, 101, 102, 123

C

Cabbage
- about, 120, 139
- Colourful Coleslaw, 101, 120

Caffeine and stress, 80
Cakes
- angel food cakes, 171
- Chocolate Snacking Cake, 101, 125
- Vanilla Angel Food Cake, 170–171

Calcium
- calcium-rich snacks, 45
- in dairy products, 34
- role in weight loss, 34, 45

Cancer and obesity, 68
Carbohydrates
- low-fat, high-carb diets, 38–39
- mood-enhancing effects, 44
- simple carbs, 39
- *See also* Breads; Cereals; Grains; Pasta; Potatoes; Rice

Carrots
- Moroccan Spiced Carrots, 159

Casseroles
- Homestyle Tuna Casserole, 103, 117
- Shrimp and Orzo Casserole, 155

Center for Preventive Cardiology, 81
Center for Science in the Public Interest (CSPI), 54–55
Cereals
- Cranberry Trail Mix, 103, 124
- Fresh Fruit Muesli, 132–133
- Oatmeal-Peanut Butter Trail Bars, 174
- Oatmeal with Apple and Flaxseeds, 128
- options, 35

Cheese
- Bean and Halloumi Soup, 142
- cottage cheese, 105
- Cottage Cheese Melba, 99, 105
- feta cheese, 148
- Lemony Blueberry Cheesecake Bars, 172
- Meatless Chili Pots with Cheddar, 102, 111
- Neufchâtel vs cream cheese, 172
- ricotta cheese, 105
- right-sizing portions, guide, 24–25
- Shrimp and Orzo Casserole, 155
- Spinach and Goat Cheese Omelette, 134
- Sugar Snap Peas with Grapes and Feta, 148
- Vegetable-Cheddar Omelette, 99, 104

Cheesecake
  Lemony Blueberry Cheesecake Bars, 172
Cherry-Almond Gratin, 178
Cherry Clafouti, 179
Chewing gum, 51
Chicken
  Chicken and Broccoli Stir-Fry, Italian Style, 102, 112
  Chicken Breasts with Peaches and Ginger, 152–153
  Chicken Fajita Pockets, 166
  compared with salmon, 59
  cooking tip, 153
  Cottage Pie, 168
  Grilled Beer-Can Chicken, 101, 119
  Grilled Chicken Salad with Oranges, 143
  One-Crust Chicken Potpie, 101, 113
  Pesto-Stuffed Chicken Breasts with Asparagus Ragout, 164–165
  Sautéed Chicken with Carmelized Onions, 100, 113
Chickpeas
  Couscous Salad with Chickpeas, 150
  Dahl with Spinach, 160
  Tomato and Chickpea Stew, 98, 120
Chocolate
  about, 123
  antioxidants in, 47
  benefits, 47, 123
  Brownie Bites, 99, 101, 102, 123
  Chocolate Angel Food Cake, 171
  Chocolate Chip Oatmeal Cookies, 100, 123
  Chocolate Snacking Cake, 101, 125
Cholesterol
  saturated vs unsaturated fats, 39
  snacking and, 42–43
Cookies
  Chocolate Chip Oatmeal Cookies, 100, 123
  Pecan Icebox Cookies, 103, 124
Cranberries
  Cranberry Scones with Orange Glaze, 99, 107
  Cranberry Trail Mix, 103, 124

D

Dairy products
  allergies and, 34–35
  calcium in, 34
  milk, 24, 34–35, 127
  serving sizes, 24
  weight loss and, 33–34
  See also Yogourt
Davis, Adelle, 30
Depression
  help for, 87–88
  risk factor for obesity, 84
Desserts
  Blueberry Bonanza, 98, 101, 125
  Brownie Bites, 99, 101, 102, 123
  Cantaloupe and Blueberry Compote with Green Tea and Lime, 181
  Cherry-Almond Gratin, 178
  Cherry Clafouti, 179
  Chocolate Chip Oatmeal Cookies, 100, 123
  Chocolate Snacking Cake, 101, 125
  Fruit Boats with Orange-Balsamic Glaze, 100, 122
  Lemony Blueberry Cheesecake Bars, 172
  Maple-Walnut Roasted Apples, 178
  meal planner, 98–103
  Mixed-Berry Almond Gratin, 178
  Moroccan Fruit Salad, 180–181
  Peach and Blackberry Phyllo Pizzas, 173
  Pear-Berry Clafouti, 179
  Pecan Icebox Cookies, 103, 124
  Pink Grapefruit Brûlée, 174
  Pumpkin Custards, 175
  Saffron and Vanilla Grilled Fruit, 176–177
  Sorbet, 103, 122
  Swap & Drop ideas, 188
  Vanilla Angel Food Cake, 170–171
Diabetes
  obesity as risk factor, 68
  weight loss, effect on risk, 37
Diet plans
  fad diets, 5–6
  high-protein diets, 52
  low-fat, high-carb diets, 38–39
  "low-glycemic-index" (low-GI) diets, 52–53
  motivation key to success, 20
  protein diet for older women, 53
  spending on weight-loss programs, 53
  See also Swap & Drop plan
Dining out
  alcohol and, 59, 62, 63, 65
  controlling what you eat, 28, 54–59, 67, 183
  decoding cooking terms, 56
  fast-food restaurants, 39, 56, 59
  fat in restaurant food, 54
  house salad dressings, 58
  Japanese food, 55
  olive oil, 57
  pizzas, 56
  portion sizes, 54–55
  questions to ask before ordering, 55
  restaurants to avoid, 56
  salads and salad bars, 39, 54, 56, 110, 183
  snack beforehand, 54
  strategies for dining well, 57
  tapas, pros and cons, 58
  See also Fast-food restaurants; Social events
Dinner
  countering boredom, 91–93, 94
  "dinner belt" to gauge fullness, 85
  family dinners, 49–50
  homemade appetizer dinner, 92
  meal planning, 51, 53, 98–103
  more leisurely dinners, 48–50, 53
  pizza crusts, 92
  Swap & Drop ideas, 50, 186–187
  times for dinner, 48
  vegetarian dinner parties, 63
  See also Dinner dishes
Dinner dishes
  Barbecue Beef on a Bun, 101, 118
  Barbecued Halibut Steaks, 98, 118
  Beef Stew, 98, 115
  Black Bean and Sweet Potato Burritos, 162
  Bulgur with Ginger and Orange, 167
  Chicken and Broccoli Stir-Fry, Italian Style, 102, 112
  Chicken Breasts with Peaches and Ginger, 152–153
  Chicken Fajita Pockets, 166
  Cottage Pie, 168
  fruit added to, 152
  Greek-Style Shrimp Skillet, 161
  Grilled Beer-Can Chicken, 101, 119
  Homestyle Tuna Casserole, 103, 117
  Mushroom and Herb Pizza, 157
  One-Crust Chicken Potpie, 101, 113
  Orange Beef Stir-Fry with Broccoli and Red Pepper, 163
  Pasta Primavera, 100, 116
  Penne with Zucchini, 98, 120
  Pesto-Stuffed Chicken Breasts with Asparagus Ragout, 164–165
  Pot Roast with Braised Vegetables, 100, 114
  Quick Black Beans and Rice, 103, 117
  Salmon and Peas in a Packet, 102, 117
  Sautéed Chicken with Carmelized Onions, 100, 113
  Seared Fish Steaks with Tomato-Olive Sauce, 156
  Shanghai Tofu "Steaks" on Kale, 168–169
  Shrimp and Orzo Casserole, 155
  Speedy Steak Stroganoff, 158–159
  Sweet-and-Sour Pork with Pineapple, 99, 115

Tomato and Chickpea Stew, 98, 120
Turkey and Bean Chili with Avocado Salsa, 154
Whole-Wheat Pizza with Broccoli and Olives, 157
Zesty Meat Loaf, 99, 114
Duke University study, 59

E

East Side Mario's, 102, 192–193
Eating alone, 51
Eating out. See Dining out; Fast-food restaurants; Social events
Eggplant & Tomato Salad, 146–147
Eggs
Eggs Benedict, 136
Herbed French Toast with Mushrooms, 128
Huevos Rancheros, 127
nutritional content, 30
omega-3 eggs, 134
Pumpkin Custards, 175
Spinach and Goat Cheese Omelette, 134
Vegetable-Cheddar Omelette, 99, 104
Vegetable Frittata, 103, 107
Exercise
adding muscle, 14, 66
attitude toward, 15
benefits, 87
calories burned, 68, 87, 89
compensating for indulgences, 60, 62
cycling, 87, 89
de-stressor, 68, 79
effect on dementia, 218
gym memberships, 212, 214
interval training, 228–231
keeping track of, 85–87
MET (Metabolic Equivalent of Task), 228–229
as natural part of day, 211, 213–214, 216–219
stair-climbing, 87
strengthening exercises, 238–249
time of day for, 86
time spent sitting, 89
in winter, 71, 213
yoga, 80
See also Walking program

F

Fast-food restaurants
Boston Pizza, 99, 190–191
drive-thrus, 59
East Side Mario's, 102, 192–193
Harvey's, 98, 194–195
healthier alternatives, 56
The Keg, 99, 103, 196–197
KFC (Kentucky Fried Chicken), 198–199
McDonald's, 102, 200–201
salads at, 39, 56
Starbucks, 202–203
Subway, 204–205
Taco Bell, 101, 206–207
Tim Hortons, 208–209
Fats
benefits of fats in moderation, 14, 39, 41, 51
in dinner menus, 51
low-fat, high-carb diets, 38–39
olive oils, 57
omega-3 fatty acids, 39, 134
percentage of average daily diet, 51
in restaurant food, 54
restaurants' house dressings, 58
saturated and unsaturated, 38–39
in Swap & Drop diet, 38, 41, 51
Fennel
about, 138
Radicchio and Fennel Salad with Oranges, 141
Rainbow Salad, 139
Fibre
benefits of, 32–33
recommended amount per day, 32
Fish. *See* Seafood
Flatbreads
Black Bean and Sweet Potato Burritos, 162
Chicken Fajita Pockets, 166
Huevos Rancheros, 127
as pizza crusts, 92
tortillas, 126, 162
Food shopping
avoiding shopping while hungry, 52, 61, 73
buying in bulk, 28, 72, 74
non-purchase of problem foods, 73, 74
nutrition in fresh vs processed food, 75
nutritional labels, 74
shopping lists to avoid impulse buys, 52, 73
supermarket layouts, 52, 73–74
whole foods, rather than processed, 74
Free radicals, 68
Fruit
added to dinner dishes, 152
at breakfast, 33
Cantaloupe and Blueberry Compote with Green Tea and Lime, 181
dried fruit, 130
freezing fruit, 137
Fresh Fruit Muesli, 132–133
Fruit Boats with Orange-Balsamic Glaze, 100, 122
fruit juices, 32, 33
kiwis, 176
Lemon-Lime Angel Food Cake, 171
Mixed-Berry Almond Gratin, 178
Moroccan Fruit Salad, 180–181
Peach and Blackberry Phyllo Pizzas, 173
Pear-Berry Clafouti, 179
right-sizing portions, guide, 26–27
Saffron and Vanilla Grilled Fruit, 176–177
Sorbet, 103, 122
zesters, 163
See also specific fruits

G

Gandhi, Mahatma, 228
Ginger
Bulgur with Ginger and Orange, 167
Chicken Breasts with Peaches and Ginger, 152–153
Rice Salad with Ginger Soy Dressing, 149
Sauteed Spinach with Ginger and Soy Sauce, 167
Glycemic index, 52–53
Grains
Bean and Barley Soup, 142
Bulgur with Ginger and Orange, 167
Couscous Salad with Chickpeas, 150
Couscous Salad with Tuna, 150
Multi-Grain Waffles, 135
serving size, 24
Shrimp and Orzo Casserole, 155
Tabbouleh with Romaine, 151
See also Rice
Grapefruit
Pink Grapefruit Brûlée, 174
Spinach, Grapefruit and Avocado Salad, 147
Grapes
Sugar Snap Peas with Grapes and Feta, 148
Green tea
benefits, 31, 32
Cantaloupe and Blueberry Compote with Green Tea and Lime, 181

H

Harvard Medical School study, 7, 87
Harvard School of Public Health, 33
Harvey's, 98, 194–195
Heart disease
benefits of whole-wheat breads, 37
laughing as protection against, 81
obesity as risk factor, 68
saturated fats and, 38–39
Hedberg, Mitch, 42
Human adenovirus-36 and obesity, 71
Hunger
"dinner belt" to gauge fullness, 85
emotional eating, 44, 62, 87–89
environmental cues, 44
hunger cues, 43–45
importance of breakfast, 30–32
satiety signals, 48–49, 50
snacking to deal with, 42–43, 68, 85
stress as trigger, 78

time for body to register fullness, 7, 24, 39, 49
See also Portion control

J

Johns Hopkins study, 87
Johnson, Samuel, 48
Journal of the American Medical Association, 6

K

Kale
- Shanghai Tofu "Steaks" on Kale, 168–169

The Keg, 99, 103, 196–197
KFC (Kentucky Fried Chicken), 198–199
Kitchen
- buying in bulk, 28, 72, 74
- clearing out the pantry, 72–73, 75
- diet-friendliness of kitchen, 76
- pantry essentials, 77
- places for healthy snacks, 74–75
- refrigerator essentials, 77
- storage containers, 74
- temptations placed out of sight, 68–69, 71, 75
- whole foods, rather than processed, 74

Kiwis, 176

L

Legumes. *See* Beans and legumes
Lemons
- Blueberry Muffins with Lemon Glaze, 101, 102, 106
- Lemon-Lime Angel Food Cake, 171
- Lemony Blueberry Cheesecake Bars, 172

Lentils
- about, 145
- Curried Red Lentil Soup, 145

Limes
- Cantaloupe and Blueberry Compote with Green Tea and Lime, 181
- Lemon-Lime Angel Food Cake, 171

Low-GI index diet, 52–53
Lunch
- breakfast for, 34
- brown-bagging, 37–38
- eating at home, 37
- eating out, 36
- at food courts, 41
- leftovers for, 39
- lunching IQ, 40
- meal planner, 38, 41, 98–103
- sandwich-filling ideas, 39
- side salad ideas, 41
- Swap & Drop ideas, 38, 185
- tips for a healthy lunch, 37
- *See also* Lunch dishes

Lunch dishes
- Bean and Barley Soup, 142
- Bean and Halloumi Soup, 142
- Black-Bean Salad, 101, 109
- Couscous Salad with Chickpeas, 150
- Couscous Salad with Tuna, 150
- Curried Red Lentil Soup, 145
- Eggplant & Tomato Salad, 146–147
- Grilled Chicken Salad with Oranges, 143
- Grilled Turkey Caesar Salad, 98, 100, 110
- Hearty Split-Pea Soup, 98, 102, 111
- Meatless Chili Pots with Cheddar, 102, 111
- Mint and Berry-Scented Melon Cup, 129
- Pita Pizza, 99, 101, 103, 108
- Radicchio and Fennel Salad with Oranges, 141
- Radish and Cucumber Salad, 140
- Rainbow Salad, 139
- Red Pepper Crab Cakes, 103, 110
- Rice Salad with Ginger Soy Dressing, 149
- Roasted Vegetable Wraps, 101, 109
- Smoked Haddock and Cannellini Bean Soup, 142
- Spinach, Grapefruit and Avocado Salad, 147
- Sugar Snap Peas with Grapes and Feta, 148
- Summer Beef Salad, 144
- Tabbouleh with Romaine, 151

M

Maintaining weight loss. *See* Weight loss maintenance
Marinades, 119, 143
Mayo Clinic, 218
McDonald's, 102, 200–201
Meal planner
- description, 14–15
- meal planner, 97–103
- meal planner recipes, 104–125

Meat
- lunch meats (for sandwiches), 24
- right-sizing portions, guide, 18–19, 24
- *See also* Beef; Pork

Melons
- Cantaloupe and Blueberry Compote with Green Tea and Lime, 181
- Mint and Berry-Scented Melon Cup, 129

Michaels, Jillian, 84
Milk
- benefits of calcium, 34
- managing allergies to, 34–35
- recommended servings, 127
- serving size, 24
- swapping whole milk for skim, 34

Monitoring progress
- diagnostic checklist, 86
- fit of clothes, 88
- keeping track of exercise, 85–87
- monitoring moods, 87–88
- reality check, 84

Montclair State University, 80
Motivation
- alcohol and, 62, 63
- celebrating small victories, 67
- diagnosing problem areas, 86
- fighting fatigue, 66–67
- hitting a plateau, 67
- keeping on track, 84–89
- key to success, 20
- managing cravings, 51, 68, 94
- managing negativity, 64
- myths re: weight loss, 69
- personal reasons for losing/maintaining weight, 88, 94
- planning ahead, 61–62, 67–68
- positive attitude, 6
- putting tempting foods out of sight, 68–69, 74
- quiz about feelings on progress, 88
- quiz about motivation level, 70
- realistic goals for weight loss, 69, 71
- rewards for reaching goals, 62
- setting milestones and goals, 66, 69
- staying motivated in social settings, 60
- weighing yourself, 89
- *See also* Weight loss maintenance

Muffins
- Apricot-Pecan Muffins, 131
- Blueberry Muffins with Lemon Glaze, 101, 102, 106
- Upside-Down Nectarine Muffins, 137

Mushrooms
- Herbed French Toast with Mushrooms, 128
- Mushroom and Herb Pizza, 157
- shiitake mushrooms, 166

N

National Cancer Institute study, 50
National Institutes of Health, 95
National Weight Control Registry, 32, 43
Nectarines
- Upside-Down Nectarine Muffins, 137

Nuts
- Apricot-Pecan Muffins, 131
- Cherry-Almond Gratin, 178
- Mixed-Berry Almond Gratin, 178
- right-sizing portions, guide, 28–29
- toasting almonds, 167

O

Obesity
- belly (intra-abdominal) fat, 89
- childhood obesity, 7
- depression as risk factor, 84

human adenovirus-36 and, 71
obesity epidemic, 5–6, 212–213
risk for heart disease and diabetes, 68
risk of cancer, 68
soft drinks and, 86
See also Weight
Obesity Research Center study, 33
Olives
Greek-Style Shrimp Skillet, 161
Seared Fish Steaks with Tomato-Olive Sauce, 156
selecting, 161
Whole-Wheat Pizza with Broccoli and Olives, 157
Onions
Sautéed Chicken with Carmelized Onions, 100, 113
Oranges
Bulgur with Ginger and Orange, 167
Cranberry Scones with Orange Glaze, 99, 107
Fruit Boats with Orange-Balsamic Glaze, 100, 122
Grilled Chicken Salad with Oranges, 143
Mint and Berry-Scented Melon Cup, 129
Moroccan Fruit Salad, 180–181
Orange Beef Stir-Fry with Broccoli and Red Pepper, 163
Radicchio and Fennel Salad with Oranges, 141

P

Pancakes
Multi-Grain Pancakes, 135
Silver Dollar Pancakes, 99, 101, 103, 105
Parsley, 151
ParticipACTION, 216
Pasta
Pasta Primavera, 100, 116
Penne with Zucchini, 98, 120
right-sizing portions, guide, 20–21, 24
Shrimp and Orzo Casserole, 155
Thai Noodle Salad, 103, 121
tips for a healthy dinner, 20
Peaches
Chicken Breasts with Peaches and Ginger, 152–153
Peach and Blackberry Phyllo Pizzas, 173
Peach Quick Bread, 102, 106
peeling, 153
Peanut butter
Oatmeal-Peanut Butter Trail Bars, 174
Pear-Berry Clafouti, 179
Peas
Hearty Split-Pea Soup, 98, 102, 111
Salmon and Peas in a Packet, 102, 117
Sugar Snap Peas with Grapes and Feta, 148
See also Chickpeas
Peppers
Orange Beef Stir-Fry with Broccoli and Red Pepper, 163
Red Pepper Crab Cakes, 103, 110
Pilates, Joseph, 212
Pineapple
Sweet-and-Sour Pork with Pineapple, 99, 115
Pizza
Boston Pizza restaurant, 99, 190–191
flatbreads as pizza crusts, 92
Mushroom and Herb Pizza, 157
Peach and Blackberry Phyllo Pizzas, 173
Pita Pizza, 99, 101, 103, 108
Whole-Wheat Pizza with Broccoli and Olives, 157
Pollan, Michael, 24
Pork
bacon vs sausages, 32
fat content, 115
Sweet-and-Sour Pork with Pineapple, 99, 115
Porter, John, 8
Portion control
50-percent trick, 20, 24
downsizing plate sizes, 28
portions today compared with past, 24
right-sizing portions, visual guide, 18–29
in the supermarket, 28
See also Hunger
Potatoes
about, 121
Black Bean and Sweet Potato Burritos, 162
German Potato Salad with Dijon Vinaigrette, 101, 121
potato chips, baked vs fried, 45
serving size, 24
Poultry. *See* Chicken; Turkey
Processed foods, 38
Proteins
high-protein diets, 52
protein diet for older women, 53
Public Health Agency of Canada, 213
Pumpkin Custards, 175

Q

Queen's University study, 226

R

Restaurant meals. *See* Dining out
Rice
Quick Black Beans and Rice, 103, 117
Rice Salad with Ginger Soy Dressing, 149
serving size, 24
Spanish Rice, 102, 116

S

Salads
Black-Bean Salad, 101, 109
Colourful Coleslaw, 101, 120
Couscous Salad with Chickpeas, 150
Couscous Salad with Tuna, 150
cucumber salads, 140
Eggplant & Tomato Salad, 146–147
at fast-food restaurants, 39, 56
German Potato Salad with Dijon Vinaigrette, 101, 121
Grilled Chicken Salad with Oranges, 143
Grilled Turkey Caesar Salad, 98, 100, 110
house dressings at restaurants, 58
Italian Salad, 100, 120
Mint and Berry-Scented Melon Cup, 129
Radicchio and Fennel Salad with Oranges, 141
Radish and Cucumber Salad, 140
Rainbow Salad, 139
Rice Salad with Ginger Soy Dressing, 149
salad bars at restaurants, 54
Spinach, Grapefruit and Avocado Salad, 147
Sugar Snap Peas with Grapes and Feta, 148
Summer Beef Salad, 144
Tabbouleh with Romaine, 151
Thai Noodle Salad, 103, 121
"virtuous" feeling, 59
Salsa
Huevos Rancheros, 127
Turkey and Bean Chili with Avocado Salsa, 154
Salt in prepared foods, 51
San Diego State University study, 228–229
Sandwiches
fillings, 39
grilled chicken, tomato and Swiss cheese, 103
lunch meats, 24
prosciutto, tomato and provolone cheese, 101
Roasted Vegetable Wraps, 101, 109
turkey, tomato and Swiss cheese, 99
Scones
Cranberry Scones with Orange Glaze, 99, 107
Seafood
Barbecued Halibut Steaks, 98, 118
buying fish, 156
cooking shrimp, 155
Couscous Salad with Tuna, 150
fish, serving size, 24
Greek-Style Shrimp Skillet, 161
Homestyle Tuna Casserole, 103, 117
Red Pepper Crab Cakes, 103, 110

Salmon and Peas in a Packet, 102, 117
salmon compared with chicken, 59
Seared Fish Steaks with Tomato-Olive Sauce, 156
Shrimp and Orzo Casserole, 155
Smoked Haddock and Cannellini Bean Soup, 142
switching from beef to fish, 52
Shopping. See Food shopping
Sleep and weight loss, 49
Snacks
Baked Apple, 98, 124
benefits of dark chocolate, 47, 123
Cranberry Trail Mix, 103, 124
dealing with hunger, 42–43, 68, 85
before dining out, 54
fighting fatigue, 66–67
"flat-tummy" foods, 47
hunger cues, 43–45
jicama "fries," 47
managing cravings, 51, 68, 94
for mid-afternoon slump, 36
Oatmeal-Peanut Butter Trail Bars, 174
options instead of snacking, 45–46
planning, 46–47, 98–103
popcorn, 44
potato chips, baked vs fried, 45
quiz about snacking habits, 46
recipes, 122–125
savoury snacks, 45
Swap & Drop ideas, 44, 47, 189
weight loss and, 42, 68
Social events
birthday cakes at work, 61
chocolates as gifts, 63
managing alcohol intake, 62, 63
need for support from others, 63, 64
planning for, 61–62
sad "chick flicks" and snacking, 65
staying motivated, 60
vegetarian dinner parties, 63
See also Dining out
Social network
benefits of group dieting, 63
diet saboteurs, 63–64, 75
help with dieting and motivation, 62–63, 68
help with stress reduction, 81
quiz re need for support, 64
Soups
Bean and Barley Soup, 142
Bean and Halloumi Soup, 142
Curried Red Lentil Soup, 145
Hearty Split-Pea Soup, 98, 102, 111
Smoked Haddock and Cannellini Bean Soup, 142
Soy sauce, 118
Spinach
Dahl with Spinach, 160
Sauteed Spinach with Ginger and Soy Sauce, 167
Spinach, Grapefruit and Avocado Salad, 147
Spinach and Goat Cheese Omelette, 134
St. Luke's-Roosevelt Hospital study, 33
St. Michael's Hospital study, 42–43
Starbucks, 202–203
Stress
addressing solvable problems, 79
crying as stress reliever, 83
definition, 78
exercise as de-stressor, 68, 79, 80
in the family, 79, 83
food as comfort, 78, 80
kitchen organization for stress relief, 73
laughing as de-stressor, 81, 82
multivitamin and mineral supplements, 83
relaxation as de-stressor, 68, 82–83
strategies to lessen stress at work, 79, 81, 83
stress quiz, 82
tips for stress reduction, 80–82
yoga to de-stress, 80
Subway, 204–205
Swap & Drop plan
benefits of, 6–7, 20, 53
description, 14–15
meal planner, 96–103
meal planner recipes, 104–125
Swap & Drop breakfast ideas, 32, 184
Swap & Drop dessert ideas, 188
Swap & Drop dinner ideas, 50, 186–187
Swap & Drop ideas for fast-food restaurants, 190–209
Swap & Drop ideas for walking, 218, 229
Swap & Drop lunch ideas, 38, 185
Swap & Drop snack ideas, 44, 47, 189
Sweet potatoes
Black Bean and Sweet Potato Burritos, 162

T

Taco Bell, 101, 206–207
Tacos, 93
Tim Hortons, 208–209
Tofu (bean curd)
Shanghai Tofu "Steaks" on Kale, 168–169
Tomatoes
Eggplant & Tomato Salad, 146–147
grilled chicken, tomato and Swiss cheese sandwich, 103
prosciutto, tomato and provolone cheese sandwich, 101
Seared Fish Steaks with Tomato-Olive Sauce, 156
Tomato and Chickpea Stew, 98, 120
turkey, tomato and Swiss cheese sandwich, 99
Turkey
Cottage Pie, 168
Grilled Turkey Caesar Salad, 98, 100, 110
Turkey and Bean Chili with Avocado Salsa, 154
Zesty Meat Loaf, 99, 114

U

University of Colorado study, 32
University of Pittsburgh study, 32
University of Rhode Island study, 41
University of South Carolina, 216–217
University of South Wales study, 229
University of Sydney study, 32–33
University of the West of England study, 92
University of Toronto study, 33

V

Vegetables
benefits, 41
at breakfast, 132
Cottage Pie, 168
Grilled Summer Vegetables, 101, 119
Pasta Primavera, 100, 116
Pot Roast with Braised Vegetables, 100, 114
Pumpkin Custards, 175
Rainbow Salad, 139
recommended servings per day, 22
right-sizing portions, guide, 22–23
Roasted Vegetable Wraps, 101, 109
vegetarian dinner parties, 63
See also specific vegetables

W

Waffles
Multi-Grain Waffles, 135
Walking program
10,000-step rule, 86–87, 216–219
12-week walking plan, 224–227
benefits of walking, 212, 219
description, 15
getting in more steps, 223
heart rate, 220–221, 222
in hot weather, 225
interval training, 228–231
mechanics of walking, 215, 229–230
MET (Metabolic Equivalent of Task), 228–229
as natural part of day, 211, 213–214, 216–219

pedometers, 85–87, 216–219
playlist for walking, 222
starting out, 220–222
staying motivated, 69
steps per minute (spm), 229–230
strengthening exercises, 238–249
stretches after walking, 232–237
in suburbia, 226
Swap & Drop ideas, 218, 229
walking missteps, 221–222
walking to de-stress, 68, 79
warm-up, 221
in winter, 213

Water
correct size of glass, 23
with dinner, 50, 57–58
for weight loss and health, 50, 95

Weight
history of, 212–213
influence of friend or spouse' weight, 20

Weight loss
controlling weekend eating, 60
diet saboteurs, 63–64, 75
"dinner belt" to gauge fullness, 85
eating only in designated places, 43, 69
eating slowly, 24, 41, 48, 62
effect on risk for diabetes, 37
emotional eating, 44, 62, 87–89
group dieting, 63
importance of breakfast, 30–32
motivation key to success, 20
muscle vs fat, 14, 66
myths re: weight loss, 69
putting problem foods out of sight, 68–69, 74
realistic goals, 69, 71
satiety signals, 28, 48–49, 50
sleep and, 49
snacking and, 42
strategies for, 15
thin-obsessed society, 69, 71, 87, 92
time for body to register fullness, 7, 24, 39, 49
weighing yourself, 14
See also Monitoring progress; Portion control; Weight loss maintenance

Weight-loss maintenance
adding humour to the day, 94–95
balancing calories in and out, 93–94, 95
celebrating success, 90
countering boredom, 91–93, 94
"dinner belt" to gauge fullness, 85
exercise as natural part of day, 211, 213–214, 216–219
getting back on track, 94
in holidays, 95
monitoring fluid intake, 95
new exercise activities, 93, 94
satiety signals, 28, 48–49, 50
time for body to register fullness, 7, 24, 39, 49
See also Monitoring progress; Walking program

White, E. B., 72
White, Paul Dudley, 216
Winfrey, Oprah, 60

Y

Yoga, 80
Yogourt
benefits of calcium, 34
benefits of probiotics, 31
Eggs Benedict, 136
Fresh Fruit Muesli and, 132–133
raita, 160
serving size, 24
Tropical Smoothie, 100, 105, 107
Yogourt Parfait, 98, 101, 102, 104

Z

Zucchini
Penne with Zucchini, 98, 120